HEALTH COMMUNICATION

A
Multicultural
Perspective

Edited by

Snehendu B. Kar
Rina Alcalay

with Shana Alex

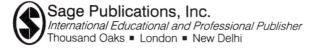
Sage Publications, Inc.
International Educational and Professional Publisher
Thousand Oaks ▪ London ▪ New Delhi

For information:

Sage Publications, Inc.
2455 Teller Road
Thousand Oaks, California 91320
E-mail: order@sagepub.com

Sage Publications Ltd.
6 Bonhill Street
London EC2A 4PU
United Kingdom

Sage Publications India Pvt. Ltd.
M-32 Market
Greater Kailash I
New Delhi 110 048 India

Printed in the United States of America

Library of Congress Cataloging-in-Publication Data

Main entry under title:

Health communication: A multicultural perspective/edited by Snehendu B. Kar,
    Rina Alcalay, with Shana Alex.
        p.   cm.
    Includes bibliographical references and index.
    ISBN 0-8039-7367-5 (pbk.: alk. paper)
    1. Health—Social aspects—United States—Cross-cultural studies.
    2. Health promotion—United States—Cross-cultural studies.
    3. Medical care—United States—Cross-cultural studies.
    4. Social medicine—United States—Cross-cultural studies.
    5. Health risk communication—United States—Cross-cultural studies.
    6. Community health services—United States—Cross-cultural studies.
    I. Kar, Snehendu B.   II. Alcalay, Rina.   III. Alex, Shana.
    RA423.2.H42 2000
    613'.089—dc21   00-009518

01   02   03   04   05   06   07   7   6   5   4   3   2   1

Acquiring Editor:	Margaret H. Seawell
Editorial Assistant:	Heidi Van Middlesworth
Production Editor:	Diana E. Axelsen
Editorial Assistant:	Victoria Cheng
Typesetter/Designer:	Tina M. Hill
Indexer:	Jeanne Busemeyer
Cover Designer:	Michelle Lee

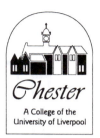
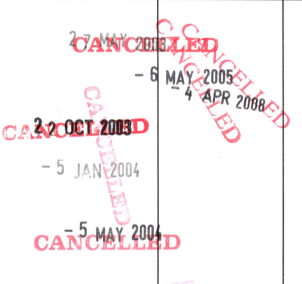
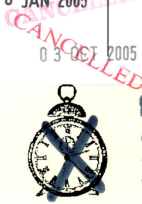

Contents

Preface   ix

Introduction   xiii

PART I: Conceptual Framework

1. Changing Health Needs:
   The Imperative for a Multicultural Paradigm   3

   Snehendu B. Kar
   Rina Alcalay
   with Shana Alex

2. The Emergence of a New Public Health Paradigm in the
   United States   21

   Snehendu B. Kar
   Rina Alcalay
   with Shana Alex

3. The Evolution of Health Communication in the United States   45

   Snehendu B. Kar
   Rina Alcalay
   with Shana Alex

4. A Multicultural Society: Facing a New Culture   79

   Snehendu B. Kar
   Rina Alcalay
   with Shana Alex

5. Communicating With Multicultural Populations:
   A Theoretical Framework   109

   Snehendu B. Kar
   Rina Alcalay
   with Shana Alex

PART II: Health Communication in High-Risk Multicultural Populations

6. Childhood Unintentional Injury Prevention:
   Multicultural Perspectives   141

   Deborah Glik
   Angela Mickalide

7. The Usefulness of the *Health Diary:*
   Findings From a Case Study of Six Healthy Start Sites   165

   Karen Thiel Raykovich
   James A. Wells
   Clifford Binder

8. Parent-Child Communication in Drug Abuse Prevention
   Among Adolescents   193

   Gauri Bhattacharya

9. The Effectiveness of Peer Education in STD/HIV Prevention   211

   Donald E. Morisky
   Vicki J. Ebin

10. Health Communication for HIV Risk Reduction
   Among Homeless Youth   235

   Lisa A. Russell

11. The Community as Classroom: A Health Communication
    Program Among Older Samoan and American Indian Women   251

    Lené Levy-Storms
    Steven P. Wallace
    Fran Goldfarb
    Linda Burhansstipanov

12. Health Communication Campaign Design:
    Lessons From the California *Wellness Guide* Distribution Project   281

    Robert A. Bell
    Rina Alcalay

PART III: Evaluation of Health Communication in Multicultural Populations

13. Evaluation of Multicultural Health Communication   311

    Snehendu B. Kar
    Rina Alcalay
    with Shana Alex

14. Lessons Learned and Implications   333

    Snehendu B. Kar
    Rina Alcalay
    with Shana Alex

Index   359

About the Contributors   375

Preface

The primary aim of this volume is to critically review issues and approaches to health communication, with special reference to public health interventions in multicultural communities. As a scientific and professional specialty, multicultural communication is in its infancy. The theories and models presented in communication textbooks and mainstream literature and often used for intervention planning are almost always based upon research done with the dominant white population and from the perspective of evaluating media effects on a target population (see Chapter 1 for examples). These theories and models are valuable conceptual tools for designing interventions in populations similar to those used for original research that served as their basis. But these theories and models are generally color-blind and gender-blind; they do not inform us about the key issues, factors, and forces intrinsic to cultures and genders that affect effective health communication in multicultural community. In this volume, we focus on key issues, factors, forces, and challenges in health communication from a multicultural perspective. We define *multicultural community* as a community where people from distinctly different cultures live, come into contact, and interact with one another to form a new way of life, both dynamic and different from each of its parts or cultures.

We have entered the third millennium with unprecedented scientific and technological innovations that have profoundly changed our societies and lives beyond our expectations. Science and technology have enabled us to eradicate or control epidemics, which killed millions and disabled many more. They have enabled us to travel in space, unravel the secrets of atoms, map every human gene, clone living beings, and amass wealth at an unprecedented level. Innovations in industrial development, medicine, and public health have prolonged human life and have significantly reduced mortality and morbidity rates due to major infectious diseases and epidemics. Consequently, world population has been growing at increasing rates. People are living longer, and women are living longer than men, especially in the older age groups.

At the same time, multiculturalism has emerged as a major challenge in social planning, both globally and nationally. But our understanding of the dynamics of multicultural communities as they affect planned social change remains at a very rudimentary level. Rapid globalization (including increased international travel, trade, education, migration, and entertainment) and the communication revolution have transformed our social realities fundamentally. At the international level, rapid globalization and the communication revolution have blurred national and cultural boundaries. We can instantly observe and participate in events across the globe, share our experiences with people around the world, and live like members of a vast and complex global village. This globalization of information exchange, travel, education, communication, commerce, and entertainment has produced dual effects. First, the younger generation is becoming more similar across cultures. The emerging global youth culture includes rock music and blue jeans, shared preferences in movies, TV programs, videos, and Internet activites, and other commonalities in lifestyle and even in political and personal aspirations. Second, an increasing cultural gap between the younger and older generations is leading to greater inter-generation and inter-gender tensions and conflicts within families and communities. Rapid industrialization and globalization have also significantly increased the gaps between the "haves" and the "have-nots" in terms of access to the benefits of these progress, including access to communication hardware and content.

On the domestic front, many urban areas are rapidly becoming demographically multicultural. For instance, in 1990, the 15 largest metropolitan areas in the United States became truly multicultural; that is, there was no single ethnic majority. The United States Census Bureau projects that by the year 2050, whites will be reduced to 52% of our national population. By another decade, whites will be one of several minorities. Our communities have also become more complex and multicultural. Increasingly, people in our communities live, work, eat, play, and form personal and family ties with people from cultures that are distant geographically (originating from tens of thousands of miles across the globe) and fundamentally dissimilar (e.g., in language, religion, identity, and tradition). This new multicultural reality means that in planning social policy and interventions, we can no longer assume a homogenous population. Theories and methods that were effective in monocultural settings or in communities with one dominant culture may not be as effective for social change in multicultural communities. We need to understand the realities of multicultural communities and build our social policies and prevention intervention on that understanding.

Effective health communication is more than disseminating health messages using popular media or enhancing people's compliance with medical regimens. It involves initiating and sustaining fundamental changes at individual and societal levels. At the individual level, it requires changing personal lifestyle and risk behaviors that are deeply rooted in culturally conditioned beliefs, attitudes, practices, norms, and patterns of personal relations (e.g., behavior related to food and nutrition, sex and reproduction, health care utilization, and personal safety). At the societal level, it requires changing cultural values, social norms, customs and practices, social organizations, and intercultural relations (including communication systems) that directly affect health-related behavior and status. Finally, multicultural communities consist of minorities and high-risk groups who are most likely to be poor, underserved, and powerless. Poverty, prejudice, and exclusion from social policy and governance that adversely affect their health and quality of life are major barriers to effective health promotion interventions in multicultural communities. Lack of multicultural competency among policy planners and professionals further aggravates the problem. Effective disease prevention and health promotion interventions for and in such communities must extend beyond communication of health information and education and deal with issues of community empowerment and participation. Athough in recent years there has been a growing recognition of the importance of multicultural health communication, there is a paucity of research-based literature and exemplary case studies that can provide adequate guidance to professionals who are involved with health promotion in multicultural communities. In this volume, we present our critical analysis of multicultural health communication issues and exemplary case studies as a contribution to our collective understanding.

There are many persons, too many to name individually, who have directly or indirectly contributed to this volume. First: Years of communication and interactions with our numerous colleagues and graduate students have significantly helped us in clarifying the issues we have presented in this volume. Second: Countless national and international health-related organizations have provided us with invaluable opportunities, as consultants and collaborators, to work and gain firsthand experience in health communication in distant and disparate cultures. They also are too numerous to mention. Third: we must acknowledge our indebtedness to the editorial team at Sage Publications. Acquiring Editor Margaret H. Seawell made a critical contribution by her efforts that led to Sage's decision to publish the volume. Heidi Van Middlesworth assisted in making sure all tables, figures, and other major elements were complete and ready to use. Linda Gray has meticulously edited the manuscript for clarity, consistency, and completeness of the text; her editorial help has been invaluable. Diana E. Axelsen played a major role by expediting the production of this volume. Finally, words cannot express the depth of support received from and sacrifice made by our family members as we worked on this volume.

Introduction

When races come together, as in the present age, it should not be
merely the gathering of a crowd; there must be a bond of
relation, or they will collide with each other.

—Rabindranath Tagore (1925/1966, p. 216)

Many Indians and Turks speak the same tongue;
Yet many pairs of Turks find they're foreigners.
The tongue of mutual understanding is quite special:
To be one of heart is better than to have a common tongue.

—Rumi (1994, p. 37)

Effective multicultural communication is much more than the use of a common language or media. The primary objective of this volume is to examine the role of health communication within the context of health promotion and disease prevention (HPDP), which make up the new public health paradigm for achieving the health objectives of our nation.

A major paradigm shift in the health care ideology and system is in process both globally and nationally. At the global level, the Alma-Ata Declaration of 1978, endorsed by over 160 nations, formally recognized that a new primary health care (PHC) paradigm should replace current emphasis and dependence on expensive tertiary clinical care in both rich and poor nations (WHO/ UNICEF, 1978). The PHC strategy focuses on primary prevention through "active community participation"; health information education and communication (IEC) is a key strategy for promoting and sustaining community participation. According to the PHC paradigm, communities must be active partners in the planning and implementation of health care policies and services, not passive beneficiaries of health services planned and provided by professionals.

Within the United States, a consensus currently exists among scholars, planners, and professionals that our continued emphasis on sophisticated and expensive tertiary care will not improve the overall quality of health of Americans. This new consensus and paradigm is described in detail in the landmark document titled *Healthy People 2000: National Health Promotion and Disease Prevention Objectives* (U.S. Department of Health and Human Services [DHHS], 1991). This HPDP paradigm identifies 22 areas of national priority and emphasizes effective applications of the public health model for achieving health objectives for the nation. In contrast to the medical paradigm, the distinctive features of the public health paradigm are that (a) its goal is prevention of disease and promotion of positive health rather than treatment of the sick, (b) its unit of intervention is the public (community) not individual patients, and (c) its strategy is to facilitate lifestyle and societal changes necessary for reduction of risks and promotion of health for communities as a whole. The public health model focuses on promoting and sustaining desired changes through effective partnerships between health planners, providers, and the public. Within this new paradigm of HPDP, health communication emerges as a vital component with vastly expanded roles extending far beyond the traditional emphasis on communication and education for patient compliance or for timely use of health services.

The HPDP paradigm requires effective use of communication interventions for achieving additional objectives, including *empowerment* of communities at risk, *advocacy* on behalf of the underserved groups for affecting policy and services, and *coalition and consensus* building for social actions for better health. According to the Ottawa Charter, which helped revolutionize health promotion globally, "Health promotion is the process of enabling people to increase control over, and to improve, their health. . . . Health promotion goes beyond health care. . . . At the heart of this process is the empowerment of communities, their ownership and control of their own endeavours and destinies ("Ottawa Charter," 1996, pp. 329, 330, 331). This includes the education and re-education of millions of health professionals of our nation to prepare them to be more responsive to the needs of the communities as defined by them (the new public health paradigm and its implications for multicultural communities are discussed in Chapter 2 of this volume). This is admittedly a formidable challenge, but the challenge of developing effective health promotion and communication strategies is far greater in multicultural and disadvantaged communities for reasons explained in the following section.

Our population also is increasingly becoming multicultural. The first U.S. census in 1790 recorded 81% of the population as white; in 1900, the population of whites had actually grown to 88% (U.S. Department of Commerce and Labor, 1909). In contrast, the 1990 census showed a decline in the non-Hispanic white population to 75% (U.S. Department of Commerce, 1998a); according to the latest projection, by 2050 the non-Hispanic white population will be reduced to 53% (U.S. Department of Commerce, 1998b). In another decade, non-Hispanic whites will be one of many minorities of our nation.

Until recently, the United States based its social policy on the "melting-pot" paradigm. This assimilationist view held that all ethnic minorities should and do desire to blend into the mainstream dominant culture; therefore, social policies should be based on the reality of one population, and the emphasis should be on designing the most effective standard intervention paradigm that would best serve most people's needs. It has become clear, especially during the last two decades, that a multicultural reality has replaced the melting-pot metaphor. One prominent sociologist and a strong proponent of the assimilationist position summed up the current situation best in his recent book *We Are All Multiculturalists Now* (Glazer, 1997). This aptly titled new demographic reality predicates that, to be effective, health promotion and communication interventions must be responsive to the needs and dynamics of multicultural communities.

Over 70 years ago, the philosopher-poet Rabindranath Tagore (1925/1966) cautioned Indian political and educational leaders with these words: "When races come together, as in the present age, it should not be merely the gathering of a crowd; there must be a bond of relation, or they will collide with each other" (p. 216). The last Los Angeles riot proved how prophetic he was. Rodney King summarized our national frustration in five words: "Can't we all get along?" The central premise of this volume is that effective health promotion communication in multicultural and underserved communities must go beyond dissemination of health information and promotion of an agenda set by outside experts using a common language—that in order to be effective, it must first establish "a bond of relation" with people from dissimilar cultures and then channel this force to build bridges between peoples' priorities, aspirations, and resources.

Multicultural, multiethnic communities consist of culturally diverse groups that vary significantly from one another in terms of their (a) objective needs and subjective priorities, (b) interethnic stereotypes and relations affecting social participation (c) culturally rooted beliefs and values affecting health-related practices, (d) language and communication behavior, (e) social networks, and (f) leadership structures. Cultures may also vary significantly from one another in terms of the values and beliefs they hold about birth, death, illness, and major life events; meanings, causes, and consequences of these events; and appropriate preventive and healing practices. Finally, multicultural and disadvantaged urban communities consist of high-risk groups with special needs. Effective health communication strategy in such communities must be based on a sound understanding of the way a culture affects health and related behavior as well as an understanding of the special needs of various groups.

In recognition of the needs of special populations, the landmark report that defined our national strategy for HPDP states: "Special population groups often need targeted preventive efforts, and such efforts require understanding the needs and the disparities experienced by these groups. General solutions cannot always be used to solve specific problems" (U.S. DHHS, 1991, p. 29). There is no standard model of effective health communication, and even if there were one, it is not likely to be effective among all ethnic groups. Typically, social science theories and methods that guide communication policy and strategies are based on research conducted primarily among the dominant segment of the white population; it would be unwise to assume that what is true for a majority would be equally valid for other groups. The social reality is more complex in communities where there is no single dominant majority (e.g., South Central Los Angeles; the UCLA School of Public Health, which has five academic departments, each with its own ideology and priorities). In such diverse communities, an effective health promotion communication will require a "bottom-up" planning process in partnership with the diverse segments of the community and the organizations serving them. This new disease HPDP paradigm requires a new philosophy of prevention, new communication strategies, and new leadership responsive to the needs of multicultural communities.

Available literature on communication theory and practice in general and on health communication is impressive and is rapidly expanding, but the literature is very weak in dealing with communication and health promotion issues of multiethnic and disadvantaged communities. As Huston et al. (1992) write, "We know a great deal about the functions of television for children, a modest amount about those for the elderly and women, and relatively little about those for many ethnic minorities" (p. 132). Although one can identify excellent text and reference books on communication in general and mass media campaigns in particular (see below under "Scope of This Volume"), our recent on-line search failed to identify a single book with its primary focus on community-based HPDP communication in multicultural communities. The authors of this volume have been teaching required graduate courses on health behavior and health communication at several leading schools of public health in the nation over two decades; throughout this period, they were unable to find a suitable text or reference book that focuses on health communication from a multicultural context. This book addresses this serious gap in the literature. It presents an analysis of key issues and factors affecting health promotion interventions in general and the role of health communication within the context of the new paradigm of HPDP in multiethnic communities in particular. The book examines communication processes and their influence on health-related behavior from a "cultural diversity" or a "multicultural" perspective rather than from the commonly used "technocentric" (or "media effects") perspective. The technocentric perspective uses a "media effects on the dominant majority (MEDM)" paradigm; it selects a popular media technology (e.g., TV, printed media, interactive network) and examines its effects on a specific behavior or group (e.g., violence, substance abuse among adults, children).

The cultural diversity perspective—hereafter, multicultural perspective—begins with the premise that ethnic groups have unique and culturally conditioned beliefs, values, knowledge, attitudes, practices (BVKAP), and ethnic communication patterns that affect their health-related behavior. Effective health communication must be based on the positive "cultural capitals" of various groups, and it requires an emphasis on local solutions rather than solutions through national media. Reports of various commissions and study groups on the effects of TV violence and pornography in mass media on aggression and antisocial behavior are examples of a "technocentric" approach looking at the effects of media on target behavior. This approach may be valid when one deals with a culturally homogeneous population in which the impacts of cultural diversity on health behavior and media use may not be a critical issue. But in a culturally diverse community, the differences among ethnic groups in their culturally anchored values, beliefs, and preferred communication behavior may have independent effects on health communication and health behavior of the members of various groups. The "cultural relativity" approach begins with the salient cultural attributes or givens of distinct ethnic groups and examines how these givens interact with modern communication media and the existing health care system in affecting health-related decisions and action within and between groups.

Scope of This Volume

This book does not attempt to review the entire field of health communication theories and research. For that purpose, there are excellent reviews of health communication from the MEDM perspective. These include Atkin and Wallack (1990); Backer, Rogers, and Sopory (1992); Bennet and Calman (1999); DeFleur and Ball-Rokeach (1995); Harris (1995); Huston et al. (1992); Kreps and Kunimoto (1994); Oskamp (1989); Rice and Atkin (1989); Rogers (1973); Tulloch and Lupton (1997); and Wallack, Dorfman, Jernigan, and Themba (1993). Our volume does not intend to duplicate these valuable works. Instead, we focus on a multicultural health communication perspective and process, emphasizing our HPDP objectives for the nation and consequently on community-based *primary prevention*—that is, community-based actions to prevent people from illness and injury in the first place. Our aim is to identify forces and factors in multicultural communities as they affect health communication.

Organization of the Text

The text is organized into three parts. Part I deals with major trends affecting public health and theoretical, conceptual, and empirical literature germane to health communication in multicultural communities (Chapters 1-5). The second part includes in-depth analyses of seven case studies on health communication interventions in high-risk populations (Chapters 6-12). Part III deals with the lessons learned and issues raised in evaluation of health communication in multicultural communities (Chapters 13-14).

Chapter 1 deals with the changing dynamics of the health needs of populations and the emergence, over the last century, of the new public health paradigm. Chapter 2 is on the global responses to the changing health needs in populations, including the evolution of the PHC paradigm globally and the emergence of the HPDP strategy for the nation. Chapter 3 looks at the changing roles of health promotion, public health organizations, and health communication in professional education and in health promotion interventions. Next, Chapter 4 discusses major theories and models of health behavior that guide health communication interventions and their implications in multicultural populations and the issue of "cultural competence." The concluding chapter in Part I, Chapter 5, looks at the realities of working in a multicultural society, and at cultural similarities and differences among minority groups.

Part II deals with seven exemplary case studies dealing with health communication in different ethnic communities. Chapter 6 begins with a discussion of childhood injuries from a multicultural perspective. Chapter 7 reviews evaluation of the usefulness of the *Health Diary* in six Healthy Start sites. Chapter 8 looks at parent-child communication, particularly as it relates to the issue of substance abuse prevention. Continuing with child-based prevention strategies, Chapter 9 considers the effectiveness of peer education as it relates to STD/HIV prevention. Chapter 10 expands on this topic, looking at HIV prevention among homeless youth. Chapter 11 discusses a community-based health promotion program for American Indian and Samoan older women. The section ends with Chapter 12, which evaluates health communication campaign design, drawing lessons from a distribution campaign of the *Wellness Guide* in California.

In conclusion of the volume, Chapters 13 and 14 summarize the implications of our analysis in all chapters and of the case studies in this volume, findings derived from the authors original research, and health communication evaluation issues particular to multicultural communities.

Summary

The authors of this volume address three key questions: What are the realities of multicultural communities? What are the roles and limitations of mainstream communication media in these settings? What are the unique forces and factors that determine effective health communication in multicultural communities. To illustrate the current demographic shifts, the *Los Angeles Times* recently reported that "José" was the most popular name for newborn baby boys in Texas and California for 1998; for the first time, a Hispanic name replaced the usual John and Michael ("José Moves Into Top Spot," 1999). This signifies two major social trends underscored in this book: (a) The proportion of minorities in the general population is growing faster than whites, and (b) society is becoming more multicultural as minorities choose not to melt into the mainstream by choosing English names—that is, increased pride in ethnic identity now overrides assimilationist hopes. Given these realities, we hope that our volume will at least raise important issues for active deliberation by researchers, policy planners, and the community alike. Through critical analyses of communication studies literature and primary experience from health communication case studies in multicultural communities, the authors of this volume illustrate what works and what does not, the problems encountered, and their implications for multicultural health communication.

References

Atkin, C., & Wallack, L. (Eds.). (1990). *Mass communication and public health: Complexities and conflicts.* Newbury Park, CA: Sage.

Backer, T. E., Rogers, E. M., & Sopory, P. (1992). *Designing health communication campaigns: What works?* Newbury Park, CA: Sage.

Bennet, P., & Calman, K., Eds. (1999). *Risk communication and public health.* New York: Oxford University Press.

DeFleur, M. L., & Ball-Rokeach, S. (1995). *Theories of mass communication* (5th ed.). New York: Longman.

Glazer, N. (1997). *We are all multiculturalists now.* Cambridge, MA: Harvard University Press.

Harris, L. (Ed.). (1995). *Health and the new media: Technologies transforming personal and public health.* Mahwah, NJ: Lawrence Erlbaum.

Huston, A., Donnerstein, E., Fairchild, H., Feshbach, N., Katz, P., Murry, J., Rubinstein, E., Wilcox, B., & Zukerman, D. (1992). *Big world, small screen: The role of television in American society.* Lincoln: University of Nebraska Press.

José moves into top spot in name game. (1999, January 8). *Los Angeles Times* (State & Local News Section).

Kreps, G., & Kunimoto, E. (1994). *Effective communication in multicultural health care settings.* Thousand Oaks, CA: Sage.

Oskamp, S. (Ed.). (1989). *Television as a social issue.* Newbury Park, CA: Sage.

The Ottawa Charter for Health Promotion (17-21 November 1986). (1996). In *Health promotion anthology* (Scientific Publication No. 557). Washington, DC: World Health Organization, Pan American Health Organization.

Rice, R. E., & Atkin, C. K. (Eds.). (1989). *Public communication campaigns* (2nd ed.). Newbury Park, CA: Sage.

Rogers E. M. (1973). *Communication strategies for family planning.* New York: Free Press.

Rumi, J. (1994). *Rumi: Daylight* (C. Helminsky & K. Helminsky, Trans.). Putney, VT: Threshold.

Tagore, R. (1966). Talks in China. In A. Chakravarty (Ed.), *A Tagore reader.* Boston: Beacon. (Original work published 1925, Visva-Bharati, India)

Tulloch, J., & Lupton, D. (1997). *Television, AIDS, and risk: A cultural studies approach to health communication.* St. Leonards, NSW, Australia: Allen & Unwin

U.S. Department of Commerce and Labor, Bureau of the Census. (1909). *A century of population growth: From the first census of the United States to the twelfth, 1790-1900.* Washington, DC: Government Printing Office.

U.S. Department of Commerce, Bureau of the Census. (1998a). *Population estimates.* Retrieved June 12, 2000 from the World Wide Web: www.census.gov/population/ www/estimates/popest.html

U.S. Department of Commerce, Bureau of the Census. (1998b). *Population projections.* Retrieved June 12, 2000 from the World Wide Web: http://www.census.gov/population/www/projections/popproj.html

U.S. Department of Health and Human Services. (1991) *Healthy people 2000: National health promotion and disease prevention objectives* (DHHS Publication No. PHS 91-50212). Washington, DC: Government Printing Office.

Wallack, L., Dorfman, L., Jernigan, D., & Themba, M. (1993). *Media advocacy and public health: Power for prevention.* Newbury Park, CA: Sage.

World Health Organization/United Nations International Children's Emergency Fund. (1978). *ALMA-ATA 1978 primary health care: Report of the International Conference on Primary Health Care.* Geneva, Switzerland: Author.

PART I

CONCEPTUAL FRAMEWORK

1

Changing Health Needs

The Imperative for a Multicultural Paradigm

Snehendu B. Kar
Rina Alcalay
with Shana Alex

This chapter follows the history of the modern practice of public health as it has evolved globally and how this has led to the adoption of the concept of multiculturalism in the United States. Since the end of World War II, major political and social forces have joined together to recognize the importance of public health as necessary to creating successful societies in all parts of the world. Although public health already had strong roots in epidemic control, the modern role of public health as a means to combat all preventable diseases did not emerge until the latter half of the 20th century. In this chapter, the underlying forces and eventual shape of the international discipline of public health will be discussed.

3

Global Issues in Public Health

The latter half of the 20th century ushered in an era of the "dual epidemic," during which countries were still plagued by the infectious diseases and problems attributable to poor sanitation and the like but also had to deal with chronic diseases caused mainly by unhealthy lifestyle choices, such as smoking. The modern mission of public health evolved largely out of a growing realization during the last three decades that, for varying reasons, the current paradigm of clinical health care could not fully address the needs of the nations of the world. For less industrialized countries, the costs associated with attempting to cover the health care needs of the entire population, much of which lived in rural settings, became overwhelming. There was a dearth of professionals who would live and work for little pay in mainly agricultural societies; to achieve the normally expected status and wealth, most health care professionals concentrated in the larger cities, leaving rural areas understaffed and without adequate health care facilities. This problem led directly to the construction of a method of improving health while keeping clinical visits (and therefore costs) to a minimum—that is, attempts at reaching the needy population through preventive medicine and public health.

In a similar manner, more urban, industrialized nations also faced a crisis of health care stemming from different causes. The increased compensation associated with providing specialized clinical care drew many health care professionals out of the primary care field and into areas of specialization that offered greater prestige. In addition, health care organizations and the medical industry found the provision of expensive care highly profitable and were therefore less inclined to provide preventive care services, many of which were not covered by health insurance agencies. This, in turn, created a bias toward clinical treatments that required higher costs, because the specialists naturally wished to use all the tools available to them. In this upward spiral, however, many primary care concerns were lost, allowing preventable chronic diseases (such as coronary disease caused by lack of exercise and poor diet) to run rampant through society. Therefore, industrialized nations also recognized the need for preventive measures throughout their populations, although for different initial purposes than the less wealthy nations of the world.

Rising health care costs and demonstrated benefits of community-based prevention added impetus to the growth of interest in the public health paradigm. First, with the introduction of antibiotics and inoculations, massive campaigns to eradicate infectious diseases were launched. Smallpox remains the most famous case in which the health field managed to entirely wipe out a

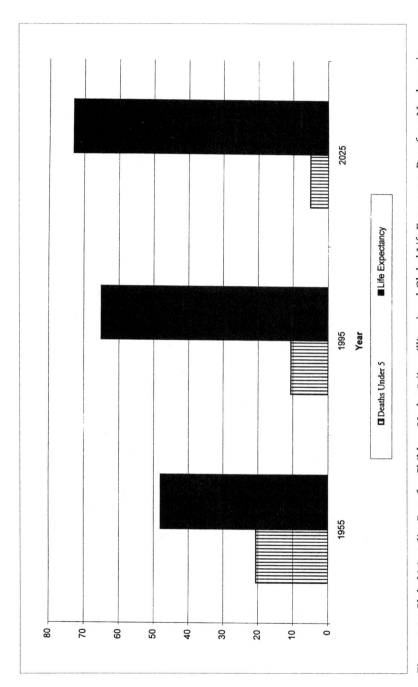

Figure 1.1. Global Mortality Rate for Children Under 5 (in millions) and Global Life Expectancy Rate for a Newborn, in Number of Years (1955, 1995, and 2025, projected)

disease and thus bring hope to suffering populations that such a feat could be accomplished. Other public health works also occurred around this time: (a) The higher quality of life with urbanization reduced the chances of contracting a deadly infectious disease from natural sources, and (b) the proliferation of sanitation reduced the chances of infection from sewage matter. When these factors combined with antibiotics and inoculations to drastically reduce the rate of infection for previously deadly and widespread diseases, this reinforced the idea that public health methods had the power to permanently help humanity. Figure 1.1 shows the decline since 1955 in the global death rate for children under 5 years of age, which mirrors the rising life expectancy, illustrating the incredible social benefits of public health works. Note that these figures are global; discrepancies among countries still exist.

Second, control of communicable diseases along with increased life expectancy brought more problems associated with chronic illness rooted in behavioral patterns and lifestyles over a long period of time. These problems are exacerbated by what the World Health Organization (WHO) calls the "population aging" trend around the world. That is, the world's populace both lives longer and has a lower rate of fertility, creating an overall older global population (WHO, 1996), although this phenomenon affects different regions of the globe with varying levels of intensity. Estimates from the United Nations show that in 1998, 16% of member countries already have at least one fifth of their female population at age 60 years and older; with the exception of Japan, every one of these countries is located in Europe (Statistics Division and Population Division of the United Nations Secretariat, 1998).

By the year 2025, however, three fourths of the world's elderly will be living in the poorer countries of the world, including the poorer European nations, all of which may lack the resources to effectively practice clinical medicine (Kumar, 1997). Richer countries are also experiencing population aging, causing foreseeable health problems that they may not have the resources to cope with, even with their comparatively greater wealth. By 2030, approximately one third of the U.S. population will be 65 and older (Gutheil, 1996). These figures are aggregates for the entire population of the world; the disparity between the life spans of the people of the developed countries as opposed to the people in the less developed nations will remain.

By the time individuals experience a chronic disease, it is often too late to cure or reverse the bodily damage that accumulated over the course of a lifetime. Therefore, any help given to alleviate the disease must start before the damage occurs—a compelling reason to practice preventive care.

The legitimization of public health as its own discipline has been percolating through the world since the early part of the 20th century; as early as 1909, in fact, Ludwig Teleky of Vienna declared that health professionals must examine the health of populations within the context of the environment surrounding that population and take steps to clean up pollution (Terris, 1992). In the 1970s, however, the idea of public health as a philosophy and a method gained acceptance throughout the world, as shown by the many documents produced during that era that outlined preventive care as necessary to human survival. Three major developments helped institutionalize public health promotion throughout the world in its modern form. First, the *Alma-Ata 1978 Primary Health Care* (PHC) publication, jointly created by WHO and UNICEF (United Nations International Children's Emergency Fund) created the strategies forming the basis that future work would build on. To summarize, it emphasized three main points:

1. That all human beings are entitled to accessible, acceptable, and afford-able primary care
2. That to be effective, prevention programs should be community based
3. That the public or community must be active participants and not simply receivers of outside information and assistance.

It was clear that the implementation of this strategy would help alleviate the financial strain on the clinical systems of both the industrialized and the rural nations and at the same time increase the quality and quantity of care received (WHO/UNICEF, 1978).

Until this point, the necessity of engaging the community as an active part-ner to further the goals of the health of the public was not a central theme of health policies. The PHC declaration emphasized that partnership was neces-sary to change those behavior patterns of community members that cause ill-ness. In other words, communities had to be (a) willing to change some behav-iors in order to become more healthy and (b) willing to create the conditions required to make the desired behavior a permanent practice. The Alma-Ata declaration, mentioned in the Introduction, states unequivocally that "pri-mary health care is essential health care based on . . . acceptable methods and technology made universally accessible to individuals and families in the com-munity through their full participation" (WHO/UNICEF, 1978, p. 3). This rep-resented a growing shift in the preventive health care paradigm, moving away from clinical practice and toward the more inclusive viewpoint of public health.

Following in the same vein as the Alma-Ata paper, WHO convened the First International Conference on Health Promotion in Ottawa, Canada, in November of 1986. During this conference, however, *advocacy* and *community empowerment* emerged for the first time as the major methods to implement the goals outlined in the Alma-Ata publication. According to the Ottawa Charter, which helped revolutionize health promotion globally, "Health promotion is the process of enabling people to increase control over, and to improve, their health. . . . Health promotion goes beyond health care. . . . At the heart of this process is the empowerment of communities, their ownership and control of their own endeavours and destinies ("The Ottawa Charter for Health Promotion," 1996, pp. 329, 330, 331). This document recognized the important contributions of government policy as an agent of change in health but then named *community action,* with the community as the unit of intervention, the most important instrument of health promotion. "Health promotion works through concrete and effective community action in setting priorities, making decisions, planning strategies and implementing them to achieve better health" (WHO, 1986, p. 2). The field of health promotion had broadened to include community partnerships as essential components to effectively achieving the desired change in the community.

The third major document, the Adelaide Declaration, emerged 2 years later from the Second International Conference on Health Promotion, held in Adelaide, Australia. Through discussion of key "action areas," the Adelaide Declaration emphasized, for the first time, the need to recognize the differing health status of women compared with men. Acknowledging that women are often treated as second-class citizens around the world, the Adelaide Declaration stated, "All women, especially those from ethnic, indigenous, and minority groups, have the right to self-determination of their health, and should be full partners in the formulations of public health policy to ensure its cultural relevance" (WHO, 1988, p. 2). This statement helped legitimize the growing movement toward using public health methods to alleviate the unjust inequalities in women's health, as well as in the health of minority groups.

In addition to these three important documents, the United Nations has also periodically convened the International Conference on Population and Development, the last of which was held in March 1993. Relating to the advancement of public health, the conferences helped institutionalize the redefinition of population control in terms of family planning and well-being. During the expert committee preparations for the conference, the secretary-general of the conference, Dr. Nafis Sadik, placed a great deal of emphasis on achieving population control goals through family planning within the broad context of addressing the quality of life for women and children around the world. Dr. Sadik called on international organizations to collaborate with national organizations, the private sector, nongovernmental organizations (NGOs), and local communities to implement the family planning techniques discussed. Hers was another voice added to the global outcry that to have successful societies, public health must be addressed (Preparatory Committee for the International Conference, 1992).

All these developments contributed to the legitimization of public health as a discipline separate from medicine in its mission and operational paradigm. The public health paradigm differs from clinical medicine in three important aspects:

1. Public health's mission is prevention rather than the treatment of disease.
2. Public health's unit of measurement is the community as a whole rather than individual cases.
3. Public health's mode of operation is prevention through active participation and partnership with the public.

Therefore, public health fundamentally requires different training than does the practice of medicine. This necessity for a different type of training created the preconditions necessary for the formation of specialized public health training centers. However, for the most part, public health training centers began internationally as adjuncts to schools of medicine. Two types of public health schools emerged: (a) "preventive medicine" training received from an established school of medicine and (b) separate public health schools that followed their own prevailing methods of training.

Internationally, the first model quickly became the norm. Preventive medicine departments remained closely connected to the original medical schools, creating a new paradigm that focused on preventing disease rather than simply curing it once contracted. However, because of their close ties to medical training, these departments often kept a strong focus on the individual as the unit of measurement and treatment rather than on primary prevention in the community. True, international organizations had led the way for recognizing the community as the vital unit for public health programs, but public health programs internationally have not completely moved away from the clinical paradigm.

Demographic Imperatives
for a Multicultural Perspective

With public health becoming its own discipline internationally, the United States followed suit (as discussed in detail in Chapter 3). During the last century, however, the U.S. population has become increasingly multicultural compared with other nations, highlighting the complexities *within* a community that intensify the need for a multicultural focus. Because of both increased immigration and higher fertility rates for nonwhites, minority populations have grown enormously compared with the rate of growth for whites in the United States. For example, according to 1990 census data, in 186 U.S. counties, whites did not constitute a majority of the population. In addition, 40 counties were split evenly between the white and nonwhite population. In 1990, non-Hispanic whites made up 75.9% of the national population, meaning minorities make up almost one quarter of the U.S. population; that number will only become larger with the dual effects of increased minority immigration and higher rates fertility among minorities. By 2050, projections state that non-Hispanic whites will constitute only 52.8% of the population. With the increased urbanization of the United States, as well as the immigrant and ethnic minority movement into the cities, it is hardly surprising to note that of the 50 most diverse counties, 33 contained major metropolises (U.S. Department of Commerce, 1998a).

As more and more people of different ethnic backgrounds have made the United States their home, mainstream society has also changed its perceptions of itself, acknowledging the new multicultural mixture of the population. Census data, and the ethnic categories under which it is gathered and categorized, clearly show this progression (see Table 1.1).

In the first census taken in 1790, the only categories that existed were "White" and "Colored," meaning "black"; the Native American population was not counted (they were not citizens of the United States), and virtually no other ethnic minorities existed in the country at this time (U.S. Department of Commerce and Labor, 1909). By 1900, the census categories had increased to include Native American and Asian, combined under the name "Indians and Mongolians" (U.S. Department of Commerce, 1953). Only recently has the

Table 1.1   Ethnic Composition of the Population:
            Census Information 1790 to 2050 (in percentages)

Year of Census	White	Asian American	American Indian	Black	Latino	Total
1790[a]	80.7	N/A	N/A	19.3	N/A	100
1850[a]	84.3	N/A	N/A	15.7	N/A	100
1900[a]	87.8	0.1b	0.5[b]	11.6	N/A	100
1950[c]	89.5	0.3d	0.2	10	N/A	100
1990[e]	75.6	2.8	0.7	11.8	9.1	100
2000[f] (proj.)	71.8	3.9	0.7	12.2	11.4	100
2050[f] (proj.)	52.8	8.2	0.9	13.6	24.5	100

a. Department of Commerce and Labor, Bureau of the Census (1909, pp. 222-223).
b. Combined into a single category—"Indian and Mongolian."
c. Department of Commerce, Bureau of the Census (1953, table 36).
d. Includes "all other" nonwhite category.
e. Department of Commerce, Bureau of the Census, 1998a.
f. Department of Commerce, Bureau of the Census, 1998b.

census begun to count "Hispanic" as an option, with fully 9% of the population identifying themselves as such in 1990 (U.S. Department of Commerce, 1998a). By 2050, it is projected that Hispanics will count as the largest minority group in the United States, with 25% of the population. Blacks will constitute 14%, Asians 9%, American Indians 1%, and whites the remaining 53% (U.S. Department of Commerce, 1998b).

These demographic realities have serious implications for the practice of public health into the 21st century. With (a) the increase in the proportion of youth and children of color, (b) the increase in proportion of white elderly, and (c) the increase in proportion of foreign-born citizens, public health practitioners must address the problems of expanding multicultural communities. First, higher birth rates will make minority children a higher proportion of the youth population. This trend is already well advance in many metropolitan areas in the United States. To illustrate, in the Los Angeles Unified School District (LAUSD), English is only one of 86 native languages spoken at home by the student population (LAUSD Survey, 1993). Second, the proportions of elderly population among whites and minorities will become even more unbalanced because whites have longer life spans than do minorities (see Figure 1.2). As

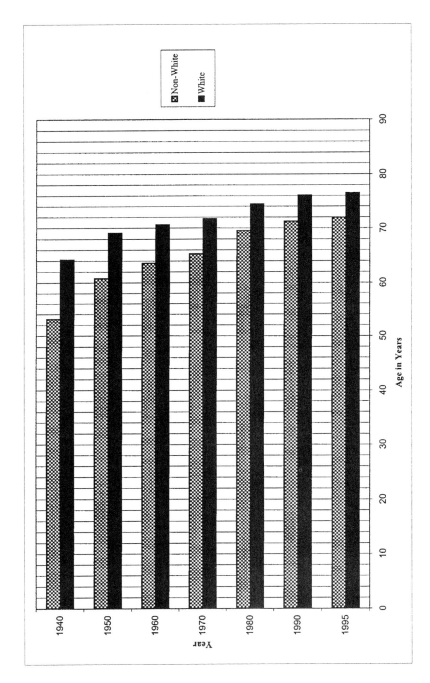

Figure 1.2. Life Expectancy at Birth, by Race, in the United States, 1940 to 1995

shown in Figure 1.2, as far back as 1940, nonwhites have had shorter life spans than whites. Judging by the uniformity of the gap between life spans for minorities and whites, it can be surmised that this pattern also existed before the data were collected, perhaps in 1930. The children born in that year and before make up today's elderly population. Not only were whites the majority in 1930, but they also tend to live longer. Therefore, today's elderly population contains proportionately fewer minority persons than it did when the cohort was born.

This trend will tend to make elderly persons less likely to be of a minority group than the general population and certainly more white than the current younger population, which contains many first-generation immigrants.

Third, as trade barriers drop and the need for workers increases, immigration restraints are loosening to allow both unskilled and highly skilled workers to come into the United States to fill vacant jobs in certain industries, such as the computer industry. On September 24, 1998, the House passed a bill to allow 142,500 additional foreign-born skilled workers into the country under the H-1B Visa (U.S. House of Representatives, 1998). However, the Senate never took up the measure, allowing it to expire at the end of the legislative session.

All these trends point to more multicultural communities appearing across the nation. Increased interaction between whites and nonwhites will also lead to more intercultural encounters, marriages, and acculturation stress, further highlighting the need for people within the field of public health who can communicate effectively with multicultural groups. Public health professionals *must* gain multicultural communication skills because of two imperatives: (a) the *deantological imperative* and (b) the *utilitarian imperative.*

The deantological imperative rests on the ideological foundations of the United States. Founding documents—the Constitution and the Declaration of Independence—unequivocally state this nation's commitment to uphold the human rights of its people. As the Declaration of Independence states, "We hold these truths to be self-evident, that all men are created equal, that they are endowed by their Creator with certain unalienable rights, that among these are life, liberty and the pursuit of happiness." According to contemporary interpretations, these rights apply to all ethnic minority citizens, as well as to undocumented immigrants who require health care. Therefore, taking into account the changing demographics of the United States, public health practitioners have a moral obligation to learn to communicate with multicultural communities to treat all people equally in regard to equal access to preventive care. Taking a more practical, self-interest approach, the utilitarian imperative states that it is in society's own best interests to provide preventive care for all people.

High rates of immigration and the growing disparity between rich and poor has led to a resurgence of the diseases (e.g., tuberculosis) that were previously thought to be under control, as discussed previously in this chapter. Also, new infectious diseases, such as AIDS, have emerged in recent decades. The United States, therefore, is undergoing a "dual-epidemic" period, during which society experiences the gamut of preventable infections and chronic diseases. If a minority population that suffers from a preventable disease is ignored, then the majority puts itself at unnecessary risk. It is in the majority's best interest, therefore, to provide access to preventive health care to minorities, to avoid future epidemics (Kar & Alex, 1999).

Looking at the leading causes of death from a multicultural perspective, some interesting differences emerge (see Table 1.2). Non-Hispanic whites constitute such a huge majority in the United States that the total causes of death nearly mimics exactly their group's causes, obscuring the differences between ethnicities. For example, although HIV infection has just this year dropped off of the top 10 list of causes of death for the total population, Hispanics, African Americans, and Asian Americans are still grappling with this pervasive infectious disease (see Table 1.2). Also, note the exceptionally low death rates for Asian Americans overall, although the factors listed in Table 1.2 are their leading causes of death. In this group, heart disease is exceptionally low; although it remains the second-highest cause of death, heart disease is the first cause of death in every other group, with some groups doubling the Asian American rate of deaths per 100,000 persons.

To effectively promote public health within a multicultural community and reduce these risks, therefore, it is not enough to simply make services available. A partnership must be formed with the minority population, from which they will gain (a) the knowledge of public health practices to avoid being a source of health risk and (b) active participation in choosing their own prevention methods. The former has been common practice for decades, but the latter actually holds the key to successful preventive care. If the communication is not congruent or consistent with the population's accepted norms, the message will be lost. An effective strategy to mobilize the public for collective action should use three necessary components:

1. Participation by the targeted population

2. Partnership with the targeted population

3. Empowerment of the target population

Table 1.2   Top Ten Causes of Death, by Ethnicity (1997)

Top 10 Causes of Death	Total Death Rate per 100,000	Non-Hispanic White Death Rate	Hispanic Death Rate	African American Death Rate	Asian or Pacific Islander Death Rate	Native American Death Rate
Heart diseases	130.5	127.5	86.8	185.7	69.8	102.6
Cancer	125.6	125.3	76.4	165.2	75.4	86.6
Unintentional injuries	30.1	29.4	27.7	36.1	16.7	58.5
Cerebrovascular diseases	25.9	24.0	19.4	42.5	24.4	19.9
Chronic obstructive pulmonary diseases	21.1	22.4	8.7	17.4	8.6	15.3
Diabetes	13.5	11.8	18.7	28.9	9.3	30.4
Pneumonia and influenza	12.9	12.4	10.0	17.2	10.1	13.4
Suicide	10.6	11.3	6.1	6.3	6.2	12.9
Homicide and legal intervention	8.0	6.7	11.1	28.1	4.3	11.0
Chronic liver diseases	7.4	3.5	12.0	8.7	2.7	20.6
HIV infection	5.8	2.6	8.2	24.9	0.9	2.4

SOURCE: National Center for Health Statistics (1999, table 30).

To gain the acceptance of the community for the public health measures, the population in question must have active *participation* in the process. However, this could become a mere didactic exercise if the community has no say in the selection of priorities and the form or content of their own participation. Therefore, a *partnership* must be formed, giving the community both a stake and a role in making decisions about taking action to enhance their health. Last, *empowerment* of the community entails creating a self-sustaining program that will outlive the direct assistance and supervision of the public health professionals (Fetterman et al., 1996). Research has previously found that "involvement in social action movements, regardless of their specific goals, methods used, or outcomes, has strong empowering effects" (Kar et al., 1999, p. 1438). Thus, the processes of partnership and participation will foster an empowerment environment that, with community support, could launch the institutionalization of the health promotion program in question.

A New Public Health Paradigm for Multicultural Settings

In sum, a new public health paradigm is needed, one that combines traditional health care with modern techniques, recognizing cultural buffers and using them in modern ways. This new model would include three major components:

1. Recognition of alternative healing practices, as well as a higher regard for modern preventive care of all forms

2. Use of traditional communication systems

3. Use of modern technological advances to dispense health-related information to a multicultural populace. Blending natural and positive (cultural capitals) practices from different cultures would enhance the health of all, and the best aspects of each could be effectively mixed to help prevent disease and infection. To put it bluntly, Western medicine and Anglo-Saxon culture do not always have all the answers to better health.

Cultural Paradoxes and Capital

The following three apparent paradoxes illustrate that some cultures have unique characteristics—or "cultural capital"—that serve as buffers to health risks: (a) Latino paradox: low rates of infant mortality among Latinos (Kar, Jimenez, Campbell, & Sze, 1998; Zambrana, Scrimshaw, Collins, & Dunkel-Schetter, 1997); (b) French paradox: low rates of heart attacks among French men (Constant, 1997); and (c) Asian paradox: low rates of adolescent risks and mortality (Kar & Alex, 1999).

The Latino paradox exists in the clash between what mainstream data predict and the actuality as it exists in the Latino population. Epidemiological data show that prenatal care correlates positively with the birth outcome. In other words, an increase in rates of prenatal care should accompany lower rates of infant mortality. Use of prenatal care, in turn, depends on access to health care, usually measured by rates of health insurance. However, the Latino population in California brings that conclusion into question. Fully 40% of Latinos do not have health insurance, compared with 20% of African Americans in the same state. Latinos also have the highest rate of poverty. Therefore, they lack access to modern, hospital-provided prenatal care. The infant mortality rate among Latinos therefore is expected to be much higher than among African Americans. Paradoxically, the African American population has 4 *times* the infant mortality rate of the Latino population. Therefore, the Latino culture must contain some attributes that negate the lack of access to prenatal care among Latina women. We call this the Latino paradox. Although definitive explanation is lacking, it can be hypothesized that (a) the Latino culture sees motherhood more positively than does the African American culture and therefore offers more institutional and social support; (b) extended and stronger family ties exist in Latino families, giving the mother greater access to health-related information; and (c) Latino women have lower rates of smoking and drinking, leading to better birth outcomes. A multicultural paradigm allows us to identify and incorporate this positive cultural capital into a more expansive prenatal program that could reach out to lower-income, minority women of other ethnicities who may not have adequate health care.

The French paradox comes from the lower rates of heart attacks among the middle-aged French men, who otherwise have every high risk compared with middle-class U.S. white men. On average, French men smoke more, eat more fatty food, and exercise less than do U.S. men. Yet middle-aged French men have a rate of heart attacks that is *one third* less than do U.S. men of the same age group. Studies have hypothesized that drinking red wine regularly in moderation underlies this buffer to heart attacks; that conclusion remains controversial as a perfect preventive measure, because moderation must be achieved to garner the beneficial effects of the wine with few of the long-term negative effects (Finkel, 1995).

Last, the Asian paradox contradicts evidence relating to adolescent risk-taking behaviors. Studies show that acculturation stress and intergenerational conflict weakens parent-child relationships; these lead to deviant behavior among young children and adolescents. In other words, the stress of assimilating into a new society while going through adolescence may push many teenagers to lower academic performance, substance abuse, and other personally detrimental behaviors. Studies show the opposite for Asian immigrant children, who in fact have greater rates of educational success than do children from the white majority (Kar et al., 1998). Other factors in their culture, such as a high value on education as a social tool for success, respect for parental authority, and greater parental supervision, counteract the negative effects of acculturation stress. This kind of knowledge can help us understand the cultural buffer that one group has successfully taken advantage of to overcome obstacles to physical and mental health.

Summary

In conclusion, the importance of the field of public health has been steadily growing internationally and in the United States since the turn of the century. The last two decades, however, have closed the century with major changes in how public health views its work. There is a greater agreement that the field must have a multicultural and community focus to effectively serve the population, particularly within the United States and in other multicultural societies. The following chapters delve more deeply into the importance of multicultural health communication.

References

Constant, J. (1997). Alcohol, ischemic heart disease, and the French paradox. *Coronary Artery Disease, 8*(10), 645-649.

Fetterman, D. M., Kaftarian, S. J., & Wandersman, A. (Eds.). (1996). *Empowerment evaluation: Knowledge and tools for self-assessment and accountability.* Thousand Oaks, CA: Sage.

Finkel, H. E. (1995). To your health! Two physicians explore the benefits of wine. *New England Journal of Medicine, 332*(5). Retrieved June 12, 2000, from the World Wide Web: www.nejm.org/content/1995/0332/0005/0339b.asp

Gutheil, I. A. (1996). Introduction: The many faces of aging: Challenges for the future. *The Gerontologist, 36*(1), 13-14.

Kar, S. B., & Alex, S. B. (1999). Public health approaches to substance abuse prevention: A multicultural perspective. In S. B. Kar (Ed.), *Substance abuse prevention in multicultural communities.* Amityville, NY: Baywood.

Kar, S., Jimenez, A., Campbell, K., & Sze, F. (1998). Acculturation and quality of life: A comparative study of Japanese-Americans and Indo-Americans. *Amerasia Journal, 24*(10), 129-142.

Kar, S. B., Pascual, C., & Chickering, K. (1999). Empowerment of women for health promotion: A meta-analysis. *Social Science & Medicine, 49,* 1431-1460.

Kumar, V. (1997). Ageing in India—An overview. *Indian Journal of Medical Research, 106,* 257-264.

Los Angeles Unified School District Survey. (1993). Back to the barricades. *The Economist, 328*(7824), A26-A27.

National Center for Health Statistics. (1999). *Health, United States, 1999.* Retrieved June 12, 2000, from the World Wide Web: http://www.cdc.gov/nchs/products/pubs/pubd/hus/hus.htm

The Ottawa Charter for Health Promotion (17-21 November 1986). (1996). In *Health promotion anthology* (Scientific Publication No. 557). Washington, DC: World Health Organization, Pan American Health Organization.

Preparatory Committee for the International Conference on Population and Development. (1992). *Preparations for the conference, recommendations of the Expert Group Meeting on Family Planning, Health and Family Well-being, report of the secretary-general of the conference.* Second Session, International Conference on Population and Development, Bangalore, India.

Statistics Division and Population Division of the United Nations Secretariat. (1998). *Indicators on youth and elderly populations.* Retrieved June 12, 2000, from the World Wide Web: http://www.un.org/depts/unsd/social/youth.htm

Terris, M. (1992). Concepts of health promotion: Dualities in pubic health theory. *Journal of Public Health Policy, 13*(3), 267-276.

U.S. Department of Commerce, Bureau of the Census. (1953). *Census of the population: 1950* (Vol. II, part I). Washington, DC: Government Printing Office.

U.S. Department of Commerce, Bureau of the Census. (1998a). *Population estimates.* Retrieved June 12, 2000, from the World Wide Web: http://www.census.gov/population/www/estimates/popest.html

U.S. Department of Commerce, Bureau of the Census. (1998b). *Population projections.* Retrieved June 12, 2000, from the World Wide Web: http://www.census.gov/population/www/projections/popproj.html

U.S. Department of Commerce and Labor, Bureau of the Census. (1909). *A century of population growth: From the first census of the United States to the twelfth 1790-1900.* Washington, DC: Government Printing Office.

U.S. House of Representatives. (1998). H.R. 3736, 105th Cong. Retrieved June 12, 2000, on the World Wide Web: http://thomas.loc.gov

World Health Organization. (1986). *Ottawa charter.* Division of Health Promotion, Education and Communication, First International Conference on Health Promotion, Ottawa, Canada.

World Health Organization. (1996). *Fact Sheet N 131.* Retrieved June 5, 2000, from the World Wide Web: http://www.who.int/inf-fs/en/fact131.html

World Health Organization. (1998). *The world health report 1998: Life in the 21st century, a vision for all.* Geneva, Switzerland: Author.

World Health Organization/United Nations International Children's Emergency Fund. (1978). *ALMA-ATA 1978 primary health care: Report of the International Conference on Primary Health Care.* Geneva, Switzerland: Author.

Zambrana, R. E., Scrimshaw, S. C. M., Collins, N., & Dunkel-Schetter, C. (1997). Prenatal health behaviors and psychosocial risk factors in pregnant women of Mexican origin: The role of acculturation. *American Journal of Public Health, 87*(6), 1022-1027.

2

The Emergence of a New Public Health Paradigm in the United States

Snehendu B. Kar
Rina Alcalay
with Shana Alex

This chapter reviews the mission and imperatives of public and the major social trends that may affect the success of health communications as we enter the 21st century. Because the aim of this volume is to review public health communication needs from a multicultural perspective, we begin with an enunciation of the mission of public health and health communication in a new world of changing technology.

Changing Health Needs and the Double Burden

Public health in its modern form has evolved over time from the mid-19th century, encompassing three main phases: (a) the struggle against infectious diseases, (b) the rise and subsequent fight against chronic diseases, and (c) the dual-epidemic control period, characterized by simultaneous battles against both chronic and infectious diseases. Although we in the United States are currently in the dual-epidemic period, to understand the nature of this era of public health, we must look first at the two eras that preceded it. Many less industrialized parts of the world still remain mired in the infectious disease stage, but they are rapidly encountering dual epidemics due to aging of the population.

The Infectious Disease Period

In the 1870s, the mechanism by which bacteria and germs spread disease became known. At that point, the world remained locked in the grip of infectious diseases, with no effective method of battling large-scale epidemics. The momentous development of combating infectious disease rested largely on the work of medical biologists, who worked tirelessly to discover how disease is caused by microorganisms in order to halt infectious diseases such as anthrax and cholera (Rosen, 1993). Between the two decades spanning 1877 and 1897, the foundations of the modern understanding of pathogen microbiology were laid. Armed with this new knowledge, the first modern public health practitioners battled epidemics around the world, taking on infectious diseases ranging from cholera to smallpox (Rosen, 1993).

Although the campaign against smallpox through vaccination has earned a great deal of recognition for public health work (especially because it was so successful and actually eradicated the disease), much of the public health work focused on increasing sanitation measures as a way to combat the spread of disease. The motto, "A clean city is a healthy city," had taken root in the health field, even before the exact nature of the transmission of disease was known (Rosen, 1993). Sanitation work earned many public health practitioners the name "sanitarian" in the United States, and much of public health's main work was performed under this title during the last decades of the 19th century and the dawn of the 20th century (Duffy, 1990).

The improvement of housing, cleaning of water, and disposal of waste materials brought about a highly reduced rate of cholera, yellow fever, and typhoid fever all over the municipalities of Western Europe and America, the areas where the improvements were mainly implemented. For example, the rate of typhoid fever in England and Wales plummeted during this time period (see Figure 2.1).

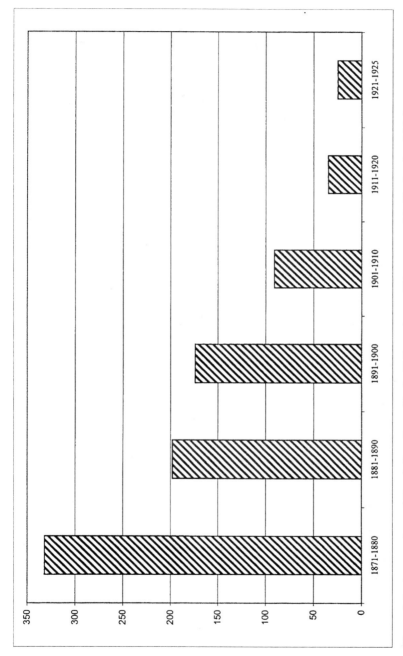

Figure 2.1. Average Annual Death Rate From Typhoid Fever (per million persons) in England and Wales

SOURCE: Rosen (1993, p. 316).

In the United States, the trend mirrored that of England, with the death rate from typhoid fever dropping from 313 cases per million in 1900 to 76 cases per million in 1920. In the case of typhoid, a combination of vaccination, increased chlorination of the water supply, and diversion of the sewers explains the sudden drop in the death rate (Duffy, 1990; Sterling, 1920). Overall in the United States, deaths from all infectious diseases fell from 797 deaths per 100,000 in 1990 to just under 100 deaths per 100,000 in 1950 (with a brief but deadly interruption by the 1918 influenza epidemic) (Armstrong, Conn, & Pinner, 1999).

However, these reductions in death and disability caused by infectious diseases brought with them two major changes in the population: (a) emergence of noncommunicable diseases as the leading causes of death and (b) increased life expectancy and changes in demographic composition, along with an aging population.

Chronic and Lifestyle Diseases Period

As more people than ever before in human history survived to old age, the diseases caused by accumulated stress to the body over a long period of time began to take their toll. Even with all our current knowledge and efforts, heart disease, a mostly preventable condition, remains the chief killer in the United States (National Center for Health Statistics [NCHS], 1998).

Beginning in the mid-20th century, public health scientists began to study the conditions that led up to heart disease and other chronic conditions that emerged as the leading causes of death and disability in industrialized societies. For example, the Framingham Heart Study launched its first program of study in 1948 in Framingham, Massachusetts. These scientists began with the healthy people in the town of Framington; still ongoing, they have now studied four generations of people. By analyzing the lifestyles of those who ended up with serious chronic conditions, the scientists found that high-fat diets and smoking do, in fact, lead to earlier death because of heart disease as well as to various types of cancer (Castelli, 1996). When the study began, society assumed that smoking and high-fat diets were not only harmless but could also have beneficial effects. Society now is fully aware of the dangers of both, and yet a significant number of people continue to engage in self-destructive behaviors.

Those behaviors have led to the second phase of public health—namely, attempting to prevent disease through changing the lifestyle or behavior patterns of individuals and environmental factors and stress. With this goal in mind, public health practitioners have necessarily embraced communication as a method with which to influence the behavior patterns of populations. As examples, the North Karelia Project, a comprehensive community program for control of cardiovascular diseases in Finland (National Public Health Laboratory of Finland, 1981; Rice & Atkin, 1989), and the University of Texas Health Science Center Campaign (Rice & Atkin, 1989) both used television broadcasts with measurable rates of success. More about the use of mass communication, both its advantages and its limitations, will be discussed in detail in Chapter 5.

Dual-Epidemic Period

Although still having to deal with these problems of chronic diseases, much of the industrialized world, particularly the United States, has found itself dealing with infectious diseases long thought eliminated in the earlier part of the century. Emergence of new infectious diseases (e.g., HIV/AIDS) further compounds the situation (Afifi & Breslow, 1994; NCHS, 1996). Nonwhites have a much higher rate of infectious disease death in the United States than do whites; the figures show a clear rise in infectious disease morbidity, particularly among the nonwhite populations (see Figure 2.2).

Figure 2.2 starkly illustrates the unique problems of the dual-epidemic period, especially in multicultural communities. With the rise of infectious diseases, public health practitioners can no longer assume that the deadly problems of the infectious disease period have passed. Simultaneously, public health must also deal with the chronic diseases that still take millions of lives. Figure 2.3, below, illustrates the trends in morbidity from cardiovascular disease during the same time period as Figure 2.2.

Note that in Figure 2.3, unlike Figure 2.2, the general trend is toward a reduction in the mortality rate, for both whites and nonwhites. However, it must also be noted that the two figures do not use the same scale; rates in Figure 2.3 range from approximately 155 to 315 deaths per 100,000 persons, whereas rates in Figure 2.2 range from approximately 1 to 43 deaths per 100,000 persons. In other words, although cardiovascular disease remains the major public health threat in the United States, the rate of death by infectious disease is rising, forcing public health practitioners to deal with both problems simultaneously rather than sequentially (see Figure 2.4).

Also noteworthy is the repeated higher rate of morbidity among nonwhite populations; minorities tend to be at higher risk than whites for many health problems. These findings add weight to the argument that the future of public

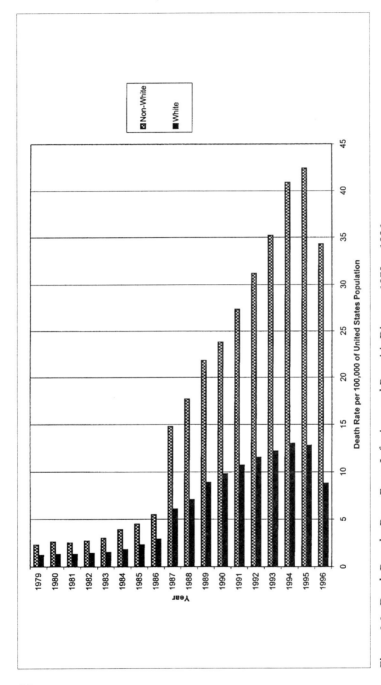

Figure 2.2. Death Rate, by Race, From Infectious and Parasitic Diseases, 1979 to 1996

SOURCE: National Center for Health Statistics (1996, p. 293, table 15).

NOTE: Excludes tuberculosis, shigellosis and amebiasis, whooping cough, streptococcus, meningococcus, septicemia, poliomyelitis, measles, viral hepatitis, and syphilis.

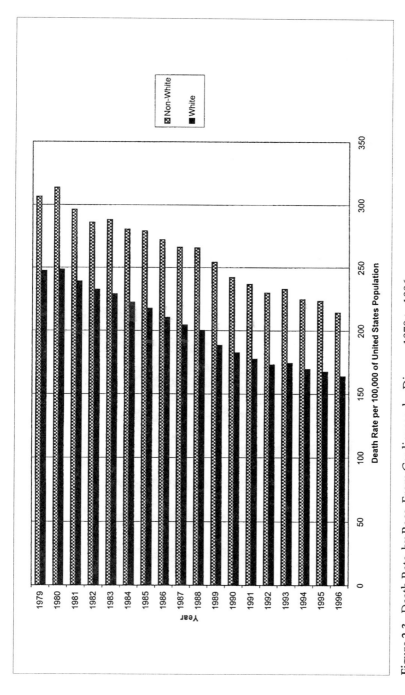

Figure 2.3. Death Rate, by Race, From Cardiovascular Disease, 1979 to 1996

SOURCE: National Center for Health Statistics (1996, p. 293, table 31).

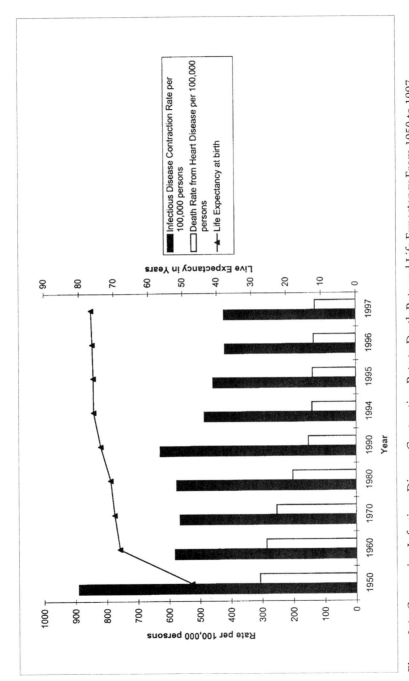

Figure 2.4. Comparing Infectious Disease Contraction Rate to Death Rate and Life Expectancy From 1950 to 1997

SOURCE: National Center for Health Statistics (1999, tables 28, 37, & 53).

health, particularly in the United States, will be in dealing with increasingly diverse populations who have varying risk factors and buffers.

Mission and Significance of the Public Health Model

There are numerous statements on the mission of public health. The three common elements of these mission statements are to aim at the following:

1. Health promotion and disease prevention (HPDP) rather than treatment of illness or injuries

2. HPDP for the public or community as a whole rather than for individual clients

3. HPDP with active participation rather than through passive compliance of the public or community at risk (Institute of Medicine, 1988; "Ottawa Charter," 1996; U.S. Department of Health and Human Services, 1991; World Health Organization/UNICEF, 1978)

Unlike modern Western medicine's focus on clinical and medical interventions for diagnosis and treatment of diseases of individual patients, public health uses a multidisciplinary and nonclinical preventive approach, a combination of medicine, engineering, education, and management that combines to create a new discipline that is both dynamic and proactive (Afifi & Breslow, 1994). Public health contains five core disciplines for HPDP with the public or the community as the unit of its intervention: (a) biostatistics, (b) epidemiology, (c) behavioral sciences and health education, (d) environmental health sciences, and (e) health policy and management.

According to the Institute of Medicine (IOM) (1988), the role of government in public health is to facilitate three functions:

1. *Assessment,* which includes diagnosis, surveillance, needs assessment, collection and analyses of data, research, and evaluation of outcome

2. *Policy development,* which includes policy analyses and formulation, setting priorities and goals, defining means to reach them, handling of conflicting views and allocating resources, policy leadership and advocacy, public policy development, and encouragement of public and private sector action through incentives and persuasion

3. *Ensurance,* which includes actions to ensure that necessary health care services are provided to reach agreed goals, implementation of legislative and statutory responsibilities, developing appropriate responses to crises and supporting critical services, regulation of services, and ensuring accountability (pp. 44-47)

We conceptualize health communication as a critical domain of public health that includes all process and actions supporting the overall mission and the three key functions of public health delineated above.

To enact health communication in a multicultural setting, however, it is first necessary to define the concept of multiculturalism as it relates to public health. We define multiculturalism as the conscious practice of recognizing "transcultural absolutes," which all human beings share (Phillips, 1997), but we realize that they come clothed in different forms in different cultures. For example, the need to protect and promote the health of children traverses all cultural boundaries and can become a powerful motivator to take action, particularly in communities that have few other resources (Kar, Pascual, & Chickering, 1999). However, the harnessing of this force must take different forms for different communities and must address the needs in understandable means for the community at large to gain the institutionalization of the action in question. In short, multicultural health communication rests on an understanding that (a) other cultures exist, (b) they contain valid aspects, and (c) they have particular methods for transmitting values to their adherents (Appiah, 1994). The next step entails using these realizations to develop effective and relevant health promotion communication.

Nature of the Health Care System

Health care in the United States has become a primarily managed care system with a predominantly clinical focus. Despite research showing that preventive care reduces health care costs in the long term, less than 2% of care expenditures go toward preventive care (Lee & Paxman, 1997). Under the clinical paradigm, care is given only after an illness, injury, or infection, by which time the harm has already occurred. However, people of all social statuses are still suffering from preventable illnesses. Therefore, the system, as it stands today, practices methods incongruent with the health needs of many ethnic minority communities, who require preventive care. In addition, an unacceptably large proportion of people in the United States do not have health insurance (estimates range from 35-45 million people). Consequently, they do not have regular access to health care services; most cannot afford preventive services and so suffer from preventable illnesses. Three major trends appear to clearly influence the necessary future of public health care: (a) the emergence of diseases that defy clinical preventive practices, (b) increased emphasis on reducing health care costs, and (c) increased use of alternative forms of medicine. Taken together, these trends point to a new direction for public health communication.

First, diseases that cannot be prevented clinically are becoming more common in the United States, because people continue to voluntarily engage in activities that damage their health. For example, although information regarding the hazards of smoking has been widely disseminated, over 1 million teenagers still start smoking every year (Shalala, 1998). These kinds of activities lead to high rates of preventable diseases that nonetheless cannot be cured once they begin, such as lung and throat cancer. Also, new diseases such as AIDS illustrate that prevention acts as the only effective measure against them. Although clinical treatment exists, it can only keep the disease in check for an indefinite period of time rather than curing the illness.

Second, health maintenance organizations (HMOs) have shifted their focus from delivering all available forms of health care to emphasizing cost-effectiveness in health care for plan members. This mind-set clashes harshly with the reality of lack of access to health insurance for many minority citizens. In 1995, only 47% of Hispanics and 54% of blacks were covered by private health insurance, compared with 78% of whites. That same year, 32% of Hispanics and 20% of blacks remained uninsured, compared with only 13% of whites (NCHS, 1998). Rather than engaging in regular checkups and preventive measures, which they would have to pay for out of pocket, they wait to ask for health care until they are in the emergency room with a painful and costly problem. Using the emergency room as the health care giver, unfortunately, remains common.

The lack of affordability creates gaps in health care coverage that affect not only the health of the adult population but the health of their children as well. About one fourth of U.S. children have no health insurance for at least 1 month during their first 3 years of life, with over half of these having a gap in their coverage that lasts over 6 months. Research has shown that children with a regular source of medical attention have 25% lower costs of overall care than do children without, because of timely immunizations and fewer emergency room visits (Kogan et al., 1995). Therefore, preventive care in multicultural communities also makes good fiscal sense.

Third, many people seek more methods of "alternative" medicine based on traditional practices. A study performed in 1990 found that 34% of those surveyed had used one or more forms of alternative medicine, or "unconventional therapy" as the survey stated, in the past 12 months, with the mean number of visits per person at 19 for the same time period (Gordon, 1996). In 1998, a survey found that 42% of the population had used alternative therapies in the past year (Eisenberg et al., 1998). A 1996 study projected that the demand for these therapies would spark a growth in the number of alternative medicine practitioners: The supply will grow by 88% between 1994 and 2010, compared with projected growth of 16% in the supply of physicians (Yankauer, 1997).

Interestingly, consumers earning over $50,000 per year had a higher prevalence of use of alternative therapies in 1997 (48%) than did those with less income (43%) (Eisenberg et al., 1998). This statistic of alternative medicine use rates belies the common stereotype that those who use alternative medicines are poor immigrants who trust only their traditional forms of medicine. That people with some college education have a higher proportion of use (51%) than those without (27%) further demolishes this common misconception (Eisenberg et al., 1998). Women also use alternative therapies with higher prevalence than do men, 49% to 38%, respectively (Eisenberg et al., 1998).

According to the Landmark Healthcare Study performed in 1998, a significant portion of the U.S. population as a whole (40%) has developed a more positive opinion of alternative medicine within the last 5 years. Of this group, 47% stated that they came to this conclusion "after learning more about it," and 41% stated that they "had a positive experience," compared with the mere 11% who said that they were "not satisfied with traditional care" (Landmark Healthcare, 1998). This trend has led some hospitals and medical schools to relabel alternative medicine as *complementary* or *integrative* medicine, emphasizing in word and in practice that these should be and often are used in conjunction with Western clinical techniques (Fontanarosa & Lundberg, 1998; Monmaney & Roan, 1998; Wetzel, Eisenberg, & Kaptchuk, 1998).

However, it must also be noted that fully 58% of respondents stated that they were using alternative medicine to "prevent future illness from occurring or to maintain health and vitality" (Eisenberg et al., 1998). This high rate of use points to a significant amount of dissatisfaction with the preventive care offered through the current clinical paradigm.

Integration of Alternative Medicine

As yet, despite the growing interest in alternative forms of medicine, much of the health care community remains opposed to the use of treatments such as the ingestion of herbs or a visit to a chiropractor. For example, although the *Journal of the American Medical Association (JAMA)* recently dedicated an entire issue to alternative medicine and whether or not it may have a scientific basis, the well-respected editors of *JAMA* took the opportunity to deride any practice of "alternative therapies [that] have not been evaluated using rigorously conducted scientific tests of efficacy based on accepted rules of evidence" (Fontanarosa & Lundberg, 1998, p. 1618). The articles published in their own journal contained mixed results; some alternative therapies achieved the desired results better than a placebo, whereas others did not. Proclamations such as, "However, until solid evidence is available that demonstrates the safety, efficacy, and effectiveness of specific alternative medicine interventions, uncritical acceptance of untested and unproven alternative medicine therapies must stop" (Fontanarosa & Lundberg, 1998, p. 1619), represents a prevalent mood in the medical community and ignores the very real reasons that people turn to alternative medicines. In addition, some of these therapies have been in practice for millennia and are not entirely "untested," although they do not use the standard drug development practices of Western medicine.

It must be noted, however, that the medical community has reasons, too, for its caution. Self-medicating is becoming more prevalent, with people ingesting substances labeled "natural" that may contain dangerous chemicals. For example, the California Department of Health Services has found imported "herbal medication" packets in Los Angeles' Chinatown that also contained mercury sulfide in 1,000 times the dosage mandated for safety in drugs in the United States (Monmaney, 1998). Despite these dangers, sales of herbal remedies continue to rise. As reported in the *Los Angeles Times,* many popular herbal remedies saw a huge increases in sales over the 2 years before the article was published (Monmaney, 1998). Echinacea increased in sales by 72%, bringing in $310 million dollars in sales in 1997; St. John's wort increased by 1,900%, accounting for $200 million in sales in 1997 (Monmaney, 1998). These figures point to the disjunction between the medical profession and the general population, as people ignore the warnings and take their preventive care into their own hands (recall from earlier in the chapter that one fourth of the U.S. population uses alternative medicine for preventive purposes).

Considered simultaneously, these trends point to a common conclusion: With a multicultural population, the need for a new health promotion paradigm emerges. Rather than focusing on clinical treatment after the fact, health care should spend more efforts on preventive care. Because many ethnic minorities have higher rates of preventable diseases than do whites, to prevent future problems the public health community must learn how to communicate with these different groups. Making the preventive measures of public health more prevalent and more communicable to minority populations would help alleviate these problems.

The Communication Revolution

A communication revolution has been sweeping both rich and poor nations of the world since the advent of electronic media and computers. This revolution has three main characteristics: (a) rapid increase in sheer volume of media and programs, (b) diversity of media, and (c) new and faster and cheaper communications. For instance, air transport cost between New York and London per passenger mile decreased by more than half between 1960 and 1990 (from 0.24 to 0.11 cents; United Nations Development Programme [UNDP] 1999, p. 30). A 3-minute phone call from New York to London for the same period was reduced to less than 1/15th ($46 in 1960 to $3.00 in 1990). The cost of a computer dropped from $12,500 in 1960 to less than $100 in 1990 (UNDP, 1999, p. 30). In addition, globalization, international migration, and travel and trade have significantly increased exposure to different cultures, worldviews, and health-related beliefs and practices. At the same time, the global market for communication and cultural products is becoming concentrated in a few countries. "At the core of the entertainment industry—film, music, and television—there is a dominance of US products. . . . For the United States the largest single export industry is not an aircraft, computers or automobiles—it is entertainment, in films and television programmes" (UNDP, 1999, p. 33). Poor people and people who do not participate in production decisions are the majority of consumers of programs designed by a very small number of persons, mostly men from the dominant culture who have a monopoly over both access (hardwire) and the content (programs) of communication media.

Different ethnic groups receive and process health information from different sources (see Table 2.1); therefore, health promotion campaigns should go beyond the standard television ads now considered essential by many for an

Table 2.1   Sources of Health-Related Information in Los Angeles (in percentages)

	Total (N = 2,054)	Non-Hispanic White (n = 924)	Hispanic (n = 679)	African American (n = 200)	Asian American (n = 251)
Television	33.7	27.5	44.3	28.5	32.1
Doctors	31.5	37.3	24.9	42.5	19.1
Newspapers	31.4	33.5	28.3	20.5	40.6
Printed materials (books, magazines, pamphlets, etc.)	31.0	31.5	29.8	37.8	26.7
Family	12.3	12.6	14.1	6.0	11.6
Friends	12.2	10.2	16.1	7.5	12.7
Radio	5.6	4.4	7.7	5.0	7.1
Hotlines	1.7	2.1	1.3	1.0	1.6
Other	7.3	7.5	9.0	3.5	5.2

SOURCE: Los Angeles County Department of Health Services (1994).
NOTE: Due to multiple respondent answers concerning media use, the percentages in the table exceed 100.

effective campaign and move into reaching multicultural communities through other means. Concurrent with the increase in use of traditional medicine, there is also greater access and use of traditional communication media (e.g., ethnic radio, newspapers) and information-sharing systems, particularly among new immigrants. Overall, different ethnic groups have different methods by which to find out health-related information (see Table 2.1).

The Los Angeles County Department of Health Services conducted a study that revealed the differences among ethnic groups in sources for health-related information (see Table 2.1). If only the overall total is looked at, it appears that people use television, doctors, newspapers, and printed materials equally as the source of health information. However, a very different picture emerges when we examine the responses by ethnicity. Non-Hispanic whites rely mainly on (in order) doctors, newspapers, and printed materials for their health information (37.3%, 33.5%, and 31.5%, respectively). In contrast, television is the most frequent source of health information among Hispanics (44.3%), with printed materials and newspapers following as the next most used sources (29.3% and 28.3%, respectively). African Americans, however, rely just as frequently on information from doctors (42.5%), with printed materials closely following (37.8%), and television coming in third (28.5%). For Asian Americans, information comes mainly from newspapers (40.6%), television (32.1%), and printed materials (26.7%). Family members and friends are also important sources of health information. With different ethnic groups using different sources of information, it can be difficult to rely on only one communication method for health promotion in a multicultural community.

Along with the traditional forms of printed materials and interpersonal networks, the Internet has joined the ranks as a new form of communication media. First, there has been a rapid expansion in the total volume of media in a population in a given area. News can also be viewed simultaneously across the world. Second, there has been a rapid diversification in media designed to serve a wide range of population segments, including many ethnic groups. More TV programs, newspapers, and communication materials are now produced and distributed to serve an increasingly diverse audience, both globally and locally. Because of these trends, the media have themselves become a risk factor for unhealthy behaviors that lead to chronic conditions. Public health promoters must recognize the limitations of and risks associated with the mass media, tailoring their programs in multicultural communities accordingly.

Expansion in the Total Volume of the Media

Since television's inception and popularization in the mid-1950s in the United States, the medium has captured the adoration of the public across ethnic lines. As of mid-1998, an estimated 98 million households in the United States had a television (Nielsen Media Research, 1998b). With the immediacy of news and the flood of information, what Marshall McLuhan termed a "global village" has come into being, bringing immediacy to news from around the globe. However, the three major networks (ABC, CBS, and NBC) now do not wield the monopoly that they once had. With the explosive growth in cable and pay channels that have turned the major metropolis areas into veritable cornucopias of entertainment with over 100 channels on nearly every television set, the viewing audience for any one particular channel is becoming increasingly fragmented. No one standard TV channel can be used to reach all segments of a multicultural population.

Television has become ubiquitous, a daily activity in almost every person's life in the United States. According to Nielsen Media Research (NMR), Hispanic children, Hispanic teenagers, and all black age groups watch more television per day than the general viewing public (NMR, 1997, 1998a). Data were unavailable for Asian American viewers. Looking back at Table 2.1, however, note that only Hispanics received most of their health-related information from television. Therefore, despite the hours per day spent viewing television, most ethnic groups do not see that medium as a consistent and competent method of finding out health-related information.

New forms of media have also emerged over the last decade, such as the Internet and interactive media. Studies show that nearly two thirds of American children have used the Internet at some point in their lives (Hertzel, 2000). As Chamberlain wrote in 1996, just as the Internet was beginning to seriously percolate through society and become a useful form of mass media, "We are moving from the Age of Mass Communication to the Age of Interactive Communication, in which many of the old communication models will be insufficient or redundant" (p. 43). Health promoters must keep the expansion and diversification of media in mind when designing a health promotion communication program.

Rapid Diversification of Media

The media's need to cater to the viewing preferences of different groups has caused this fragmentation. Major broadcast network channels appeal mostly to the white, middle-class viewing audience, for the simple reason of demographics; this group remains the most populous and therefore has the most clout and buying power. In addition, mostly white male media executives, producers, and directors make media programming decisions. However, this group has become a much smaller proportion of the overall population, leaving many audiences starved for television programs that serve their needs. Since 1970, network TV viewership among the general population has declined from 90% to only 60% in the 1990s (UCLA Center for Communication Policy, 1997). When the audience of the network channels is broken down by ethnicity, it becomes clear that different ethnic groups have different viewing patterns. Among English-language shows, the highest-ranked program for the 1996-97 season among Hispanic viewers was *Ellen* on ABC (NMR, 1997); this show was canceled the following season for overall low ratings. According to NMR (1998a), for the full 1996-97 season, the overall top rated show for Hispanic households was *Maria La Del Barrio,* a Spanish-language program broadcast on Univision.

A look at the data for black viewership compared with the general audience also reveals some disparities. The networks are ranked as follows (from highest to lowest) for the 1998 fall season among the general viewing population: CBS,

NBC, ABC, FOX, UPN, and WB. Among the black viewing population, the ranking is as follows: UPN, WB, FOX, CBS, ABC, NBC (NMR, 1998c). To further highlight this gap between black viewers and the general population (composed mainly of white viewers across the nation), the top 10 shows between the two groups for the full 1997-98 season share only two shows in common; both were specials, not regular programming. Although 9 of the 10 top programs for the general public were aired on NBC, the top 10 shows for blacks included broadcasts on FOX, WB, ABC, and NBC (NMR, 1998c). Unfortunately, no data were available for the viewing preferences of Asian Americans, but the above data clearly illustrate how different television viewing can be by ethnicity, and consequently, how difficult it can be to use television as a medium for effectively reaching a multicultural community. Similarly, newspapers, which serve as an important source of information for many ethnic groups, are freely distributed to diverse interests in diverse languages, creating a uniquely multicultural medium.

Media as a Risk Factor

Although all forms of mass communication have the potential for imparting health-promoting messages, the commercial media as a whole has actually become a separate health risk factor, for two reasons: (a) the cumulative effects of repeated exposure to glamorization of health-damaging activities and (b) use of the media by industries with significant capital to spend on commercials, promoting products that are detrimental to the overall health of the population. The Center for Media Education (CME) has found that children who watch TV excessively are more likely to be obese, more likely to abuse alcohol and drugs within their lifetime, and more likely to engage in sexual activities earlier in life (CME, 1998b). The CME also discovered that alcohol and tobacco companies, longtime promoters of their products through billboards and television, are now using online media to further promote their brands (CME, 1998a). Because of these increasingly aggressive media tactics on the part of industries whose products can harm a person's health, such as cigarettes, alcohol, and fatty foods, the mass media has become in and of itself a health risk factor.

Consolidation of the mainstream media into fewer and fewer large conglomerates has also become a fact of life over the past 5 years. With the upcoming merger of America Online and Time Warner creating the biggest multimedia company in the world, consumer groups have begun focusing their attention on keeping access to information as open as possible to preempt the stifling of smaller media outlets (CME, 2000a). America Online, previously an outspoken advocate of open access, has since become a believer in letting the "free market" decide—that is, in leaving Time Warner with sole control of the high-speed Internet cable it currently operates, now that its partner can share that access (CME, 2000b).

The role of media in society in general, and in women's persistent inequality, is an area of global concern. There is a global consensus that news and entertainment perpetuate gender inequality by (a) portraying women in subordinate positions and as sex objects, (b) depicting violence against women as a way of life, and (c) excluding women's perspective in programs by denying women policy-making positions in media establishments. The 1995 Fourth World Conference on status of women adopted a platform for a global agenda for the advancement of women forward. The Beijing +5 meeting, which took place in June 2000 at the United Nations headquarters in New York, was a special session of the U.N. General Assembly titled "Women: 2000: Gender Equality, Development and Peace for the Twenty-First Century" (see the Beijing +5 Web site at http://www.un.org/womenwatch/followup/beijing5/about.htm; United Nations, 1999). In addition, with increasing globalization of commercial and entertainment industries, people in poor countries and communities are being increasingly exposed to media programs produced by richer countries and alien cultures. A UNESCO (United Nations Educational, Scientific, and Cultural Organization) study shows that trade of media materials with "cultural content" (printed matter, music, visual arts, movies, photography, radio, TV,) almost tripled between 1980 and 1991, from $67 billion to $200 billion" (UNDP, 1999, p. 33). Modern communication technology via satellite has expanded very rapidly; the number of TV sets per 1,000 population worldwide doubled between 1980 and 1995 from 121 to 235. Multimedia industries have experienced a boom in their trades in the 1990s; sales for the largest 50 multimedia companies reached $110 billion in 1993 (UNDP, 1999, p. 33). That is more than the gross domestic product (1997 figures) of many countries, including Malaysia, Israel, Colombia, the Philippines, and Venezuela (UNDP, 1999, p. 323). Media production and sales are also becoming the monopoly of a few rich nations; there is a growing dominance of U.S. products. The impacts of such rapid expansion of modern media propagating sex, violence, and hazardous lifestyle (e.g., MTV, CNN, movies, videos, western TV) on Third World cultures, and generation and gender role conflicts everywhere is unknown (Kar & Alex, 1999). Clearly, commercial media do not act as a welfare system, and democratic societies uphold the value of freedom of media. Consequently, we cannot demand that media must educate and reform our societies, and we cannot control the media through draconian measures. At the same time, all freedoms of action and expression have their limits that must be balanced against collective interests and utility. Rather than introducing sanctions, it is more desirable to rigorously apply two widely accepted principles for media reform—"gender equity" and protection of minors from media violence and pornography.

The question remains: How can health promoters counter these effects? A media war would be impossible, because no public health program would ever have the funds necessary to compete with commercial monies. Furthermore, the media, as a business industry, will not donate a sufficient amount of their valuable advertising time to health promotion campaigns. Therefore, the most appealing option that remains is to mobilize community-based communication resources to counter the harmful messages in the mass media. With the knowledge that multicultural and ethnic communities use a greater variety of communication sources than more homogeneous groups, health promoters can create programs that take advantage of, rather than marginalize, local and ethnic networks for health communication.

Implications for
Public Health Communication

In summary, as a consequence of the diversification of popular media and the communication explosion, public health practitioners have both a moral and a practical justification to adopt a multicultural perspective in health communication. However, with the changing demographics of the nation, many may not realize that using standard television or newspapers to reach out to multicultural communities may actually sabotage their own efforts. Public health communication must be progressive and creative in identifying an array of community-based ethnic networks to present information in a format that is accessible and acceptable to ethnic communities. The communication flow should also go both ways, because other cultures have much to teach Western medicine about risk prevention and health care. A new public health communication paradigm should be developed that combines ethnic communication networks with modern communication methods and incorporates alternative forms of medicine and Western practices.

References

Afifi, A., & Breslow, L. (1994). The maturing paradigm of public health. *Annual Review of Public Health, 15,* 223-235.

Armstrong, G. L., Conn, L. A., & Pinner, R. W. (1999). Trends in infectious disease mortality in the United States during the 20th century. *JAMA, 281,* 61-66.

Appiah, K. A. (1994, September 12). *Identity against culture.* Avenali Lecture, University of California, Berkeley.

Castelli, W. (1996). Take this letter to your doctor (measuring cholesterol in people over age 65). *Prevention, 48*(11), 61.

Center for Media Education. (1998a). *Alcohol and tobacco on the Web: New threats to youth* (Executive summary). Retrieved June 9, 2000 from the World Wide Web: http://www.cme.org/children/marketing/execsum.html

Center for Media Education. (1998b). *Frequently asked questions.* Retrieved in February 1999 from the World Wide Web: http://www.cme.org

Center for Media Education. (2000a, January 10). *Consumer groups respond to AOL-Time Warner deal.* Retrieved June 9, 2000 from the World Wide Web: http://www.cme.org/press/000110pr.html

Center for Media Education (2000b, January 25). *Open access: The campaign continues.* Retrieved June 9, 2000 from the World Wide Web: http://www.cme.org/access/broadband/campaigncontinues.html

Chamberlain, M. A. (1996). Health communication: Making the most of new media technologies—An international overview. *Journal of Health Communication, 1,* 43-50.

Duffy, J. (1990). *The sanitarians: A history of American public health.* Urbana and Chicago: University of Illinois Press.

Eisenberg, D. M., Davis, R. B., Ettner, S. L., Appel, S., Wilkey, S., Van Rompay, M., & Kessler, R. C. (1998). Trends in alternative medicine use in the United States, 1990-1997: Results of a follow-up national survey. *JAMA, 280,* 1569-1575.

Fontanarosa, P. B., & Lundberg, G. D. (1998). Alternative medicine meets science. *JAMA, 280,* 1618-1619.

Gordon, J. S. (1996). Alternative medicine & the family physician. *American Family Physician, 54*(7), 2205-2212.

Hertzel, D. (2000). Don't talk to strangers: An analysis of government and industry efforts to protect a child's privacy online. *Federal Communication Law Journal, 52*(2), 429.

Institute of Medicine. (1988). *The future of public health.* Washington, DC: National Academy Press.

Kar, S. B., & Alex, S. B. (1999). Public health approaches to substance abuse prevention: A multicultural perspective. In S. B. Kar (Ed.), *Substance abuse prevention in multicultural communities.* Amityville, NY: Baywood.

Kar, S. B., Pascual, C., & Chickering, K. (1999). Empowerment of women for health promotion: A meta-analysis. *Social Science & Medicine, 49,* 1431-1460.

Kogan, M. D., Alexander, G. R., Teitelbaum, M. A., Jack, B. W., Kotelchuck, M., & Pappas,
G. (1995). The effect of gaps in health insurance on continuity of a regular source of
care among preschool-aged children in the United States. *JAMA, 274*(18), 1429-
1435.

Landmark Healthcare. (1998). *The Landmark report on public perceptions of alternative
care.* Sacramento, CA: Landmark Healthcare.

Lee, P., & Paxman, D. (1997). Reinventing public health. *Annual Review of Public Health,
18,* 1-35.

Los Angeles County Department of Health Services. (1994). LA County annual health
risk assessment. Information from data on CD-ROM.

Monmaney, T. (1998, August 31). *A dose of caution.* Retrieved June 13, 2000 from the
World Wide Web: http://www.loop.com/bkrentzman/sup.vitamin.alt/supplements/
caution.ethnic.meds.html

Monmaney, T., & Roan, S. (1998). Hope or hype? Retrieved June 13, 2000 from the
World Wide Web: http://www.latimes.com/news/timespoll/stories/19980830/
t000078986.html

National Center for Health Statistics. (1996). *FASTATS—A-Z.* Retrieved June 13, 2000
from the World Wide Web: http://www.cdc.gov/nchswww/fastats/deaths.htm

National Center for Health Statistics. (1998). *Health, United States, 1998.* Hyattsville,
MD: U.S. Department of Health and Human Services.

National Center for Health Statistics. (1999). *Health, United States, 1999* (PHS 19-
1232). Atlanta, GA: Centers for Disease Control.

National Public Health Laboratory of Finland. (1981). *Community control of cardiovascular diseases.* Copenhagen, Denmark: World Health Organization, Regional Office
for Europe.

Nielsen Media Research. (1997). *General market sample—Hispanic household viewing.*
New York: Nielsen Media Research.

Nielsen Media Research. (1998a, November). *African American household viewership.*
Presentation given to The Summit, New York.

Nielsen Media Research. (1998b). *Household network primetime report for the week of
7/6/98–7/12/98.* Retrieved June 13, 2000 from the World Wide Web: http://tv.zap2it.
com/news/ratings/networks/980706networks.html

Nielsen Media Research. (1998c). *1998 report on television.* New York: Nielsen Media
Research.

The Ottawa Charter for Health Promotion (17-21 November 1986). (1996). In *Health
promotion anthology* (Scientific Publication No. 557). Washington, DC: World
Health Organization, Pan American Health Organization.

Phillips, A. (1997). Why worry about multiculturalism? *Dissent, 44*(1), 57-63.

Rice, R. E., & Atkin, C. K. (Eds.). (1989). *Public communication campaigns* (2nd ed.).
Newbury Park, CA: Sage.

Rosen, G. (1993). *A history of public health* (Expanded ed.). Baltimore, MD: Johns Hopkins University Press.

Shalala, D. E. (1998). Testimony before the Senate Labor and Human Resources Committee on September 25, 1997, Washington, D.C. In *Targeting tobacco use: The nation's leading cause of death.* Rockville, MD: Centers for Disease Control.

Sterling, L. G. (1920). Tendencies of the times: Medical and otherwise. *New Orleans Journal of Medical and Surgical Journal, 72,* 218-220.

UCLA Center for Communication Policy. (1997). *The UCLA television violence report 1997.* Los Angeles: University of California.

United Nations. (1999). *Beijing declaration.* Retrieved June 13, 2000 from the World Wide Web: http://www.un.org/womenwatch/followup/beijing5/about.htm

United Nations Development Programme. (1999). *Human development report 1999.* New York: Author.

U.S. Department of Health and Human Services. (1991). *Healthy people 2000: National Health promotion and disease prevention objectives* (DHHS Publication No. PHS 91-50212). Washington, DC: Government Printing Office.

Wetzel, M. S., Eisenberg, D. M., & Kaptchuk, T. J. (1998). Courses involving complementary and alternative medicine at US medical schools. *JAMA, 280,* 784-787.

World Health Organization/United Nations International Children's Emergency Fund. (1978). *ALMA-ATA 1978 primary health care: Report of the International Conference on Primary Health Care.* Geneva, Switzerland: Author.

Yankauer, A. (1997). The recurring popularity of alternative medicine. *Perspectives in Biology and Medicine, 41*(1), 132-137.

3

The Evolution of Health Communication in the United States

Snehendu B. Kar
Rina Alcalay
with Shana Alex

This chapter focuses on the evolution of health communication as a field in its own right, distinct both in research and in practice from other aspects of public health. At the outset, it is important to recognize the growth of secular social trends, particularly the increased health consciousness of the general population of the United States, which has played a supporting role in the development of health communication. Concurrently, the number of academic institutions offering degrees in health education, communication, and promotion (including social and preventive medicine) has increased exponentially in the last 50 years. Our focus here is on the development of and interaction between health-related organizations and the field of health education, communication, and promotion.

This field as we know it today (hereafter, *health communication* but including, in actuality, health education and promotion as well) has grown from a confluence of six interrelated developments discussed below, not necessarily in order of importance:

45

1. The evolution of communication studies into a discipline

2. The growth in research on human behavior and relations

3. The development of action research for health and human services pro-grams globally

4. The proliferation of schools of public health

5. The initiation by nonprofit and governmental institutions of agenda-setting and funding-prevention programs

6. The explosive growth in targeted health promotion communication campaigns

Health communication exists as the synthesis of these six trends.

The Evolution of Communication Studies

With the advent of electronic mass media, all aspects of American society be-gan using media to promote themselves. Commercial corporations and the en-tertainment industry obviously saw the advantage in increasing their commer-cial markets, but other sectors, such as political parties, also realized the advantage of reaching a mass audience through a persuasive communication medium. Communication studies emerged through efforts by academia and the advertising industry to examine the role of media in these exchanges. As early as the 1930s, researchers began studying the effects of the new media of movies and radio on the public (Cantril & Allport, 1935; Charters, 1933).

The federal government, by funding projects in both public and private uni-versities, also played a role in the creation of communication studies as a field in its own right. During World War II, the Allies recruited psychologists to study strategies to promote morale among the troops, mainly through the use of communication methods that both psychologically inoculated our troops against enemy propaganda and attempted to demoralize enemy forces. Also, these scientists studied methods of deterrence to counter propaganda from the Axis governments. Early applications of interpersonal and behavioral research by psychologists and sociologists led to communication studies' inherent in-terdisciplinary focus.

One of the earliest systematic studies of communication emerged from Yale University in the 1940s, concerning the role of mass media (radio, that is, because this occurs before television existed) on presidential elections (Lazarsfeld, Berelson, & Gaudet, 1944). These works led to the development of the famous "two-step" model of the flow of communication. In a parallel mode of thought, researchers at Iowa University were studying the diffusion of innovations in the agricultural and medical fields. This two-step flow of communication became the foundation for the diffusion of the innovation model subsequently popularized by Rogers and others (Beal, Blount, Powers, & Johnson, 1966; Coleman, Katz, & Menzel, 1966; Katz & Lazarsfeld, 1964; Rogers, 1995).

The increased interest in communication as a separate field led to the institutionalization of departments of journalism, mass media, and interpersonal communication at many prestigious universities around the country. Large grants from both public and private agencies supported this process. As Everett Rogers pointed out, large grants from private sources have complemented government funds to help establish departments around the country. The National Institute of Drug Abuse, the National Institute of Alcoholism and Alcohol Addiction, and the National Cancer Institute monies have joined with the Rockefeller Foundation, the Robert Wood Johnson Foundation, the Kauffman Foundation, the Annenberg Foundation, and the Kaiser Family Foundation to fund communication studies not only in the United States but also internationally to study health communication ideas abroad (Rogers, 1994). Such actions helped the disparate modes of communication theory merge into a single discipline, although like many fields, different schools concentrate their strengths on different research aspects.

Academic Research on
Human Relations and Behavior

Within the fields of various social sciences, studies on group dynamics and influence began to gain in popularity in the mid-20th century, particularly in psychology circles (Cartwright & Zander, 1968; Lewin, 1964). Beginning this trend, Kurt Lewin conducted particularly telling studies during the 1940s, in which he illustrated that group behavior can have a great deal of impact on personal choices. Through the use of comparing a discussion group that arrived at its own conclusions through a discussion led by a moderator with a lecture group that simply received health-related information regarding the same desired behavior, those who felt empowered and supported by the group tended to not only change their behavior in the desirable fashion but also to maintain that change over a longer period of time (Lewin, 1947, 1948).

Similarly, psychological studies delved into questions of persuasion and attitude change (Ajzen & Fishbein, 1980; Bandura, 1986; Festinger & Kelley, 1951). This research included communication as a necessary variable, the only means through which persuasion is possible. Studies found that the initial attitude of an individual or group greatly affected how a communication message was received, whether to blunt, enhance, or simply distort the meaning of the original missive (Ball-Rokeach & Cantor, 1986; Berger & Burgoon, 1995; DeFleur & Ball-Rokeach, 1995; National Cancer Institute, 1980). The initial knowledge and attitudes of the audience, it was found, played a key element in persuasion.

Other social sciences followed similar research patterns, each in its own domain but all recognizing the importance of communication. In political science, the impact of mass media on the voting public remains a heavily researched field. Samuel Kernell (1997) has stipulated that a new culture of mass media has emerged, in which politicians, particularly visible leaders such as the president, can use mass communication techniques to bypass the old methods of interpersonal discussion and create direct public support for their ideas, thus forcing their political opponents to bow before the seeming "will of the people." Public opinion research also often focuses on how communication can set the national agenda, moving the public debate from one issue to another (Iyengar, 1994).

Marketing and economic studies have likewise studied communication in regard to marketing and its media effects, attempting to maximize profits by tailoring advertising messages to audiences to increase the likelihood of positive reception. In actuality, little difference exists at the theoretical level between studying the marketing techniques underlying the sale of a product and studying the marketing techniques underlying the sale of a candidate. The obvious parallel nature of this research nurtured independent communication studies research and programs that explored theories applicable across disciplinary lines.

Developments in several related fields also contributed directly to the growth of health communication, specifically, as an interdisciplinary field of study. The medical- and biological-based health sciences began to look more seriously at the psychosocial determinants of health and health behavior to maximize knowledge and promote compliance of medical regimens. For example, health psychology, medical sociology, and medical anthropology emerged as established subfields in the 1970s. According to the American Psychological Association's (APA, 1996) official literature, the goals of health psychology are these:

- To promote education and services in the psychology of health and illness
- To inform the psychological and biomedical community, as well as the general public, on the results of current research and service activities in this area

These goals explicitly recognize the importance of communication, by stating that the promotion of education and the proliferation of information exist as necessary goals to the successful practice of health psychology.

The medical professions have followed the same pattern in overtly stating that health communication underlies their work. As Wies Weijts (1994) states, "Health communication is currently a significant topic in medical training programs and in research in clinical practice" (p. 257). Fueled by the rapid expansion of health maintenance organizations (HMOs), health care and its related fields have, through necessity, turned to the practice of preventive care (Marwick, 1996; Niles, Alemagno, & Stricklin, 1997). By nature, preventive medicine includes a component of health communication, because it requires the successful implementation of health promotion or individual health counseling. Therefore, the increased focus in the medical professions on preventive medicine has also supported the heightened development of the health communication field.

Other professional fields have similarly contributed to the growth of the discipline of health communication. As has been recognized by health communication specialists, the field also draws from management, marketing, social welfare, government, and education (Ratzan, 1994); the radical shift of the health care industry to HMOs has affected any field that deals with health issues. The same increasing focus on preventive care that has permeated the health professions has also percolated into other fields, depending on their focus. For example, management deals with the business aspect of health care; therefore, when faced with increasing costs, they turn to preventive care to reduce expenditures. Health communication campaigns have proven to be an effective method through which to achieve better health and preventive medicine goals. Excellent reviews of growth of communication related to public health can be found in works by DeFleur and Ball-Rokeach (1995), Rice and Atkin (1989), Rogers (1994), and Piotrow, Kincaid, Rimon, and Rinehart (1997).

Important Studies (1959-1970s)

Important studies in the United States and around the world led to the development of health communication models that have served as blueprints for health promotion campaigns throughout the country. The first occurred in 1959, studying the reasons why autoworkers in a factory would not undergo tuberculosis (TB) screening, even though it was available and they knew the benefits of the program. The findings led to the formation of the "health belief model," now widely known to health communication specialists. Others followed during the next 20 years, building health communication models that remain invaluable to the public health promoter.

1959 TB Screening Study and the Health Belief Model. In 1959, the U.S. Public Health Service (USPHS) attempted to increase the rate of TB screening among autoworkers at a factory (Hochbaum, 1958). With a target population of autoworkers at a certain factory, the researchers hypothesized that fundamental beliefs and perceptions about the disease and that the external factors of convenience and money discouraged TB screening. Therefore, they moved the screening site to the factory itself, reduced the cost to the workers, and launched a media campaign within the workplace to educate people about the seriousness of TB. Theoretically, these actions should have increased the rate of screening, but the rate actually remained fairly flat at about a third of the autoworkers.

To explain what made the difference regarding whether or not an autoworker came in for TB screening, the health practitioners conducted a series of interviews within the factory. Their findings helped develop the health belief model, with five basic reasons why people do or do not engage in health-promoting behavior, regardless of cost and convenience:

1. The person must sincerely believe that the health risk is serious.

2. The person must believe that he or she is susceptible to the health risk.

3. The person must believe in the efficacy of the proposed solution.

4. The person must be exposed to cues that trigger action.

5. The person must believe that he or she is able to effectively prevent the threat of personal injury.

These and other findings challenged the position that a health promoter only must impart correct knowledge and the public will decide, out of self-interest, to follow the desired health-promoting outcome. In the health belief model, this need to impart health beliefs remains the first key point of the model; a person must believe there is a health risk before he or she will take any corrective action. But the health belief model goes further, stating that the person must also believe that he or she is at risk. In other words, the knowledge about a general health risk phenomenon will not change behavior unless that risk is personalized to an individual. Last, the health belief model states that the person must believe that the proposed solution to alleviate the health risk will work for him or her. A person must feel empowered to change his or her own condition (personal efficacy), or he or she will not bother to change a behavior, even if changing that behavior may be more financially or physically advantageous. In the case of the TB study, the researchers found that many of the autoworkers felt that even if they found out that they were at risk or had contracted TB, there would be nothing they could do about their condition at that point anyway and therefore did not bother to undergo the initial screening.

The Stanford Heart Disease Prevention Program. During the early 1970s, a major project was launched by a multidisciplinary group from Stanford University in Stanford, California, to reduce the rate of heart disease in the study area through a mass media campaign (Pancer & Nelson, 1990; Winkleby, Feldman, & Murray, 1997; Winkleby, Taylor, Jatulis, & Fortmann, 1996). Incidentally, a concurrent and similar study was being performed in Finland, showing that the development of public health in the United States mirrored in some ways the field as it was practiced internationally (Puska et al., 1985).

These studies took the unprecedented step of using the community as the unit of measurement rather than the individual. Until this point, public health, although attempting to change the behavior patterns of large populations, did so on more of an individual scale. This program occurred in two phases (Pancer & Nelson, 1990; Winkleby et al., 1997). First, a three-community study was performed by an interdisciplinary group from Stanford University from 1972 to 1975. With one community as a control for comparison purposes, the other two towns were blanketed with extensive television, radio, and newspaper ads. Also, some particularly high-risk individuals were chosen at random and asked to participate in a group intervention consisting of meetings over a 10-week period with dietitians and project leaders who instructed the subjects on necessary life changes. Evaluation showed that the media campaign had produced a 17% reduction in risk factors in the targeted communities, whereas the control area actually saw a 6% *increase* in risk factors over the same period of time (Pancer & Nelson, 1990). Those who received face-to-face intervention had the highest risk reduction, an impressive 30% (Pancer & Nelson, 1990).

In the subsequent second phase, the researchers were careful to use only community-wide techniques to influence behavior, showing that such methods could indeed produce long-term and sustained beneficial effects on a targeted population (Winkleby et al., 1996). To test more long-term, community-based interventions, the Stanford group began a five-community study in 1978, which is still ongoing. A major goal of this program is to create a self-sustaining health promotion institution within the communities involved. Furthermore, this project focused more on community involvement with and ownership of the program, to enhance the effects of the campaign. Available interim results show that reduction in risk factors for heart diseases in intervention communities is 13% compared with 7% in control groups (Pancer & Nelson, 1990).

The North Karelia Project. Begun in 1972 under the auspices of the National Public Health Institute (Helsinki) and the University of Kuopio, the North Karelia Project endeavored to reverse the trend toward a large amount of heart disease in Finland. Using a community organization approach, the program directors used existing community structures to disseminate their message. The project gave materials that encouraged cessation of smoking and healthier eating habits to mass media, health services, industry and business sites, and other existing sources of health-related information, who would then communicate directly with their constituents (Pancer & Nelson, 1990; Puska et al., 1985).

Based on the principles of a community-based approach, the project also used collaboration rather than fear to persuade people to change their habits. Rather than scaring the public with horrific details of the damage that high-fat food and smoking can do, people were given practical solutions and ideas for quitting smoking and changing their diets (Pancer & Nelson, 1990; Puska et al., 1985). Also, the project enlisted the help of a national housewives' organization that included over 300 local clubs in order to teach people how to cook low-fat recipes (Pancer & Nelson, 1990). A 10-year evaluation showed long-term reductions in all risk factors, including smoking, blood pressure, and cholesterol levels relative to the control county in Finland (Tuomilehto et al., 1986; Vartiainen, Puska, Koskela, Nissenen, & Tuomilehto, 1986). It's important to note that, unlike urban populations in the United States, the Finnish population is largely homogeneous, which had a role in the success of the program.

The Minnesota Heart Health Program. Designed over the course of 3 years by the School of Public Health at the University of Minnesota, this program was funded by the National Institutes for Health in 1980 for a 9-year duration (Pancer &

Nelson, 1990; Winkleby et al., 1997). It used three communities of different sizes for interventions, matching each to a comparable community that would not receive the program for control purposes. Using media techniques, direct education, and community organization, the program involved more than simple blanketing of communication sources with information. Community task forces not only involved the target population in their own intervention but also allowed the researchers to target those segments of the population in a manner that they would recognize as legitimate. The final data showed reductions in risk, but not as much as had been hoped (Winkleby et al., 1997).

The Pennsylvania County Health Improvement Program (CHIP). After almost 3 years of planning and careful research of the most current results coming from the North Karelia Project, CHIP began in 1980 in Lycoming County in Pennsylvania. The steering committee included Pennsylvania Secretary of Health, Dr. Albert Stunkard, representatives from Williamsport hospital, and community leaders from various organizations within the target population. Operating through mass media, worksites, schools, and the health sector, this campaign distributed information mainly from other sources, such as the American Lung Association through events and a media campaign. An interesting result of this study was the indication that despite smaller than expected reductions in health risks (Winkleby et al., 1997), the number of organizations that were involved in health promotion activities in the county doubled from 1980 to 1983, whereas the same number decreased by 42% in the control county over the same time period (Pancer & Nelson, 1990). This shows one long-term positive effect of community-based prevention; organizations within the community itself become accustomed to engaging in health promotion and will likely continue these activities after the study itself has ceased. In this manner, the community creates a more receptive atmosphere to health-promoting messages over time.

Alcohol, Tobacco, and Other Drugs (ATOD) Prevention Programs. Since the passage of the Drug Free Schools Act in 1986, and through the 1990s, considerable efforts and resource have been invested in school-based ATOD prevention. Because of increased public concerns over high rates of drug use among children and youth, federal contributions to prevention programs at various levels increased significantly. Schools were required to introduce comprehensive drug prevention program to qualify for federal education funds. The prevailing prevention strategy shared two common elements: (a) Prevention targeted at all children, not just those who were at high risk, and (b) school-based health education and prevention became the primary modus operandi. Perhaps the best known among these is the DARE (drug abuse resistance education) program led by local police departments. Although systematic evaluation of the DARE program questioned the effectiveness of this approach, the proliferation of the program and increased public concern with ATOD abuse helped fund several prevention programs that used school-based communication and education programs. Other initiatives include QUEST: Skills for Living; Project CHARLIE; Here's Looking at You; 2000; BABES; Project Adventure; OMBUDSMAN; and Children Are People (see Ellickson, 1999; Hansen & O'Malley, 1996). The passage of Proposition 99 (cigarette taxation to support prevention programs) in California, which became a model for others to follow, also expanded the use of mass media for tobacco prevention education in communities. A recent comprehensive state-of-the art review of substance abuse prevention from a multicultural perspective by recognized researchers have identified important elements of effective and ineffective prevention strategies (Kar, 1999). That review elaborates various risk factors and prevention strategies in schools and communities. Clearly, increased national concern about ATOD abuse among the children and youth and antitobacco campaigns have led to increased funding for ATOD prevention and expansion of health communication research and interventions.

HIV/AIDS Prevention. This campaign peaked in the 1990s as a result of several developments, including a high level of public concern, effective campaigns by HIV/AIDS activists and their sympathizers, and organized efforts of the public health community (e.g., former Surgeon General Everett Coop's daring public education campaigns). Public participation by several entertainment celebrities and local leaders in public education for HIV/AIDS prevention significantly expanded the role of mass and interpersonal communications for health promotion and disease prevention.

Action Research for Health and Human Services Programs

In the 20th century, social and human services programs, including community development, health, and agricultural programs, began to more fully develop and to apply modern media devices and techniques to maximize the effectiveness of their programs. This development gave rise to the field of "action research" in academia, pioneered by Kurt Lewin in the mid-1940s. In his publications, Lewin combined the study of a social problem with propositions for its solution, forging a new path of practical social research that focused on dealing effectively with real-world problems (Bargal, Gold, & Lewin, 1992; Deutsch, 1992). The new action research methodology provided a theoretical foundation for public health and health communication, in that its focus is on not only discovering the root of a problem but also on formulating solutions based on a diagnosis of a social problem within a specific ecological context. Within those solutions, health communication often played a major role through promoting interpersonal and governmental influences.

Poor and rich nations alike began to apply lessons learned from the growing field of communication studies to tackle profound health and social concerns. Internationally, campaigns to control malaria, smallpox, TB, typhoid, and overpopulation all contained important communication components to propagate information (Piotrow et al., 1997; Rogers, 1962, 1994). Within the United States, campaigns have included the promotion of vaccination, fluoridation, TB screening, sexually transmitted disease prevention, substance abuse prevention, and heart disease risk reduction (American Water Works Association, 1995; Barker, Strikas, & Brugliera, 1994; Bloom, 1994; Eng & Butler, 1997; Harris & Christen, 1995; Kar, 1999; MacLean, 1994; Office of Technology Assessment, 1993; Pancer & Nelson, 1990; Pirie, Stone, Assaf, Flora, & Maschewsky-Schneider, 1994; Rogers, 1973; U.S. Senate, 1996, Winkleby et al., 1997).

In particular, family planning endeavors have relied on communication, because the program must not only increase knowledge but must persuade as well, in that contraceptive use by necessity involves conscious choices by the participants (Rogers, 1973). According to Piotrow et al. (1997) in their pioneering work in this field, family planning programs from Bangladesh to Brazil must use communication to implement positive behavioral changes: "Communication is the key process underlying changes in knowledge of the means of contraception, in attitudes towards fertility control and use of contraceptives, in norms regarding ideal family size, and in the openness of local cultures to new ideas and aspirations and new health behavior" (p. 2). With monetary and programmatic support from national governments and external donors, family planning campaigns, particularly in developing nations, have achieved incredible success since 1970, when the implementation of communication strategies began to take hold (see Table 3.1).

The combined positive influences of health communication strategies along with increased access to contraceptive services are clearly shown by the data in Table 3.1. Interestingly, these nations, although all developing countries, are

Table 3.1   Changes in Contraceptive Prevalence Rates (CPR), 1970 to
              1996 (in percentages)

Country (Year National Planning Program Began)	CPR in 1970	CPR in 1996
Columbia (1967)	18	72
Egypt (1965)	9	48
Hong Kong (1956)	50	81
Indonesia (1968)	9	55
Malaysia (1966)	9	56
Morocco (1965)	3	42
South Korea (1961)	33	79
Sri Lanka (1965)	32	66
Taiwan (1964)	44	75
Turkey (1967)	9	63

SOURCE: Piotrow, Kincaid, Rimon, and Rinehart (1997, p. 10).

spread around the globe, showing the universality of underlying health communication theories, although each campaign must, of course, be tailored to
the targeted population. Quantitative results, such as those shown in Table 3.1,
have greatly added to the scientific validity of health communication as an independent discipline.

Schools of Public Health Expansion

In the fall of 1913, the first school of public health in the United States began ac-
cepting students, primarily for an ancillary education to their previous clinical
training. The School for Health Officers of Harvard University and Massachusetts Institute of Technology filled an existing lack of focus on the community,
mainly offering courses in engineering and sanitation, because the focus of
public health at the time was on literally cleaning up the sewage-filled, disease-
infested cities (Curran, 1970). Soon after, the two schools divided the School
for Health Officers into separate public health academic entities at each cam-
pus. Yale and Columbia Universities created their own public health units,
bringing the total number of public health schools to 4 by 1920. Currently,
there are 29 schools of public health accredited by the Council of Education in

Public Health (CEPH), plus 5 associate members and 6 schools currently awaiting accreditation (see the ASPH Data Center, http://www.asph.org/data.htm).

The Association of Schools of Public Health (ASPH) defined behavioral sciences and health education (which includes health behavior and health communication) as one of the five core areas of public health graduate study required for national accreditation. Along with this, health information, education, and communication are now included on the list of 10 essential public health services by all national public health organizations (Barry, Centra, Pratt, Brown, & Giordano, 1998). These developments have substantially enhanced the importance of health communication teaching, research, and practice in American universities.

In the United States, public health has emerged as not only its own discipline but as an entire field with its own schools, with core areas and departments composing the whole. During the development of public health in the United States, it became increasingly apparent that an amalgam of social and behavioral sciences buttressed the emerging field. Originally, to reduce the global problems of infectious disease, public health had been an offshoot of the field of preventive medicine, dealing with the medical causes of disease, such as raw sewage and animal vector infestation. However, with the growth of the second wave of disease, that of chronic conditions preventable only through human behavioral change, public health practitioners in the United States began to use tools from other social sciences to achieve health goals. Schools of public health in the United States, as independent centers for higher education, have played a major role in establishing health education and communication as a discipline. Through their programs in professional education, collaborative research, and community services they have prepared professional leadership and promoted the three basic functions of public health: (a) assessment of health, (b) policy development, and (c) ensurance of services and conditions necessary for better health.

Three Foundations of Public Health (1900-1950s)

In public health, the attempt to understand how and why people behave in a self-destructive manner was based on the theories and practices of epidemiology, biostatistics, medicine, and other social and behavioral sciences. The importance of using theories from other disciplines to achieve public health goals led directly to three major foundations of public health as it is practiced in the United States:

1. The codification of the original interdisciplinary focus of many public health schools

2. The emergence of the discipline of health communication and health education within the public health framework

3. The use of theories and practices from the field of communication to inform, educate, persuade, and mobilize the public

Men who had their initial roots in the medical field founded the first school of public health in the United States in 1913, the School for Health Officers of Harvard University and Massachusetts Institute of Technology. The three founders had appointments in the departments of Sanitary Engineering, Biology and Public Health, and Preventative Medicine and Hygiene, which led to the creation of their distinctly interdisciplinary program for the new school. "The plan provided for . . . a suitable program of studies, which included anatomy, physiology, pathology, biological chemistry, sanitary biology, preventative medicine, hygiene, demography, and sanitary engineering" (Curran, 1970, p. 5). This focus has continued within schools of public health all over the country (Afifi & Breslow, 1994). To paraphrase Afifi and Breslow (1994), the field of public health is an amalgam of medicine, engineering, education, and management; three of these categories encompass the exact same departments that made up the Harvard/MIT School, illustrating how the initial interdisciplinary focus of public health has remained intact throughout the century. The fourth category, health behavior and health education, has grown in importance over time, eventually becoming one of the foundations of health promotion and disease prevention in its own right.

When the U.S. government began recruiting medical practitioners and scientists for the USPHS, they discovered the benefits of fluoridation, polio vaccinations, and TB screening but could not effectively spread the use of these advances without educating the public as to the benefits of changing behavior. This led directly to the third foundation of modern health promotion in the United States: the use of health education and communication to educate the public. Through the application of communication models, health practitioners found themselves able to mobilize and notify the public on a mass scale, affecting the reach and scope of public health campaigns. In this manner, communication became inextricably intertwined with health education as a means to achieve the goals of public health—namely, to improve the quality of life for all members of a society. During the first half of the 20th century, the founda-

tions for the modern discipline of health communication developed and became institutionalized.

The field has exploded during the last two decades. According to the ASPH,
29 schools offer accredited graduate-level public health programs within the
United States. In addition, 6 schools are currently awaiting accreditation.
Taking into account the health sciences departments that offer public health
programs and the medical schools that focus on preventive medicine, the number of places to train professionals for public health and health promotion
grows exponentially.

According to the Bureau of Labor Statistics (BLS, 1998), public health-related jobs such as health services managers and social and human services as-
sistants are expected to increase in number by over 30% through the year 2006.
This boom in health field-related jobs would require an increased focus from
the schools of public health in training their graduates for real-world applications of public health and health promotion theories. The fields of health education, promotion, and communication will play a major role in this boom,
because it directly relates to dealing with the public to promote health programs, particularly in multicultural communities.

The ASPH's figures regarding the composition of the incoming student
body in public health shows that the graduates will be increasingly multicultural over time (assuming similar graduation rates among ethnicities), using
the latest available data, academic year 1993-94. This trend mirrors the general
population of the United States, which, as discussed in Chapter 1, is also becoming increasingly multicultural.

Figures 3.1 and 3.2 illustrate how the public health workforce will become
more multicultural; the trend should create a greater interest within the health
field of promoting effective communication messages to multicultural communities. In Figure 3.3, the enrollment rates over the most recent decade available for information (1987-1997) further show this multicultural trend; here,
however, these are rates for current students, who may or may not have graduated.

Currently, the field of public health as represented by every major organization in the United States has adopted a mission statement titled *Public Health in
America,* both for educational purposes for future health practitioners and
for practical purposes in daily work. It states, "Mission: Promote Physical
and Mental Health and Prevent Disease, Injury and Disability," (Barry et al.,
1998, p. 2). The six major purposes of public health are as follows (Barry et al.,
1998, p. 2):

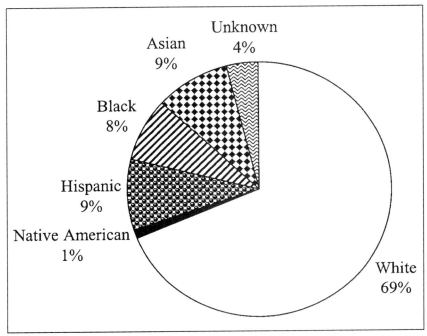

Figure 3.1. Graduates of Public Health Schools, by Ethnicity (1992-93)
SOURCE: ASPH Data Center (http://www.asph.org/data.htm).

1. Prevent epidemics and the spread of disease

2. Prevent against environmental hazards

3. Prevent injuries

4. Promote and encourage healthy behaviors

5. Respond to disasters and assist communities in recovery

6. Ensure the quality and accessibility of health services

Each of these has derived into a separate discipline within a school of public health; for our purposes in the field of health promotion, communication, and education, we focus on the methods that accomplish Numbers 1 and 4.

Also in the mission statement are 10 "essential public health services," many of which relate directly to health promotion. They are as follows (Barry et al., 1998, p. 2):

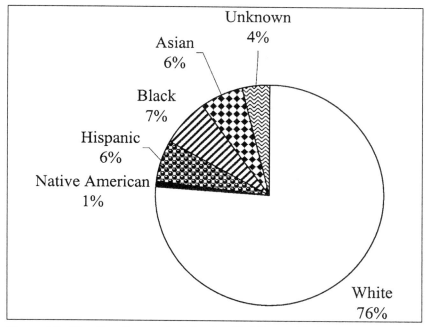

Figure 3.2. New Enrollments in Schools of Public Health, by Ethnicity (Fall 1993)
SOURCE: ASPH Data Center (http://www.asph.org/data.htm).

1. Monitor health status to identify community health problems

2. Diagnose and investigate health problems and health hazards in the community

3. Inform, educate, and empower people about health issues

4. Mobilize community partnerships to identify and solve health problems

5. Develop policies and plans that support individual and community health efforts

6. Enforce laws and regulations that protect health and ensure safety

7. Link people to needed personal health services and ensure the provision of health care when otherwise unavailable

8. Ensure a competent public health and personal health care workforce

9. Evaluate effectiveness, accessibility, and quality of personal and population-based health services

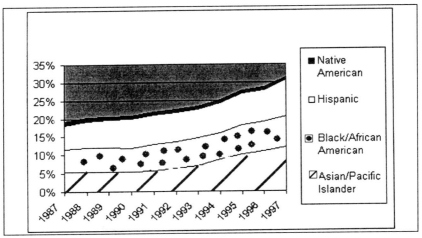

Figure 3.3. U.S. Schools of Public Health Enrollments, by Race/Ethnicity:
1987-1997
SOURCE: ASPH Data Center (http://www.asph.org/data.htm).

10. Research for new insights and innovative solutions to health problems

Since that time, departments and schools of public health have been institutionalized, training the next generation of health practitioners with an interdisciplinary focus based on a combination of medicine, engineering, and management. Also, education has become a prominent part of the public health
field, because it emerged as the most effective means by which to change the behavior patterns of a large number of people. Because of education's growth in
prominence, theories from the field of communication have become an important part of health promotion. Through communication, the public can
become educated. However, as was shown in the health belief model, to produce the desired behavior, public health practitioners often must deal with
forces acting within individuals.

Strengthening of Governmental Health Institutions

The U.S. government's role in the development of health promotion and education as a field cannot be overstated. Through creating permanent health-
related institutions, setting the national agenda, and funding research, educa-

tion, and health promotion projects, the federal government has supported and advanced health communication efforts.

Creating Permanent Health-Related Institutions

On July 16, 1798, the USPHS was created under the Treasury Department to treat sick Marines (Lundberg, 1998; National Library of Medicine [NLM], 1998). These doctors formed hospitals on both coasts (the West Coast later, in the 19th century) to provide health services to troops. Until 1870, the USPHS acted more as a cadre of doctors than as public health practitioners as we understand the field today.

From 1870 to 1916, the USPHS developed as a modern public health force, battling against the scourges of smallpox, yellow fever, typhus fever, cholera, and bubonic plague on a macrolevel. The first surgeon general, Dr. John Woodworth, took his office in 1870. In 1887, the first USPHS research center, the Hygienic Laboratory, incorporated out of a need to better understand infectious diseases, became the forerunner of the later National Institutes of Health (U.S. Public Health Service, 1998). A major paradigm shift occurred, refocusing the USPHS on the study of people and their relationship to their environment, particularly in urban centers, which began overflowing with people at this point.

With the outbreak of World War I in 1917, the USPHS once again took on the responsibility of acting as the health care provider for the military. By the early 1920s, however, this burden was lifted by the newly created Veterans Administration, which took over many of the hospitals originally managed by the USPHS. In 1930, the Hygienic Laboratory was officially renamed the National Institutes for Health. By 1939, the Federal Security Agency, later named the Department of Health, Education and Welfare, was created to house the USPHS as well as all the expanding and diversifying health services. In 1980, what had begun almost 200 years earlier with a small group of military doctors had transmogrified into the modern Department of Health and Human Services (DHHS) (Lundberg, 1998; U.S. Public Health Service, 1998).

The USPHS still makes up the major portion of the DHHS, but many if its current and former offices have now become well-known in their own right, such as the Surgeon General's office, the Office of the Secretary of Health and Human Services, the Centers for Disease Control and Prevention (CDC), and the USPHS Commissioned Corps. Although their duties overlap to some extent, each has a distinct function, many of which use health communication. The surgeon general, for example, not only administers the USPHS but also must, among other duties, (a) educate the public, (b) advocate for disease prevention, and (c) lead the efforts of Departmental health promotion campaigns (U.S. Office of the Surgeon General, 1998). The proactive role of former Surgeon General C. Everett Koop in HIV/AIDS prevention and sex education is one recent example of social activism under the auspices of this office. In other words, explicitly stated in the duties of the surgeon general, one of the most visible health-related offices in the nation, is a mandate to engage actively in effective health promotion through use of communication.

The National Center for Chronic Disease Prevention and Health Promotion also has contributed greatly to the evolution of health communication. In 1978, President Carter's Committee on Health Information and Education suggested the creation of a separate office for the dissemination of information; in 1979, the Office for Health Information, Health Promotion, Physical Fitness, and Sports Medicine was established. In 1988, the office became permanently established at the CDC in its current form. This center collects and provides information regarding effective health promotion, acting as a clearinghouse for health professionals seeking to learn more applicable and effective strategies.

Developments During the Last Two Decades (1970s-2000)

In the late 1970s, the USPHS undertook a major national consensus approach to developing health objectives for the American public. The DHHS and the USPHS led a national health campaign, called *Healthy People 2000* (U.S. DHHS, 1991). In 1979, the first national health objectives report came out of the DHHS, titled *Healthy People 2000: The Surgeon General's Report on Health Promotion and Disease Prevention.* The objectives in this report integrate health recommendations from public health and medical practitioners from around the country into a single composite document. The DHHS recognizes this movement as an ongoing goal for which to strive, and so is constantly in a state of updating and reviewing the recommendations. As we enter the 21st century, the DHHS has created a draft of *Healthy People 2010,* now circulating throughout the health community in the United States for revisions and comments (U.S. DHHS, 1998). The DHHS also held a series of public hearings and created a hotline for people to call in their comments.

Setting the National Agenda

The surgeon general's report in 1979 popularized the term *health promotion* in the United States and made it part of common public health vocabulary.

Since that time, furthering the importance of health promotion as a goal in its own right, the DHHS has attempted to achieve the goals laid out in the original report. *Healthy People 2000* (U.S. DHHS, 1991) constituted the first setting of long-term goals for the nation, many of which have already been partially reached through the combined efforts of public health organizations around the country.

Also, presidents often exercise another powerful method of setting the national agenda; by creating a commission, highlighting an issue in a speech, or implementing a program, a president can bring a particular issue to the forefront of discussion and prompt national debate (Cohen, 1997). Recent examples of this phenomenon include the summit on media violence held in 1994, at which the Clinton administration emphasized the deleterious compound effects of exposure to constant violent scenes. This summit led to a voluntary ratings system implemented by broadcasters, as well as to a strengthening of the timeliness and wording of parental warnings before objectionable shows. To use this power, however, a president must have the attention and the interest of the people, or the debate will fizzle.

Funding Research, Education, and Health Promotion Projects

Since the mid-20th century, the U.S. government has had a policy of active investment in research and development, which has laid the foundation for much public health research around the country. The DHHS, mainly through the National Institutes of Health (NIH), has become a major funder in health promotion and preventive medicine. In fiscal year 1997, the NIH supplied over $300 million (spread out among 559 research grants) to public health schools for research activities. Of these grants, 507 funded projects were presumably community based, although it is impossible to derive from the data how many of these grants went to health promotion programs (NIH, 1998). Still, the fact remains that the NIH supplies a great deal of money to research programs, institutionalizing the role of the federal government as a promoter of prevention strategies. However, as competition grows, these funds are becoming more difficult to receive; in addition, the NIH leads in emphasizing basic research in health issues. In fiscal year 1988, 40% of the applications accepted by the NIH were for public health research; in fiscal year 1997, that rate had dropped to 30% (NIH, 1998).

Another method by which government is institutionalizing health promotion is through the use of taxes that fund and subsidies to ease the cost of intervention programs. Several states around the country have instituted antismoking campaigns, for example, funded mainly through an imposed cig-

arette tax (Siegel, 1998). In California, this program has been highly scruti-
nized, particularly because the intervention had the unusual aspect of being
introduced and approved by the public directly through the proposition system (Proposition 99). Initially highly successful, the program has lost some
momentum in its later phase, in part because its own success and division of reviews to clinical services reduced the available funding for preventive education through cigarette taxes (Pierce et al., 1998). However, the passage of the
program into law boldly illustrated the public's support for health promotion
and the role of the media in cancer and cardiovascular risk reduction. That
kind of positive reinforcement and atmosphere has helped health communication further gain legitimacy both in academia and in practice.

The Growth of Health
Promotion Communication Campaigns

During the last three decades, the industrialized nations of the world have seen
a rapid expansion of the number and types of health promotion communica-
tion-based campaigns. Funded both through governments and private foundations, these community-level multidisciplinary campaigns help develop,
test, and evaluate the overall effectiveness of comprehensive prevention interventions. The campaigns themselves included several important complementary intervention modalities: (a) use of multiyear or longitudinal projects as
opposed to cross-sectional surveys, (b) use of multimedia techniques, (c) promotion of community involvement, (d) increase in preventive services and
support, (e) use of case management, and (f) systematic evaluation of impacts.
Integrating the lessons learned through health behavior and communication
studies with public health successes of the past, these campaigns embraced,
codified, and institutionalized the principles of community-based prevention
through active public participation, first enumerated in the Alma Ata Declaration and the Ottawa Charter (see Chapter 2). Cited below are a few major examples of the progression of this movement.

Emergence of Health Promotion

In 1945, medical historian Henry Sigerist coined the term *health promotion*
when he expanded on the accepted clinical definition of health care and
defined the major tasks of medicine as (a) health promotion, (b) illness preven-

tion, (c) healing the sick, and (d) rehabilitation of health-risking behaviors (Terris, 1992). Sigerist's next major publication regarding the duties of public health education further discussed his new concept, stating that health promotion precludes illness prevention and must include diverse fields such as sanitation, maternal and child health, and occupational health (Sigerist, 1946). Although health promotion had its roots in the earlier century and the growth of the urban sanitary public health practitioners (as discussed in Chapter 2 of this book), Sigerist was the first to coin the term and give it equal placement alongside the curing of the sick as a necessary factor in creating a healthy society.

In 1979, the U.S. surgeon general's report defined the national strategy for the creation of a more healthy society in a volume titled *Healthy People: The Surgeon General's Report on Health Promotion and Disease Prevention*, the first time that this term was used widely in a national strategy (Surgeon General, 1979). Since then, health promotion has become a generally accepted concept that includes strategies to both enhance health and prevent health risks. Health promotion has also been connected from the beginning with education; Sigerist himself made free education a requisite item in any national health program, because inadequate education leads to ignorance regarding preventive measures and to low compliance with needed behavioral changes (Terris, 1992).

Forty years after Sigerist coined the term, health promotion became the central message of the Ottawa Charter, in 1986. This document synthesized two major strategies: prevention of general causes (e.g., poverty, injustice) and prevention of specific causes (cancer, polio, TB), creating an integrated blueprint for the modern practice of health promotion ("Ottawa Charter," 1996). This critical document used as its foundation a previous delineation of the major principles of health promotion created by the World Health Organization (WHO) in 1984. These principles are as follows:

1. Health promotion includes the population as a whole.

2. Health promotion focuses on actions toward the causes of health problems.

3. Health promotion includes multidisciplinary and integrated methods.

4. Health promotion must entail public participation.

5. Health professionals have an important role in enabling health promotion (Kickbusch, 1986).

With these concepts in mind, the Ottawa Charter sought to affect public policy through education and advocacy to make the practice of health promotion more widespread throughout the world. The Ottawa Charter itself served as a landmark document, underscoring that health promotion had become a fully recognized field of study and practice in the international health community. Through the emphasis on advocacy as a primary modus operandi (along with education), the Ottawa Charter highlighted the importance of effective health promotion and health communication strategies and media advocacy.

Use of Communication and Behavioral Theories for Health Promotion

Concurrently with the emergence of health promotion, people in public health began to apply theories from behavioral and communication models to health-related questions. In the mid-1950s, colleagues of social psychologist Kurt Lewin (1890-1947) developed theories in the field of group dynamics that began the move toward looking at human behavior as a combination of factors within the person and in the environment. Lewin's "field theory" combined his field's major focus on outside sources (force field) with a renewed focus on subjective factors (life space); previously, these two ideas had created a schism in psychology. As one of his students, Ralph K. White (1992) described the new theory, "It was a return to common sense, and it was a much-needed corrective to the behaviorists' foolish taboo on all subjective-sounding words" (p. 46). To encapsulate the theory, a resulting behavior derives from a situation (life space) or psychological ecology that affects the behavior combined with a mix of internal, personal, and external factors (Conway, Vickers, & French, 1992).

Marc Lalonde, former Minister of National Health and Welfare of Canada, applied Lewin's field theory to health, postulating that all health-related fields should merge. Stating that both internal and external factors are integral to health promotion, Lalonde combined medicine, public health, psychology, biology, and environmental sciences (among other fields that relate peripherally to health) into one health field that would incorporate elements of each. Within the health field, there would be four domains: human biology, environment, lifestyle, and health care organization (Lalonde, 1974). *Human biology* would encompass all the physical and mental aspects of health within the human body, including genetics, psychology, clinical medicine, and pharmacology. *Environment* would contain the fields of sanitation, environmental health, epidemiology, communicable disease control, and other fields that related to external factors over which individual humans have little control.

Lifestyle fields are those that relate to health-risking behaviors over which humans have control, such as drug and alcohol abuse, lack of exercise, and poor dietary choices. Finally, *health care organization* relates to the nature of how health care is to be dispensed, containing the actual health care system along with community-based prevention strategies (Lalonde, 1974).

The health field concept's characteristics made it uniquely adaptable to modern health needs, as well as a powerful tool for controlling health costs through prevention strategies (Lalonde, 1983). First, all four domains were considered equal, making lifestyle and environmental concerns as important as the more commonly prestigious fields relating to human biology and health care organization. Second, as a comprehensive model, it can encompass any health concern and "ensures that all aspects of health will be given due consideration," (Lalonde, 1983, p. 15). Third, the concept allows analysis by which any question of health risks may be examined in terms of which domain contributes most to the cause, giving planners the ability to focus on the more directly relevant policies that will ameliorate the problem. Fourth, the health field concept remains extremely flexible, enabling a further subdivision or expansion of categories that will give health professionals a clearer idea of the causes of a health risk. Finally, by integrating the relevant health fields, one can be freed from the rigid boundaries of arbitrary disciplines and can integrate the most effective tools from every field to create a healthier society (Lalonde, 1983).

Others advocate a "beyond Lalonde" approach, emphasizing that issues such as poverty, alienation, social isolation, and powerlessness also affect health campaigns (Buck, 1995). Although Lalonde would argue that these issues would fall under his environment category, Buck states that the connection between larger societal forces/factors and their effects on personal health has not been made by health practitioners and must be taken into account. The cumulative effects of things such as unfulfilling work and discrimination, Buck argues, can be measured in their toll on personal health and should be considered part of health promotion. However, she also acknowledges the difficulty of creating reform; although Buck discusses how to implement change, she does not and cannot offer concrete solutions, because these problems are pervasive in every society on the planet. As one WHO slogan says, "All health problems are global, but the solution must be local." Buck's point that environmental concerns must be given actual equality in practice rather than mere lip service, however, should be considered when creating health promotion campaigns.

Health concerns have become more prevalent also because of the rising health consciousness of the general population that gives health messages a receptive audience. As will be discussed in Chapter 4, many communication theories discuss why and how marketing affects consumer's behavior. With the general public's increased interest in health, people are more receptive to health promotion that takes the form of marketing; in essence, the public is choosing to "buy" a certain health message when it begins changing the health risk behavior targeted by the campaign, at least among affluent population segments.

Interestingly, the increasing privatization of health care has led to health promotion campaigns led by corporations, who further contribute to the use of marketing techniques. As Nancy Milio (1988) points out, "Health promotion is literally being commodified, packaged, brand-labeled, and sold or franchised through advertising techniques," (p. 577). Also, corporations have a vested interest in keeping their employees healthy and so have become large consumers of health promotion communication campaigns themselves. Critics of this increasing corporatization argue that public policy should be dictating the content and nature of health promotion rather than the marketplace, which tends to target mostly affluent people to maximize profits (Milio, 1988).

Community-Based Health Promotion Communication Campaigns

Health promotion campaigns strive to affect the behavior of a certain community to reduce health risks. Through social action, health education, community organization, and community empowerment, the successful campaign will ultimately create healthier communities. To effect these changes, a campaign should contain the following elements for community mobilization (Pancer & Nelson, 1990):

1. *Community involvement:* Community members should be involved in the development of the program.

2. *Planning:* Development of the program should not be hurried and should be done carefully.

3. *Needs and resources assessment:* The program should address the needs identified by the community using the resources reasonably at hand.

4. *A comprehensive program:* The program should deal with multiple levels of risk factors, program delivery, and behavioral changes.

5. *An integrated program:* Each component of the program should reinforce the others.

6. *Long-term change:* This should produce stable and lasting changes in the targeted audience.

7. *Altering community norms:* The behavioral changes should be tied to altering existing norms of conduct.

8. *Research and evaluation:* Research and evaluation must occur to document successful methods for future applications.

9. *Sufficient resources:* The resources must exist for an organization to effectively conduct a campaign.

10. *Professional and community collaboration:* The program must have the active participation of health professionals.

We cite examples of successful community-based campaigns that followed the above guidelines to great success (see Chapters 6-12). Because cardiovascular disease is intimately related to diet and exercise, it remains one of the most common targets of health promotion efforts. These and other community-based prevention campaigns were theory based and tested the effectiveness of several intervention modalities that contribute to the acceptance of health communication as a major foundation of health promotion strategies. The major modalities are (a) counseling or education through interpersonal, face-to-face contact; (b) blanketing messages through the mass media; (c) using a reinforcing network of volunteers to re-create norms in the community; and (d) evaluation and feedback (Amezcua, McAlister, Ramirez, & Espinoza, 1990; McAlister, 1991; Roberts & Maccoby, 1985).

Implications

The lessons learned from the developments discussed above have formed a synergy that has recently energized health professionals into a more active approach to community-based health promotion programs using robust communication input. Communication interventions serve multiple functions, including social marketing, agenda setting, and advocacy (Ling, Franklin, Lindsteadt, & Gearon, 1992; Wallack, 1994). The following 10 elements, derived from our observations of case studies and our original research by the authors of this volume, have proven themselves integral components in successful health communication campaigns of differing types and will become the cornerstones of future programs.

1. *Perform interpersonal communication, education, and counseling.* Although this is subject to the criticism that it does not properly belong in community-wide programs, face-to-face intervention with those elements in a target population who are most at risk seems to have the strongest long-term effects in changing behavior (Pancer & Nelson, 1990; Winkleby et al., 1997).

2. *Provide social support and endorsement.* Without this crucial step, the health promotion message could simply drop into the community without any noticeable impact. The population must be receptive to listening to and processing the message; they will be more likely to do so with support from their community leaders and peers (Pancer & Nelson, 1990; Pirie et al., 1994; Winkleby et al., 1997).

3. *Set the agenda* and create public awareness using a mass media campaign. This reinforces the social support while also creating an atmosphere of awareness regarding the health risk behavior (Pancer & Nelson, 1990; Puska et al., 1985; Tuomilehto et al., 1986).

4. *Use cognitive and behavioral modeling.* Theories such as the health behavior model can provide insight into designing an effective program and should be taken into strong consideration (Amezcua et al., 1990; Hochbaum, 1958; MacLean, 1994; Pancer & Nelson, 1990). As will be discussed more in Chapter 4, an effective health promotion campaign must rest firmly on social and behavioral models.

5. *Reinforce positive changes.* Successful programs give people positive instructions on how to change their behavior rather than simply frightening them with information regarding the dangers of a certain action. Also, social support can help reinforce long-term, sustained change (Pancer & Nelson, 1990; Puska et al., 1985; Tuomilehto et al., 1986).

6. *Advocate for policy and service reform using mass media.* Governmental policies can influence certain behaviors, and advocating for positive change should be considered one aspect of a successful program. Using the mass media will create an atmosphere of urgency to the problem, placing it higher on the agenda of both the public and policymakers (McKinlay, 1992; Piotrow et al., 1997).

7. *Practice social marketing and mobilization* with health promotion concepts, services, products, programs, and practices. The goal of social marketing and mobilization is to first create the political impetus within the community to change social service policies and then to translate this force into the institutionalization of the desired change. This requires an overarching program that covers all facets of grassroots organizing, including marketing, training, community education, and advocacy (Ling et al., 1992). Tied in with the

mass media campaign mentioned above, these forces can have a powerful effect on policy.

8. *Develop leadership and empowerment of communities.* For long-term change, leadership of the project must derive from the community itself so that the program can survive in some form after the proscribed intervention ends. Empowerment of the community therefore should involve some amount of leadership training to develop the health promotion skills of community leaders (Gardner, 1993; Kar, Pascual, & Chickering, 1999; Minkler, 1997).

9. *Conduct process and impact evaluation.* Evaluation remains an imperative aspect of an intervention; without comprehensive impact evaluation, it is impossible to determine the overall methodological effectiveness and long-term impact of the health promotion program (Pancer & Nelson, 1990; Pirie et al., 1994; Winkleby et al., 1997).

10. *Support health communications with professionals.* Successful campaigns must be collaborations, not only with community leaders but also with established health professionals and their affiliated institutions, to ensure that the program fits into the community's legitimized form of health care and health information distribution. Different ethnicities receive health information from diverse sources to varying degrees, necessitating careful strategic planning on the part of the program designers (Los Angeles County Department of Health Services, 1994); to reach all aspects of the community, health professionals of all types must be involved.

References

Afifi, A., & Breslow, L. (1994). The maturing paradigm of public health. *Annual Review of Public Health, 15,* 223-235.

Ajzen, I., & Fishbein, M. (1980). *Understanding attitudes and predicting social behavior.* Englewood Cliffs, NJ: Prentice Hall.

American Psychological Association. (1996). *Health Psychology, Division 38 mission statement.* Retrieved June 24, 2000 from the World Wide Web: http://freud.apa.org/divisions/div38/mission.html

American Water Works Association. (1995). *Water fluoridation principles and practices* (4th ed.). Denver, CO: Author.

Amezcua, C., McAlister, A., Ramirez, A., & Espinoza, R. (1990). Health promotion in a Mexican-American border community: *Program a Su Salud* in Eagle Pass, Texas. In N. Bracht (Ed.), *Organizing for community health promotion: A handbook.* Newbury Park, CA: Sage.

Ball-Rokeach, S. J., & Cantor, M. G. (1986). *Media, audience, and social structure*. Beverly Hills, CA: Sage.

Bandura, A. (1986). *Social foundations of thought and action: A social cognitive theory*. Englewood Cliffs, NJ: Prentice Hall.

Bargal, D., Gold, M., & Lewin, M. (1992). Introduction: The heritage of Kurt Lewin. *Journal of Social Issues, 48*(2), 3-13.

Barker, W. H., Strikas, R. A., & Brugliera, P. D. (Eds.). (1994). *Immunization in medical education*. New York: Oxford University Press.

Barry, M. A., Centra, L., Pratt Jr., E., Brown, C. K., & Giordano, L. (1998). *Where do the dollars go? Measuring local public health expenditures* (Executive summary). Washington, DC: Public Health Foundation, National Association of County and City Health Officials, National Association of Local Boards of Health.

Beal, G. M., Blount, R. C., Powers, R. C., & Johnson, W. J. (1966). *Social action and interaction in program planning*. Ames: Iowa State University Press.

Berger, C. R., & Burgoon, M. (Eds.). (1995). *Communication and social influence processes*. East Lansing: Michigan State University Press.

Bloom, B. R. (Ed.). (1994). Tuberculosis: Pathogenesis, protection, and control. Washington, DC: ASM Press.

Buck, C. (1995). Beyond Lalonde: Creating health. In *Health promotion: An anthology* (Scientific Publication No. 557, pp. 6-13). Washington DC: World Health Organization, Pan American Health Organization.

Bureau of Labor Statistics. (1998). *1998-99 occupational outlook handbook*. Chicago: Author.

Cantril, H., & Allport, G. (1935). *The psychology of radio*. New York: Harper & Brothers.

Cartwright, D., & Zander, A. (Eds.). (1968). *Group dynamics: Research and theory* (3rd ed.). New York: Harper & Row.

Charters, W. W. (1933). *Motion pictures and youth: A summary*. New York: Macmillan.

Cohen, J. E. (1997). *Presidential responsiveness and public policy-making: The public and the policies that presidents choose*. Ann Arbor: University of Michigan Press.

Coleman, J. S., Katz, E., & Menzel, H. (1966). *Medical innovation: A diffusion study*. Indianapolis, IN: Bobbs-Merrill.

Conway, T. L., Vickers, R. R., & French, J. R. P. (1992). An application of person-environment fit theory: Perceived versus desired control. *Journal of Social Issues, 48*(2), 95-107.

Curran, J. A. (1970). *Founders of the Harvard School of Public Health*. New York: Josiah Macy, Jr., Foundation.

DeFleur, M. L., & Ball-Rokeach, S. (1995). *Theories of mass communication* (5th ed.). New York: Longman.

Deutsch, M. (1992). Kurt Lewin: The tough-minded and tender-hearted scientist. *Journal of Social Issues, 48*(2), 31-43.

Ellickson, P. (1999). School-based substance abuse prevention: What works, for whom. In S. B. Kar (Ed.), *Substance abuse prevention: A multicultural perspective* (pp. 101-130). Amityville, NY: Baywood.

Eng, T. R., & Butler, W. T. (Eds.). (1997). *The hidden epidemic: Confronting sexually transmitted diseases* (Committee on Prevention and Control of Sexually Transmitted Diseases, Institute of Medicine, Division of Health Promotion and Disease Prevention). Washington, DC: National Academy Press.

Festinger, L., & Kelley, H. H. (1951). *Changing attitudes through social contact: An experimental study of a housing project.* Ann Arbor: University of Michigan, Institute for Social Research, Research Center for Group Dynamics.

Gardner, J. W. (1993). *On leadership.* New York: Free Press.

Harris, N. O., & Christen, A. G. (Eds.). (1995). *Primary preventive dentistry* (4th ed.). Norwalk, CT: Appleton & Lange.

Hansen, W. B., & O'Malley P. M. (1996). Drug use. In R. J. D'Clemente, W. B. Hansen, & L. E. Ponton (Eds.), *Handbook of adolescent health risk behavior.* New York: Plenum.

Hochbaum, G. M. (1958). *Public participation in medical screening programs: A sociopsychological study* (Public Health Service, Bureau of State Services, Division of Special Health Services, Tuberculosis Program). Washington, DC: U.S. Department of Health, Education, and Welfare.

Iyengar, S. (1994). *Is anyone responsible? How television frames political issues.* Chicago: University of Chicago Press.

Kar, S. B. (Ed.). (1999). *Substance abuse prevention: A multicultural perspective.* Amityville, NY: Baywood.

Kar, S. B., Pascual, C., & Chickering, K. (1999). Empowerment of women for health promotion: A meta-analysis. *Social Science & Medicine, 49,* 1431-1460.

Katz, E., & Lazarsfeld, P. F. (1964). *Personal influence: The part played by people in the flow of mass communications.* New York: Free Press of Glencoe.

Kernell, S. (1997). *Going public: New strategies of presidential leadership* (3rd ed.). Washington, DC: CQ Press.

Kickbusch, I. (1986, September/October). Health promotion: A global perspective. *Canadian Journal of Public Health, 77,* 321-326.

Lalonde, M. (1974). *A new perspective on the health of Canadians.* Ottawa: Government of Canada.

Lalonde, M. (1983). The health field concept: A Canadian perspective. *Epidemiological Bulletin, 4*(3), 13-15.

Lazarsfeld, P. F., Berelson, B., & Gaudet, H. (1944). *The people's choice: How the voter makes up his mind in a presidential campaign.* New York: Duell, Sloan and Pearce.

Lewin, K. (1947). *The research center for group dynamics.* New York: Beacon House.

Lewin, K. (1948). Resolving social conflicts: Selected papers on group dynamics (G. W. Lewin, Ed.). New York: Harper.

Lewin, K. (1964). *Field theory in social science: Selected theoretical papers* (D. Cartwright, Ed.). New York: Harper & Row.

Ling, J. C., Franklin, B. A. K., Lindsteadt, J. F., & Gearon, S. A. N. (1992). Social marketing: Its place in public health. *Annual Review of Public Health, 13,* 341-362.

Los Angeles County Department of Health Services. (1994). *LA County annual health risk assessment.* Information from data on CD-ROM.

Lundberg, G. D. (1998). 200 years of protecting the public health. *JAMA, 280*(7), 592.

MacLean, D. R. (1994). Theoretical rationale of community intervention for the prevention and control of cardiovascular disease. *Health Reports, 6*(1), 174-180.

Marwick, C. (1996). Effect of managed care felt in every medical field. *JAMA, 276*(10), 768-769.

McAlister, A. L. (1991). Population behavior change: A theory-based approach. *Journal of Public Health Policy, 12*(3), 345-361.

McKinlay, J. B. (1992). Health promotion through healthy public policy: The contribution of complementary research methods. *Canadian Journal of Public Health, 83*(Suppl. 1), 811-819.

Milio, N. (1988). The profitization of health promotion. *International Journal of Health Services, 18*(4), 573-585.

Minkler, M. (Ed.). (1997). *Community organizing and community building for health.* New Brunswick, NJ: Rutgers University Press.

National Cancer Institute. (1980). *Health message testing service: A standardized approach for assessing audience response to health messages.* Bethesda, MD: Author.

National Institutes of Health. (1998). *NIH awards to U.S. institutions of higher education by component and funding mechanism, fiscal year 1997* Retrieved June 24, 2000 from the World Wide Web: http://silk.nih.gov/public/cbz2zoz.@www.trends97.school.act.fy97.dsncc

National Library of Medicine. (1998). *The history of the U.S. Public Health Service.* Retrieved June 24, 2000 from the World Wide Web: http://www.nlm.nih.gov/exhibition/phs_history/contents.html

Niles, S., Alemagno, S., & Stricklin, M. L. (1997). Healthy talk: A telecommunication model for health promotion. *Caring, 16*(7), 46-50.

Office of Technology Assessment. (1993). *The continuing challenge of tuberculosis.* Washington, DC: Author.

The Ottawa Charter for Health Promotion (17-21 November 1986). (1996). In *Health promotion anthology* (Scientific Publication No. 557). Washington, DC: World Health Organization, Pan American Health Organization.

Pancer, S. M., & Nelson, G. (1990). Community-based approaches to health promotion: Guidelines for community mobilization. *International Quarterly of Community Health Education, 10*(2), 91-111.

Pierce, J. P., Gilpin, E. A., Emery, S. L., White, M. M., Rosbrook, B., & Berry, C. C. (1998). Has the California tobacco control program reduced smoking? *JAMA, 280*(10), 893-899.

Piotrow, P. T., Kincaid, D. L., Rimon, J. G., Rinehart, W. (1997). *Health communication: Lessons from family planning and reproductive health.* Westport, CT: Praeger.

Pirie, P. L., Stone, E. J., Assaf, A. R., Flora, J. A., & Maschewsky-Schneider, U. (1994). Program evaluation strategies for community-based health promotion programs: Perspectives from the cardiovascular disease community research and demonstration studies. *Health Education Research, 9*(1), 23-36.

Puska, P., Nissinen, A., Tuomilehto, J., Salonen, J. T., Koskela, K., McAlister, A., Kottke, T. E., Maccoby, N., & Farquhar, J. W. (1985). The community-based strategy to prevent coronary heart disease: Conclusions from the 10 years of the North Karelia Project. *Annual Review of Public Health, 6.* (Reprinted in *Health promotion: An anthology,* pp. 89-125. Washington, DC: World Health Organization, Pan American Health Organization)

Ratzan, S. C. (Ed.). (1994). Health communication: Challenges for the 21st century. *American Behavioral Scientist, 38*(2).

Rice, R. E., & Atkin, C. K. (Ed.). (1989). *Mass Communication and public health: Complexities and conflicts* (2nd ed.). Newbury Park, CA: Sage.

Roberts, D. F., & Maccoby, N. (1985). Effects of mass communication. In G. Lindzey & E. Aronson (Eds.), *The handbook of social psychology* (Vol. 1; pp. 539-598). New York: Random House.

Rogers, E. M. (1962). *Diffusion of innovations.* New York: Free Press of Glencoe.

Rogers, E. M. (1973). *Communication strategies for family planning.* New York: Free Press.

Rogers, E. M. (1994). The field of health communication today. *American Behavioral Scientist, 38*(2), 208-214.

Rogers, E. M. (1995). *Diffusion of innovations* (4th ed.). New York: Free Press.

Siegel, M. (1998). Mass media antismoking campaigns: A powerful tool for health promotion. *Annals of Internal Medicine, 129*(2), 128-132.

Sigerist, H. (1946). *The university at the crossroads.* New York: Henry Schuman.

Surgeon General. (1979). *Healthy people: Surgeon general's report on health promotion and disease prevention.* Washington DC: U.S. Department of Health and Human Services, Public Health Service.

Terris, M. (1992). Concepts in health promotion: Dualities in public health theory. *Journal of Public Health Policy, 13*(3), 267-276.

Tuomilehto, J., Geours, J., Salonen, J. T., Nissinen, A., Kuudasmoa, D., & Puska, P. (1986). Decline in cardiovascular mortality in North Karelia and other parts of Finland. *British Medical Journal, 293,* 1068-1071.

U.S. Department of Health and Human Services. (1991). *Healthy people 2000: National Health promotion and disease prevention objectives* (DHHS Publication No. PHS 91-50212). Washington, DC: Government Printing Office.

U.S. Department of Health and Human Services. (1998). *Healthy People 2010 Objectives: Draft for Public Comment.* Washington, DC: U.S. DHHS, Office of Public Health and Science.

U.S. Office of the Surgeon General. (1998). *Duties of the surgeon general.* Retrieved June 24, 2000 from the World Wide Web: http://www.surgeongeneral.gov/osg/sgfunct. htm

U.S. Senate. (1996). *Improvements in U.S. childhood immunization rates. Hearing before the Subcommittee on Departments of Labor, Health and Human Services, Education, and Related Agencies of the Senate Committee on Appropriations.* 104th Cong., 1st sess., special hearing. Washington, DC: Government Printing Office.

Vartiainen, E., Puska, P., Koskela, K., Nissinen, A., & Tuomilehto, J. (1986). Ten year results of a community-based anti-smoking program (as part of the North Karelia Project in Finland). *Health Education Research: Theory and Practice, 1,* 175-184.

Wallack, L. (1994, Winter). Media advocacy: A strategy for empowering people and communities. *Journal of Public Health Policy, 2,* 420-436.

Weijts, W. (1994). Responsible health communication: Taking control of our lives. *American Behavioral Scientist, 38*(2), 257-270.

White, R. K. (1992). A personal assessment of Lewin's major contributions. *Journal of Social Issues, 48*(2), 45-50.

Winkleby, M., Taylor, C., Jatulis, D., & Fortmann, S. P. (1996). The long-term effects of a cardiovascular disease prevention trial: The Stanford Five-City Project. *American Journal of Public Health, 86*(12), 1773-1779.

Winkleby, M. A., Feldman, H. A., & Murray, D. M. (1997). Joint analysis of three U.S. community intervention trials for reduction of cardiovascular disease risk. *Journal of Clinical Epidemiology, 50*(6), 645-658.

4

A Multicultural Society
Facing a New Culture

Snehendu B. Kar
Rina Alcalay
with Shana Alex

This volume began with a discussion on the rapidly growing multicultural
population in the United States and the imperatives of this trend for public
health. In this chapter, we review the key issues in multicultural health communication for health promotion and disease prevention. A strong justification
for a multicultural approach in health communication is based on several well-
documented realities:

1. Ethnic groups significantly vary on measures of preventable deaths and
   disabilities.

2. These deaths and disabilities are largely due to personal behavioral risk
   factors, environmental risk factors, and access to health care services.

3. Behavioral risk factors are deeply rooted in culture, and access to health
   care is strongly affected by the compatibility between the cultures of the
   provider and users of health care.

Table 1.2 (Chapter 1) showed significant differences in mortality due to 10 leading causes of death in five ethnic groups. For instance, the death rate due to heart diseases (the number-one killer of our nation) among African Americans is more than 2.5 times than among Asian Indians. Ethnic differences in other causes of death are even more severe (e.g., HIV/AIDS rates range between 24.9 per 100,000 for African Americans and 0.9 per 100,000 for Asian Americans).

Other important indicators of inequality in health status across ethnic groups are measures of (a) infant mortality, often used as a primary indicator of health status of a population; (b) life expectation at birth as a summary measure of mortality risk; and (c) years of potential life lost before age 75. Statistics show significant ethnic differences in infant mortality for the country as a whole; in addition, these differences have been increasing between 1983 and 1995 (NCHS, 1998, pp. 50-51). Among the most educated mothers, black infants are nearly 3 times (2.7) more likely to die than non-Hispanic whites (NCHS, 1998, p. 50, Figure 8 p. 51). Data in Table 4.2 in this chapter for Los Angeles also show significant differences in infant mortality by four ethnic groups. Asian Americans have the lowest infant mortality rate (4.3 per thousand live births), blacks have the highest rate (11.4); interestingly, in spite of their lower education and access to health insurance, Latinos have lower infant mortality (rate 5.1) than whites (6.8). Figure 1.2 in Chapter 1, this volume, shows that life expectancy at birth has steadily risen since 1950; at the same time, ethnic differences in life expectancy continue to persist. For black men, the expectancy is just above 65 years; for white women it is about 80 years (for both white men and black women life expectancy is about 75 years (Figures 1.1 & 1.2, President's Initiative on Race, 1999). Table 4.1 presents age-adjusted rates of years of potential life lost per 100,000 population before the age of 75.

Relative Health Risks in Multicultural Communities

There are several problems with obtaining reliable and comparable data on many ethnic groups, including that data on several subgroups simply do not exist and some of the high-risk groups are not adequately represented in populations surveys. For instance, we do not have risk profiles of Asian Indians and other recent immigrants based on reliable data. In addition, aggregate data at the national level do not represent the risk profile and magnitude by ethnic groups in multicultural communities where they actually live (e.g., by catchment or service area).

	Asian American	Hispanic	Whites Non-Hispanic	Native Indians	Blacks
Table 4.1 Years of Potential Life Lost Before Age 75, by Race, 1996					
Total (all races and genders) = 7,748.0 per 100,000 population before age 75					
Female	2,949.8	4,211.4	4,899.9	6,197.2	10,012.6
Male	5,101.5	9,989.9	8,744.4	11,607.8	18,994.6

SOURCE: From data in U.S. Department of Health and Human Services (1998, table 32).

One useful way to compare ethnic variations in risk factors at the multicultural community is to review reliable data from large communities that represent all ethnic groups in sufficient numbers. Los Angeles County is one of the most multicultural communities in our nation, in which no single ethnic group has the majority. Table 4.2 contains data from Los Angeles County; it compares five major ethnic groups on 12 indicators of health and quality of life (United Way, 1999). The data show that African Americans (about 7% are foreign-born) are at greatest risk on all measures. Asian Americans (mostly foreign-born, 61%) and Latinos (35% foreign-born) have large proportions of recent immigrants and are relatively less acculturated in the United States, but they have the lowest death and infant mortality rates, the two measures most commonly used to assess health risk of populations. Yet these groups have higher rates of poverty. Asians have a higher rate of poverty than do whites, and Latinos have significantly higher poverty than do African Americans.

These data illustrate the "cultural paradoxes" we discussed in previous chapters of this volume and indicate that significant ethnic differences in deadly outcomes exist and persist over time. Culture has strong effects on personal and collective health behavior, and health communication aims to modify these culturally rooted risk factors both at the individual and collective levels. Consequently, effective health communication should be based on a sound understanding of how culture influences health risks in various groups.

The 1990 U.S. census revealed a 30% increase, from 1980, in the number of non-Anglos and persons of color living in this country. They are African Americans, Asian Americans and Pacific Islanders, Hispanics, and members of other

Table 4.2   Ethnicity, Health, and Quality of Life by Selected
Indicators, Los Angeles County, California, United States

	Los Angeles	African American	Asian American	Latinos	Whites
Population:					
1990 census	8,863,164	10.6	10.3	37.8	40.8
1998 estimate	9,649,800	9.0	12.0	44.0	34.0
Poverty rate per 1,000 people	22.1	22.3	15.9	32.6	9.5
Birth rate 1992 per 1,000 people	17.9	17.2	13.3	25.6	9.8
Infant death rate per 1,000 live births	5.9	11.4	4.3	5.1	6.8
Public school enrollment rate (%)	100.0	11.8	10.5	57.1	20.3
Graduation rate (%)	62	56	96	53	75
Uninsured (%)	29	21	23	45	16
Deaths per 100,000— all causes	494.5	774.5	368.8	439.3	471.0
Heart diseases per 100,000	135.7	218.4	102.6	112.6	136.1
Suicides per 100,000	10.2	8.4	7.0	6.2	13.9
Accidents per 100,000	24.8	34.5	16.9	27.8	22.5
AIDS cases in 1997 per 100,000	Males: 1,527	103	10	39	36
	Females: 222	25	1	5	3
AIDS deaths per 100,000	25.7	50.2	4.4	23.5	26.7

SOURCE: United Way of Greater Los Angeles (1999).

ethnic groups. The combined growth of these racial and thnic groups is more than 7 times the rate for non-Hispanic whites, leading to a new demographic reality for the 21st century—a country in which whites will no longer form a majority of the population (U.S. Bureau of the Census, 1999, http://www.census.gov/population/estimates/nation/intfile3-1.txt). Many of these groups are composed mainly of new, low-acculturated immigrants.

Acculturation and Identity

Acculturation is the process of integration of native and traditional values with the dominant culture's values (Falicov, 1983). Preference for the language of their country of origin is the strongest indicator of level of acculturation (Kar, Jimenez, Campbell, & Sze, 1998; Valdes & Seoane, 1995). People who prefer to speak their language of origin are considered to be at a low level of acculturation. Most first-generation adult immigrants will prefer to speak their language of origin rather than English, even if they are bilingual. External and internal factors affect acculturation. External factors include the size of the same-culture community or neighborhood in which the person lives, with lesser acculturation when people live in a densely populated same-culture neighborhood. This facilitates the maintenance of ties with the culture and language of origin. If the individual works in a mostly Anglo environment, this will accelerate the accuituration process. Age will also affect acculturation, with children and adolescents having an easier time adapting to new circumstances. Also, some cultures experience extreme intergenerational conflict.

The latter was the single most important source of concern adversely affecting the quality of life of Indo-Americans (persons originally from India). Issues related to dating and mating/marriage were the greatest source of conflict between generations, causing enormous mental health stress (Kar, Campbell, Jimenez, & Gupta, 1998; Kar et al., 1998). Internal factors include psychological characteristics, educational level, economic status, and the presence or absence of personal and family networks. Isolation will deter acculturation. Also, learning and adopting the English language will be easier than changing beliefs and values even among highly educated and affluent immigrants (Falicov, 1998; Gordon, 1964).

In addition, foreign-born Hispanics with low socioeconomic backgrounds tend to view more Spanish-language television. Latino women also tend to watch more Spanish-language television than do Latino men. Low-acculturated Asians tend to read more newspapers in their native language, whereas highly acculturated Asians favor newspapers such as the *New York Times* and the *Wall Street Journal*. Groups such as the Vietnamese are almost entirely first-generation immigrants and are therefore foreign-born and often non-English speakers (Pasick, Sabogal, et al., 1996). By the year 2010, foreign-born Hispanics will account for about 40% of the total Hispanic population (about 13.6 million), and second and later generations for about 60% (20.4 million) (Edmonston & Passel, 1992). This raises difficulties in communicating health-related information to these groups. For example, concepts such as Pap smears, routine checkups, clinical breast exams, and mammograms cannot be translated into

Chinese or Vietnamese. First-generation immigrants will bring with them cultural values, beliefs, and preferences that were acquired and molded in their countries of origin (Valdes & Seoane, 1995).

Culture encompasses everything a person has seen or heard from the day of birth: parents, grandparents, siblings, friends, schoolteachers, radio and TV programs, clergy, and so on. It is the deposit of knowledge, experiences, beliefs, meanings, notions of time, spatial relations, concepts of the universe, and other elements acquired in the course of generations through individuals, groups, and mass media (Valdes & Seoane, 1995). Culture is revealed through the uniquely shared values, beliefs, and practices (a) that are directly associated with a health-related behavior, (b) that are indirectly associated with a behavior, or (c) that influence acceptance and adoption of a health education message (Pasick, D'Onofrio, & Otero-Sabogal, 1996).

Immigrants had to leave their homes, either for economic or political reasons. They had to leave their families, friends, and the way they used to live. Some chose to do so; some were forced. By contrast, their children, born and raised in the United States, did not share the same experiences, and they acquire some of their values and preferences from their exposure to American culture through schools, media, and friends as well as from the beliefs and customs of their parents. Often, these ethnic groups exhibit biculturalism, whereby two distinct sets of aspirations, values, and beliefs coexist and are often a source of conflict, particularly among youth.

Structural Determinants

In addition to culture, structural factors determine the environment of multicultural populations. Even with highly motivated, U.S.-born audiences, if people have no or only limited access to health services, are uninsured, or live in environments that promote unhealthy lifestyles, there is little that communication campaigns can achieve. Structural constraints affect most multicultural groups to some degree: These groups tend to have less access to health care, to be poorer than the rest of society, and to have a larger percentage of uninsured individuals. As a matter of fact, in a multicultural study on breast and cervical cancer prevention among multicultural populations, when race/ethnicity, age, education, household income, insurance coverage, English literacy, employment status, marital status, and nativity were adjusted, the influence of race/ethnicity was seen significant only for Chinese and Vietnamese. Education and lack of insurance were consistent predictors of screening behaviors

(National Institutes of Health [NIH], 1989; Pasick, Sabogal, et al., 1996; Subervi-Velez & Colsant, 1993). Access issues associated with low income and lack of health insurance are critical to all racial/ethnic groups. Thus, socioeconomic factors as well as culture have consistently been shown to predict behavior, morbidity, and mortality across a range of risk factors and health problems (Feinstein, 1993; Pasick, Sabogal, et al., 1996).

Low-acculturated immigrants in particular have to struggle to create a "reasonably functional" new definition of reality that incorporates their country of origin experiences with the ways of the new host country. Immigrants must try to make sense from often conflicting values and patterns of behavior and create a new persona that can be functionally adapted to their new environment—not an easy task considering additional language, financial, educational, and other constraints.

Cultural Patterns of Hispanics and Asian Americans

We examine similarities and differences between two least-acculturated ethnic groups—Hispanics and Asian Americans—to identify key processes through which culture affects health and their implications for health communication. We do not suggest that whites, African Americans, and Native Indians are less important ethnic groups; however, the overwhelming majority (more than 9 of 10) of the members of these three groups have been in this country for centuries, and much has been written on them. We know less—in some cases, nothing—about recent immigrants and their experience in multicultural communities. Although generalization can be misleading and can lead to stereotyping, the following section will present some general traits associated with these two major immigrant groups. Multicultural groups are heterogeneous; there is no such thing as Hispanics or Asians as homogeneous entities. Age, gender, level of education, socioeconomic status, geographic origin and concentration, religion, circumstances for immigration, language preferences, amount of time in this country, level of identification with the culture of origin, type of migration and degree of acculturation, and presence and kinds of social support networks create great differences within groups. Health promotion campaigns must consider the specific demographic, psychographic, and cultural characteristics of the group(s) that will be the target population for an intervention.

Hispanics

According to Valdes and Seoane (1995), core Hispanic values include family loyalty and group orientation; respect for authority; difference in treatment according to social class, age, sex, and generational stratification; mostly adhering to the Catholic faith; placing importance on appearances and social graces; and having a present rather than a future orientation. Three key values of Hispanic culture—*familismo, machismo,* and *simpatía*—will be discussed briefly. The pillar of Hispanic culture is the family, which includes the extended family of grandparents, uncles, aunts, and cousins. Family needs and welfare take precedence over individual member's needs. Parents will make sacrifices for the children; in return, children are expected to show respect and gratitude and to assume responsibility for younger siblings and for the parents in their old age. Old parents, no matter how debilitated by conditions such as Alzheimer's disease, are rarely put into nursing homes. To put parents in such facilities is perceived negatively in Latino culture. Also, parenting roles are strongly internalized at a young age by Hispanic children. Hispanics tend to stress interdependence over autonomy, a characteristic often at odds with the new scripts they encounter in their adopted land. In the Latin model, parents are expected to provide for the children, and children are not pushed to act independently (Falicov, 1998). Hispanic mothers continue to cook for their adult children, Hispanic families tend to stick together on weekends, and Hispanic parents encourage their children to live with them for as long as possible (Valdes & Seoane, 1995).

Machismo goes beyond treating women in stereotypically dominating ways or being "macho." It involves men's functioning as providers, protectors, and representatives of the family to the outer world. They are responsible to uphold the honor of family members, deal effectively with the public sphere, and maintain the integrity of the family unit. Machismo also refers to having socially acceptable manly characteristics, such as being courageous, strong, and virile. It includes being respectful of women. Machismo provides much more freedom for men than women with regard to sexual activity and public-social interactions. Machismo can sometimes protect women from high-risk behaviors. For example, men are encouraged to drink and smoke in public, a behavior not acceptable among low-acculturated women. Unfortunately, smoking rates among highly acculturated Hispanic women go up dramatically.

Machismo, on the other hand, hinders women from effective AIDS prevention. This is due to Hispanic culture taboos regarding sexual matters. It is not acceptable for women to raise these issues with their partners. These taboos can have serious consequences. Compared with whites, AIDS has affected Hispanics disproportionately. The cumulative incidence for Hispanic men is 2.5 times the rate for white men (Bakeman, McCray, Lumb, Jackson, & Whitley, 1987).

Being sociable, outgoing, likable, and demonstrative are highly valued characteristics in the community (*sympatía*). Generally in Hispanic culture, social interactions are more open, less restrained, and more frequent than in the Anglo culture. Overall, Hispanics tend to be lighthearted and enjoy group activities involving relatives and friends. Latinos are also comfortable in church-related, social, and community activities and tend to live in neighborhoods densely populated by Spanish-speaking people. Special birthdays, such as quinceanera;[1] anniversaries; engagements; weddings; and religious ceremonies, such as baptisms and communions, are elaborate and well attended. These values are often shared by second- and third-generation Hispanics in the community. Hispanic women tend to characterize themselves as "romantic." This romantic mind-set may help explain the overwhelming popularity of novelas, Spanish-language TV soap operas that last a couple of months and portray highly charged romances (Valdes & Seoane, 1995). For the foreign-born Hispanic woman, especially if the extended family does not reside in the United States, there is always an element of nostalgia.

Hispanics tend to be "outer directed" and very conscious of their overall appearance, including fashion and cosmetics. Even among highly acculturated Hispanic women, the tradition of pleasing is strong. Being helpful, giving, and a good hostess are values appreciated in the Hispanic culture. Children and family are extremely important and tend to be more central to their identity than work, particularly among low-acculturated Hispanic women. Also, Hispanics have access to around-the-clock Spanish language radio and TV programs and to daily print media. This factor has been quoted as slowing down the process of acculturation. On the other hand, this fact increases the chance of effectively using media, and community-wide meetings, with much-needed health promotion messages. For example, the Hispanic Health and Nutrition Examination Survey (HHANES) showed that 40% of Mexican American women reported never having had their breasts examined by a health professional or having had a Pap smear performed (Lecca, Greenstein, & McNeil, 1987). Results from the 1987 National Health Interview Survey (NHIS) showed that 24% of Latina women never had a Pap smear, compared with 9% of Anglo American and 11.9% of African American women (Harlan, Bernstein, & Kessler, 1991). Spanish-speaking media must be used to address these and other public health issues. Chapter 5 in this volume describes in detail the presence of Spanish language/Latino media in the United States and its strong ties to Latin America.

Asian Americans

The term *Asian American* covers a broad array of diverse ethnic groups that originated in Asia and are currently residing in America. As of 1990, Asian Americans constituted 2.9% of the American population and are its fastest-growing segment. It is estimated that there were 11,022,000 Asian Americans in the United States in November 1999; compared with 7,462,000 in 1990, this represents about 48% growth in 9 years or 5.5% increase per year compared with annual U.S. growth of 0.9% per year (U.S. Bureau of the Census, 1999). The Asian American population is estimated to double to 22,020,000 by 2025 and to nearly quadruple to 37,589,000 by 2050 (U.S. Bureau of the Census, 1999, middle-series estimates, http://www.census.gov/population/estimates/nation/intfile3-1.txt). Socioeconomically (education and income) and culturally, Asian Americans are the most diverse ethnic group in the nation. Although in 1994 whites had a higher per-capita income than the average for all Asian Americans, Indo-Americans (Asian Indian) had the highest level of education and median household income of all ethnic groups at $46,912. At the same time, some Asian American ethnic groups, such as Cambodians had the lowest median household income at $17,343. Cambodians and Laotians also had the lowest per-capita income—$4,639 and $6,357, respectively (United Way, 1994). The aggregate household income data may be misleading because of the tendency of several groups to have larger families.

Asian Americans are also the most diverse ethnic group linguistically; they speak over 70 distinct languages. Asian Indians alone speak 17 languages; India is the only nation in the world that prints its currency bills in 17 languages. In addition, Asians follow all major religions of the world in large numbers (e.g., Buddhism, Hinduism, Islam, Christianity, Sikhism, Judaism). Finally, census data show that the overwhelming majority of Asian Americans (61%) are recent immigrants and foreign-born (compared with 35% Hispanics, 7% whites, 6% blacks, and 9% of the total U.S. population). Among some subgroups, over 7 of 10 are foreign-born (e.g., Vietnamese, Cambodians, Laotians, Indians, Hmong). Most families have foreign-born parents and U.S.-born children; these parents tend to be less acculturated than their children. They often hold onto their traditional values and beliefs about gender role and parental authority. In one recent survey of Asian Indians, Japanese, and Koreans in California, the majority of college students reported that intergenerational and gender role conflicts were the two most significant sources of psychological distress; they also reported higher percentages of depression than rates reported in national surveys (Kar et al., 1995; Kar et al., 1998).

As of the last official census, Chinese Americans were the largest Asian ethnic group in the United States (U.S. Bureau of the Census, 1990; Kar et al., 1998), but it is projected they will be outnumbered by Filipinos after the 2000 census. From 1980 to 1990, the Chinese population increased by 103% to 1,645,472 people (Asian and Pacific Islander Center for Census Information and Services, 1992/1993.). Of Asian Americans, 30% are linguistically isolated—that is, no one in the household aged 14 years or older reporting to speak English well or very well (U.S. Bureau of the Census, 1993). The Centers for Disease Control Behavioral Risk Factor Surveillance System survey of English-speaking Chinese in California during 1989 showed that 45% of Chinese women aged 20 to 74 reported never having had a Pap smear. Among women 40 or older, 68% reported never having had a mammogram, and 75% reported never having had a clinical breast exam (Chen et al., 1992). These low rates should not be viewed solely as a lack of preventive orientation in the Chinese culture. In fact, traditional Chinese medicine is holistic and preventive in nature. Traditional Chinese medicine focuses on the philosophical framework of balancing the two complementary body opposite properties, the *yin* and *yang* (Shi & Shi, 1992). The Chinese use a different set of preventive measures, such as herbs and acupuncture. Western medicine is mostly used when a health problem already exists. Studies with Chinese women show that language was one of the major barriers to screening use (Lovejoy, Jenkins, Wu, Shankland, & Wilson, 1989). Other barriers reported include (a) modesty, (b) having no primary physician, (c) being unaware of screening tests, (d) concern about costs, (e) getting time off from work, (f) transportation, (g) worrying about tests results, and (h) not knowing where to go for screening tests (Lovejoy et al., 1989).

Since 1975, nearly 600,000 refugees have arrived in the United States from Vietnam. The early waves (1975-1977) were typically well educated, urban, relatively young, and in good health, whereas later groups of immigrants, mainly the "boat people" (1978 and after) tended to be less educated, from rural backgrounds, less familiar with Western concepts, less fluent in English, and in poorer health (Gold, 1992; Muecke, 1983). Health statistics for this population are limited. Compared with women in California, Vietnamese women in general are about half as likely to develop breast cancer but about four times as likely to develop cervical cancer (McPhee et al., 1996). Cervical cancer is more common among Vietnamese women than among other Asian women. Cultural aspects from the Vietnamese population, relevant for designing health interventions (Pasick, D'Onofrio, & Hiatt, 1996) include the following: (a) They are likely to stay close to their neighborhoods; (b) they are unlikely to respond to health information coming from outside their family or friendship circles; (c) personal modesty among women acts as a barrier to health care (McPhee et al., 1996); (d) the disruption of family and social roles (patriarchal society) resulting from immigration tends to be manifested in a sense of isolation and alienation from the host society (Lin, Masuda, & Tazuma, 1982); (e) other survival issues are competing, and preventive health often is not a high priority; (f) cost, lack of health insurance, and language act as barriers; (g) low levels of acculturation, limited knowledge of English, and scant knowledge of Western medicine may preclude Vietnamese from understanding publicly disseminated health information. Vietnamese women have more of an Eastern medical orientation and lack Western ideas of preventive health care.

In some Southeast Asian cultures, it is not permitted to touch someone else's head, because the spirit is located in the head. Also, it is insulting to point at someone's feet, because feet are considered the lowest in value in the body. Having eye contact with someone with superior authority is considered impolite. Avoiding shame and loss of face are of great importance. Some Asian cultures may find it impolite to say they do not understand what another person is saying, so they tend not to ask for explanations so as not to lose face, a trait shared by Hispanics. Vietnamese groups value modesty, honor discretion and other people's privacy, and place great value on community solidarity, generosity and helpfulness.

Research shows that when studying different low-acculturated Asian American groups it is possible to see many similarities among them; they all face language difficulties, barriers in accessing mainstream health care system, economic hardship, changes of social status vis-á-vis their country of origin and changes in family role and family structure, psychological distress, and cultural loss. They also share an emphasis on the family unit; are grounded in the values of Confucianism, Hinduism, and Buddhism; have strong same-ethnicity group orientation; are restrained about emotional expressivity; maintain harmonious interpersonal relationships; tend to avoid confrontations; emphasize academic achievements; experience generational conflicts; face the deterioration of older people's authority; and have identity confusion among the newer generation (Wong, Lai, Nagasawa, & Lin, 1998).

Asian Americans at an aggregate level fare well on most indicators of health and quality of life. These and other findings tend to reinforce the "model minority myth," which is frequently used to divert attention form serious problems experienced by the Asian Americans. Contrary to the stereotype that Asian Americans are doing well enough because of their seemingly high socio-economic status, studies show that they experience serious physical and mental distress despite their favorable socioeconomic achievements. Unemployment among Asian Americans in 1990 was in excess of 15% (United Way, 1994). One recent study of college students and their parents reported that students were relatively more psychologically distressed than parents; they felt depressed and thought about suicide or death twice as often as did their parents (18% and 8%, respectively; Kar et al., 1995; Kar et al., 1998). One important measure of eco-nomic status is poverty level. For the country as a whole, in 1989, about 13% were defined as poor (individuals earning less than $6,451 per year). The 1990 census data show significantly higher poverty levels among several Asian In-dian immigrant groups. These include Hmongs (63%) Cambodians (40%), Laotians (33%), Vietnamese (25%), Pacific Islanders (22%), Chinese (16%), and Koreans (14%). Only Filipinos (6%), Asian Indians (10%), and Japanese and Thais (12% each) had a lower proportion of poverty (Jibou, 1996, p. 52).

Differences and Similarities Among Minorities

Collectivism is one profound difference that distinguishes other cultures from U.S. values. In Anglo-American culture, individual pursuits and needs and the pursuit of individual happiness and success are primary goals in life and often take precedence over community. Among groups as diverse as His-panics and Asians, a collectivistic outlook generally takes precedence. Collec-tivism takes the form of a heightened concern and dependency on family, an emphasis on harmony in human relations and positive interpersonal interac-tions *(simpatía),* and respect for authority figures (Pèrez-Stable, 1987; Sabogal, Marín, Otero-Sabogal, Marín, & Pèrez-Stable, 1987; Triandis, Marín, Lisansky, & Betancourt, 1984).

On the other hand, on some issues there is also great diversity among mem-bers of the same ethnic group, depending on socioeconomic strata, language, and religiosity. Other factors will vary among rich and poor, educated and un-educated, religious or not, isolated or rooted in family ties, and so on (Pasick, D'Onofrio, & Hiatt, 1996). Fatalism, for example, is often shared among Asian and Hispanic low socioeconomic groups. *Fatalismo* refers to a perception in having limited influence in the course of one's own life events, believing that those events are determined by fate or by an external force such as God (Orlandi, 1992). Fatalistic individuals feel less control over jobs, quality of life, and capacity to provide for the family. Fatalism is relevant for health promotion because it can significantly limit preventive behaviors needed, such as cancer screenings when an individual is asymptomatic. According to Pèrez-Stable and others, *fatalismo* is a cultural construct associated with behaviors that are detrimental to health. It is particularly observed among low socioeconomic groups in these cultures. Such tendencies must be challenged through culturally appropriate interventions (Pèrez-Stable, Otero-Sabogal, Sabogal, & Nápoles-Springer, 1996).

This characteristic might be more a reflection of lack of control due to low socioeconomic status than to ethnicity. It appears to be a trait reinforced by a sense of lack of control and a low sense of self-efficacy, not only toward health but toward other aspects of life. High socioeconomic groups among Hispanics, Vietnamese, and others would tend to be less fatalistic, as a result of more control over their lives. In fact, several studies have noted that once income, education, and other socioeconomic variables are included in a model, race has little explanatory power for mortality (Logue & Jarjoura, 1990). Culturally diverse groups must construct a new reality in the United States that will permit them to operate functionally and survive. Few agencies are in place, except for organized groups from their own ethnic background, to enable this process of adaptation to be a smooth one, where the member of a diverse culture will feel understood and accommodated. With the increasing presence of multicultural groups in the United States, culturally competent communication strategies must be developed. Culturally competent interventions require an understanding of interethnic group differences and levels of acculturation.

Cultural Diversity and Health Behavior

A culture affects the health of its members through five key processes or dimensions; these are health-related beliefs, values, knowledge, attitudes, and practices (BVKAP). In addition, culture affects one's time orientation, preferred decision-making modality (individual vs. collective), nature of social and political participation, and communication networks. One way to understand health risks and practices in a multicultural community is by examining how different subgroups are similar or different on these dimensions. On the basis of our literature review, we present a conceptual framework for examining the differences in the cultural and societal processes, including communication processes, that affect health behavior in a multiethnic community (see Table 4.2). This framework allows a cross-cultural comparison of groups on five

Table 4.2 Health Behavior Matrix: Modern and Traditional Societies

Cultural Beliefs, Values, Knowledge, Attitudes, and Practices	Modern Societies (e.g., United States, United Kingdom, Canada)	Traditional Societies (e.g., Japan, India)
Disease etiology	Modern scientific—believes in germs, genes, toxins, trauma	Unitary cosmic and magicoreligious—believes in chi, yin/yang, karma)—and modern scientific
Preferred treatment modality	Modern clinical and surgical specialist driven	Traditional medical, spiritual, and self-care augmented by modern medicine
Individual responsibility	Individual and personal	Collective, familial decision, hierarchic, and compliant
Communication/social relations	Mass: printed and electronic; formal and impersonal	Informal personal network augmented by modern media
Accessibility of services	Highly variable, low/no access for disadvantaged	Traditional services more accessible and affordable

SOURCE: Kar, Jimenez, Campbell, and Sze (1998).

important dimensions through which cultural and societal processes may affect health and communication behavior:

1. Cultural etiology and beliefs related to health and illness
2. Preferred modalities of treatment and prevention
3. Personal responsibility and locus of control
4. Communication and social participation
5. Accessibility of services

This comparison allows us to identify similarities and differences among the groups compared in terms of major cultural and social factors that may have profound effects on health-related behavior. This cross-cultural framework was developed by the author (Kar) through one of his assignments as a consultant with the World Health Organization; the mission was to develop a framework for planning health promotion strategies appropriate for the Western Pacific nations.

For illustrative purpose, two cultures are compared on the five dimensions: non-Hispanic white Americans (representing the Western or modern cultures) and Asian Americans (representing the Eastern or traditional cultures). They are different in many important dimensions: language, religion and philosophy, social organization, health and food habits, and important cultural practices. This comparison of two distinctly different cultures allows us to readily identify similarities and differences in health-related behavior. In reality, of course, we will expect individuals in both cultures, especially those who are more acculturated, to integrate elements from their native and host cultures. A detailed description of this cross-cultural health behavior framework has been presented elsewhere (Kar et al., 1998; Kar & Alex, 1999). Following is a brief description of each of the five dimensions.

Cultural Etiology and Beliefs Related to Health and Illness

The concept of cultural etiology includes cross-cultural differences in beliefs and meanings related to life and death, causes of diseases, definitions and significance of illness, and the meaning of various symptoms. For instance, according to Chinese etiology, *chi* is the universal and primary force, which governs every aspect of this universe. Good health is enjoyed when human mind and body are in harmony with the universal *chi*. The *chi* consists of two forces, *yin* and *yang;* when these two complementary forces are in balance, the result is harmony, good health, and happiness, whereas imbalance causes illness and misery. The purpose of a treatment is to restore balance between the *yin* and *yang* through manipulating energy forces within the body (e.g., acupuncture, tai chi, meditation, herbal medicine, etc). There is no room for germs, toxins, and genetics in this paradigm. The Vedic philosophy, which governs the Indian Ayurvedic medicine, is remarkably similar. *Prana* is the primary and ubiquitous life force, which is eternal and indestructible. This universal *prana* is temporally manifested in the human body, which is made of five elements (the Chinese system also holds that five elements combine to make everything). An imbalance among these five elements causes three types of maladies (*tridoshas*), which in turn lead to distress and diseases. The treatment objective is to restore the balance through culturally prescribed interventions—that is, traditional medical systems (Ayurveda, Chinese medicine, Unani, Yoga, meditation, diets, etc.). Cultures also vary significantly in terms of the beliefs and values related to hot and cold food, magical/metaphysical/supernatural causes of diseases, and major life events affecting health and illness (e.g., life, births, deaths, abortions, euthanasia, divorce, homicide, suicide, unwed motherhood, contraception, value of children, status of women, role of the elderly, etc). These beliefs and values lead to significant cultural differences in health practices.

Preferred Modality of Treatment and Prevention

Consistent with the culturally defined etiology of illness and health-related beliefs, treatment systems and practices vary by cultures. Traditional Chinese medicine, Indian Ayurvedic medicine, Islamic Unani medicine systems, and various folk medicine and healing practices are important living systems; they have significant influence on health-related practices among the believers. Often, people may use both systems, Western and alternative, for different types of problems. The Western system is usually preferred for acute and infectious diseases, for life-threatening situations, and by the younger generation, whereas the traditional system is preferred by many for chronic disease management and particularly by the older generations. We do not have any reliable estimate of the extent to which Americans as a whole, or by ethnicity and social class, believe and practice traditional medicine. The degree to which one believes in any one of these systems will significantly influence his or her use of modern medical services and preventive practices. Effective health communication programs cannot be oblivious to this reality; sound health communication should be based on an understanding of cultural preferences for modern and traditional practices for preventive and curative care (Eisenberg et al., 1998).

Personal Responsibility and Locus of Control

Cultures vary in terms of beliefs about individual responsibility for personal well-being, the extent to which one is able to control his or her life events, and how assertive or passive one should be in acting in self-interest in a family and social setting (especially for women and younger family members). This dimension affects the extent to which individuals depend on other members of the family and social network for their own health promotion and disease prevention needs. In several cultures from which ethnic minorities originate, aggressive pursuit of one's self-interest, be it for health or something else, is considered an offensive antifamily or anticommunity aspect of one's personality. It meets with strong social disapproval. On the contrary, Western culture underscores the importance of individualism and personal choices. This aspect of culture may cause significant differences in the expectations of care providers and the health behavior of their clients from unfamiliar ethnic groups.

Preferred Modalities Communication and Social Participation

Various ethnic groups in a multicultural community differ significantly in terms of their language preference and proficiency, level of formal education, and interpersonal network. These differences affect health and communication behavior in several important ways: (a) who communicates with whom for seeking and providing health-related information and for making decisions; (b) which mass media is used, how frequently, and for what purpose; (c) how effectively one interacts with health care professionals; and (d) how actively one participates in social and political processes that affect health needs and services.

Accessibility, Acceptability, and Affordability of Health Care Services

Accessibility and affordability of health services is a major determinant of health care use. Major ethnic minorities are poor, uninsured, and underserved by health care organizations. Over 30% of minorities in California are uninsured; the scenario is similar nationally. Ethnic minorities have an additional barrier—the cultural distance between themselves and health care providers. This is more than a language problem; it is driven by lack of mutual trust and understanding of cultural and existential realities. These aspects of cultural practices cannot be overcome by hiring bilingual providers alone (although that will help). Cultural competency of the communicators is a primary determinant of acceptability of services even when they are available. Partnership with traditional healers, community-based organizations (CBOs) dedicated to ethnic cause, and involvement of local health promoters (LHPs) can reduce the problems of accessibility and acceptability due to cultural distance between multicultural communities and health communicators and health service providers.

There are at least four models for delivering cross-cultural health care services:

1. Mainstream agencies providing outreach services to multicultural populations

2. Mainstream agencies supporting services by multicultural populations within their own communities

3. Agencies providing bilingual, bicultural services

4. Multicultural population agencies providing services to their own people independently

The basis for competency in conducting business with culturally diverse communities requires providers to (a) demonstrate knowledge of the group, (b) show respect for the community being served, (c) relate in a trusting manner, (d) establish empathy, (e) strive toward ease of rapport and mutual understanding, (f) discount stereotypes (generalizations about a group or category of people, usually unfavorable, exaggerated, and oversimplified), and (g) provide continuity of care. Also, minority community members must feel that providers are their advocates and that services are reasonably available and accessible to them. Careful attention to these provider-initiated communication components will strongly enhance not only the satisfaction of culturally diverse clients but also their empowerment. Health providers are in a privileged position to act as community advocates, encouraging and reaffirming community strengths, assisting in strengthening community networks, and building network coalitions to improve community conditions, based on principles of community building and community empowerment (Bird, Otero-Sabogal, Ngoc-The, & McPhee, 1996). Strategies that have demonstrated effectiveness include the use of lay health workers and using a chain of communication within existing social networks to maximize the number of people effectively reached.

Cultural construction of communication includes styles of communication significant to the ethnic group. The delivery of services must be done by means of appropriate messages and channels and by using appropriate language (verbal and nonverbal). It can be done through the media, family members, informal social support mechanisms, and institutional resources. An illustration of an appropriate message style to communicate with Latinos, for example, is the use of stories with strong imagery. In addition, behavioral intentions may not be relevant in cultures where planning for the future is not valued. For example, the San Francisco Smoking Cessation project found that in promoting cessation among Latinos, preparation for future quitting was ineffective and irrelevant; a do-it-right-now, cold-turkey approach to cessation was more consonant with cultural values. Talking about cancer is not accepted in certain cultures, except in the most general terms rather than personal, because personalizing can bring the evil eye.

Barriers to Competency Among Multicultural Groups

Structural factors, as well as cultural ones, influence the level of competency with which members of multiethnic groups use the health care system. Among Vietnamese women, cultural factors, such as year of immigration and English fluency, and structural factors, such as marital status, poverty status, and cost of screening, are associated with cancer-screening status (Pasick, Sabogal, et al., 1996). Among Latino women, deterrents to screening include structural factors, such as cost, lack of health insurance, and transportation. Positive cultural factors that predict cancer screening are level of acculturation, size of social network, and strength of traditional family attitudes. Barriers for both Vietnamese and Latino women who are not fluent in English include difficulty in making medical appointments and receiving appropriate medical care. Interventions must take these factors into account. Structural barriers such as poverty, crime in the neighborhood, or lack of transportation must also be taken into account in intervention planning. Other barriers—for example, lack of exposure to the concept of prevention among certain populations, such as the Vietnamese—must also be considered.

Types of Communication

Communication occurs in a cultural and social setting. Culturally competent communication requires that the sender and receiver share the same codes of language, symbols, and images. This is harder to achieve in bicultural communication. Thus, the sharing of common codes must be acquired through a conscious effort. Also, message meaning can change a lot in bicultural settings. Something that is a given for most people who grew up in the same culture is not a given for immigrants who were not exposed to that message earlier in life. Effective bicultural communication recognizes and uses cultural awareness, cultural sensitivity, and an understanding of the mind-set of clients from the conceptualization stage of the messages through strategic planning to implementation. The rest of this section will be devoted to delineating some cultural traits specific to Hispanics that can be useful to providers interested in acquiring such cultural competency.

Authors Valdes and Seoane (1995, p. 345) describe a series of approaches that do work and others that do not work with Hispanic populations. According to these authors, what does not work with Hispanics, particularly the low-acculturated, has to do with abstract or elaborate metaphors (images and messages tend to be missed or, even worse, misinterpreted), unfocused messages, too much information in one message, no emotional pull. On the other hand, what does work with Hispanics includes (a) an emotionally driven campaign (talk to the heart); (b) messages presented in simple, familiar, and realistic backgrounds; (c) messages direct and to the point; (d) enough repetition of key messages; (e) having a logo and as many concrete images as possible; (f) telling a simple story with a beginning and an end; (g) people shown in messages as "average looking" Hispanics, not too dark, mestizo, or Indian looking, but not too European or blond looking either; and (h) creating parasocial interactions—that is, a sense of vicarious intimacy between the audience and the sender of the message, either a reporter or television or radio personality. The latter benefits from the idea of *personalismo,* which can be used to promote healthy messages. There is much Hispanic consumer sensitivity in this area, and careful pretesting is advised. It is good to show family members, such as mother, father, grandfather, grandmother, teenager, and baby, preferably with happy smiling faces. Do not dwell on negative images. Among high-acculturated Hispanics, there is a conscious search for ethnic identity or roots, especially by second-, third-, or fourth- generation immigrants who have lost some or most of their cultural traits. They must learn the language, values, music, arts, and food preferences of their original culture. Messages that support this audience in their pursuit of cultural roots are appropriate.

Culturally Relevant Methods

Several methods maximize the possibility of obtaining culturally relevant information to facilitate the understanding of culturally diverse groups. The richly textured data obtained through these methodologies are essential also for the design of culturally appropriate messages that will reach the target audience. Subjective culture methodology, which combines qualitative techniques (e.g., open-ended, in-depth, individual interviews, focus groups, extensive pretesting) and quantitative approaches (e.g., survey research methodology and epidemiological data) is used to study cultural values, language, and ethnic visual symbols that need to be incorporated when developing health promotion materials. Analysis of subjective culture seeks to find general and specific culturally related elements among specific nonphysical aspects of culture (Triandis, 1972). Focus groups have been tested and accepted as valid for cross-cultural research and for eliciting culturally appropriate ways of encoding the health issue to make it relevant for the specific cultural group (Alcalay, Ghee, & Scrimshaw, 1993). Use of carefully selected and trained "key informants," a method frequently used by cultural diplomats, is another important method that deserves full consideration for formative research and evaluation of multicultural communities.

Other qualitative methods such as *semiology* (Barthes, 1957), or the analysis of people's narrative about specific subjects, and Freire's method, a verbal-visual strategy to obtain information meaningful to the group being studied are excellent strategies to provide a basis for the imagery, language, and context needed for the design of culturally competent messages. Recommendations to create cultural competence include (a) setting up a partnership between neighborhood health centers and medical schools, (b) emphasizing language and culture, (c) emphasizing primary care and family medicine, (d) having students work in teams on different outreach settings, (e) teaching people how to access health care systems, and (f) making sure that cross-cultural education occurs throughout the provider's education and practice, not just during a few lectures. Strategies for teaching cultural competence to providers include seminars, panel discussions, group discussions, self-reflection, and exercises.

Cultural Competency: Beyond Language

In this section, we look at cultural competency as a part of effective communication planning; the cultural competency of communicators can make the difference between the success and failure of a program. The word *culture* refers to integrated patterns of behavior, including thoughts, verbal and nonverbal language, actions, customs, beliefs, values, and institutions of a racial, ethnic, religious, or social group. The word *competence* refers to the capacity to function in a particular way, within the context of a culturally integrated pattern of behavior as defined by the group. Bilingual competency is often used as a proxy measure of cultural competency among communicators and educators. Although a common language is an important medium of multicultural communication, we make an important distinction between the *language competency* and the *cultural competency* of care providers and communicators. Elimination of language differences helps but does not eliminate cultural differences. For instance, African Americans and non-Hispanic whites both speak English and have lived next to each other for centuries, yet these two groups do not have the same cultural experiences and ethnic identities. Intergenerational conflict is another example in which members of a family may use the same language but do not communicate because they hold dissimilar priorities, values, and beliefs. Although knowing the language of another ethnic group can help, it does not necessarily make the communicators or providers culturally competent to deal with members of another ethnic group. Cultural competency requires a deeper understanding and behavioral skills that go beyond language competency (the two quotations at the beginning of the Introduction to this volume point to this important principle).

Levels of Cultural Competency

We identify at least three levels of cultural competency that go beyond language competency (including competency of language at four levels). The first is *cultural understanding,* which includes a working knowledge of the core beliefs, values, norms, mores, institutions, and traditions unique to another culture. Cultural understanding, however, may promote cultural acceptance or work against it. One might reject another culture based on a clear understanding of the fundamental values and proscriptions of that culture. The second level is *cultural acceptance,* including sensitivity, respect, acceptance of differences, and recognition of the right of another culture to maintain its own identity and uniqueness, insofar as that identity and uniqueness do not deprive others of basic rights. The opposite of cultural acceptance is the insistence by one culture, usually the dominant culture, that minorities assimilate into the dominant culture (the extreme would be prejudice, culture clash, and hostility, such as hate crimes). Cultural acceptance is more than cultural understanding and cultural tolerance. On the basis of one's understanding of another ethnic group and one's own ethnocentric values, one can understand another culture and yet may not accept that culture. It can, however, be argued that one cannot develop a sound cultural understanding unless there is some degree of acceptance of that culture.

The third level is *reciprocal relationship.* This is what Tagore called "a bond of relations" and what Rumi means by "to be one of heart" with others. This is the highest level of cultural competency and requires trusting and sustained communication and relationships between members of different ethnic groups (e.g., intimate friendship, trusting partnership, dating, and marriage). This level of cultural competency of providers and of health communicators may ultimately determine the effectiveness of a health communication messages. A demonstrated cultural competency of the health care providers and communicators should be an important category of indicators of a process evaluation of multicultural communication (see Chapters 1 and 5 for related discussions.) The burden to change is heavier on the communicators than on their audience.

Two models are aimed at enhancing cultural competency among health care providers and health communicators. First is the *training model,* which aims at increasing the cultural competency of providers who come from the dominant culture. The second model is *selection,* which aims at increasing cultural diversity among providers by proactively recruiting members from minority groups. The basic assumption here is that when providers and clients come from the same ethnic group, the quality of interaction should be more trusting and effective. In recognition of the importance of both models, the Pew Health Professions Commission (1998), an influential force for health professionals and the medical education policy of our nation, argued that

> the next generation of health professionals must be prepared to practice in more intensively managed and integrated systems. Specifically, the clinicians of the future will be required to use the sophisticated information and communication technology to promote health and prevent disease, to sharpen their skills in areas ranging from clinical prevention to health education to the effective use of political reforms to change the burden of disease, to be more customer or consumer-focused, and to be ready to move into new roles that ask them to strike an equitable balance between resources and needs. (p. 3)

The commission goes on to recommend actions through which a greater diversity in health professionals could be achieved. Recognizing that this goal would not be achieved immediately and that ethnic differences between providers and clients will continue, the Pew Commission further adds,

> There is substantial body of literature which concludes that culturally sensitive care is good care. This means two things for all health professional schools. First, they must continue their commitment to ensure that the students they train represent the rich ethnic diversity of our society. Second, diversifying the entering class is not sufficient to ensure understanding and appreciation of diversity. Cul-

Table 4.3   Domain and Hierarchy Matrix of Communication Effects

Domain 1	Domain 2	Domain 3
Hierarchy of Effects: Individual Level	*Communicator/Program Effects: Cultural Competency*	*Community Effects*
1. Audience *exposure*	1. Language competency or bilingual interpreter use	1. Community interest
2. Audience *awareness*	2. Cultural competency	2. Community awareness & trust
3. Audience's being *informed*	3. Participatory program planning with minority communities	3. Leadership involvement & support
4. Audience's being *persuaded*	4. Use of "cultural capital" (e.g., ethnic community network)	4. Community willingness to invest resource/volunteers
5. Audience's *intent* to act	5. Coalitions with community-based organizations.	5. Community norms change
6. Actual *change* in audience's behavior	6. Partnership for program implementation	6. Community adoption of preventive behaviors
7. Maintenance of audience's behavior	7. Institutionalized participatory planning & evaluation	7. *Community empowerment and ownership of program by the commumunity and organizations*

SOURCE: Backer, Rogers, and Sopory (1992).

tural sensitivity must be a part of the educational experience that touches the life of every student. (p. 4)

This recommendation is based on the assumption that work experience in multicultural community settings, under proper supervision, would enhance cultural competency of health professionals. These two recommendations should be equally valid for health communicators. In our "domains and hierarchy matrix" of evaluation in Table 4.3, we integrate cultural competency in program-level indicators. This is a conceptual framework derived from our review of literature; it is analogous to a hypothesis. The specific indicators or measures in each domain would have to be empirically determined.

Cultural competence involves systems, agencies, and practitioners with the capacity to respond to the unique needs of populations whose cultures are other than "mainstream" American (Georgetown University Child Development Center, 1992, p. 3). In regional communities, this can begin with a common language. Ultimately, cultural competence is a set of congruent behaviors, attitudes, and policies that come together in a system or agency, or among health professionals, that enables that system, or those professionals, to work effectively in cross-cultural situations. Simply put, it's the ability to relate with a person of another culture as ably as one can relate to a person from one's own culture.

Cultural competence may be viewed as a goal toward which professionals, agencies, and systems can strive. Therefore, becoming culturally competent is a developmental process. This process defines responses to cultural differences as a continuum, ranging from cultural destructiveness to cultural proficiency, with at least six stages between these two extremes: (a) cultural destructiveness, (b) cultural incapacity, (c) cultural blindness, (d) cultural precompetence, (e) cultural competence, and (f) cultural proficiency (Georgetown University Child Development Center, 1992). For example, providers range from culturally destructive (I have only a few rushed minutes with you) to culturally competent, uplifting, instructive, and inspirational. A culturally competent system would (a) value diversity, (b) have the capacity for cultural self-assessment, (c) be conscious of the dynamics inherent when cultures interact, (d) have institutionalized cultural knowledge, and (e) have developed an adaptation to diversity.

Note

1. The 15th birthday marks the transition from girlhood to womanhood. After the 15th birthday, Latino teenagers can date, accompanied by a chaperone.

References

Alcalay, R., Ghee, A., & Scrimshaw, S. (1993). Designing prenatal care messages for low-income Mexican women. *Public Health Reports, 108*(3), 354-363.

Asian and Pacific Islander Center for Census Information and Services. (1992/1993, Fall/Winter). Our ten years of growth: A demographic analysis on Asian and Pacific Islander Americans. *ACCIS Newsbrief,* p. 3.

Backer, T. E., Rogers, E. M., & Sopory, P. (1992). *Designing health communication campaigns: What works?* Newbury Park, CA: Sage.

Bakeman, R., McCray, E., Lumb, J. R., Jackson, R. E., & Whitley, P. N. (1987). The incidence of AIDS among blacks and Hispanics. *Journal of the National Medical Association, 79*(9), 921-928.

Barthes, R. (1957). *Mythologies.:* Paris: Editions du Seuil.

Bird, J. A., Otero-Sabogal, R., Ngoc-The, H., & McPhee, S. J. (1996). Tailoring lay health worker interventions for diverse cultures: Lessons learned from Vietnamese and Latina communities. *Health Education Quarterly, 23*(Supp.), S105-S122.

Chen, A., Lew, R., Thai, V., Ko, K., Ohara, L., Chan, S., & Wong, W. (1992). Behavioral risk factor survey of Chinese in California 1989. *Morbidity and Mortality Weekly Report, 41*(16), 266-269.

Edmonston, B., & Passel J. S. (1992). Immigration and immigrant generations in population projections. *International Journal of Forecasting, 8*(3), 459-476.

Eisenberg, D. M., Davis, R. B., Ettner, S. L., Appel, S., Wilkey, S., Van Rompay, M., & Kessler, R. C. (1998). Trends in alternative medicine use in the United States, 1990-1997: Results of a follow-up national survey. *JAMA, 280,* 1569-1575.

Falicov, C. J. (Ed.). (1983). *Cultural perspectives in family therapy.* Rockville, MD: Aspen.

Falicov, C. J. (1998). *Latino families in therapy: A guide to multicultural practice.* New York: Guilford.

Feinstein, J. S. (1993). The relationship between socioeconomic status and health: A review of the literature. *Milbank Quarterly, 71*(2), 279-323.

Freire, P. (1994). *Pedagogy of hope.* New York: Continuum.

Georgetown University Child Development Center. (1992). *Towards a culturally competent system of care.* Washington, DC: CASSP Technical Assistance Center.

Gold, S. J. (1992). Mental health and illness in Vietnamese refugees. *Western Journal of Medicine, 157*(special issue), 290-294.

Gordon, M. M. (1964). *Assimilation in American life: The role of race, religion, and national origins.* New York: Oxford University Press.

Harlan, L. C., Bernstein, A. B., & Kessler, L. G. (1991). Cervical cancer screening: Who is not screening and why? *American Journal of Public Health, 81*(7), 885-890.

Jibou, R. M. (1996). Recent Asian Pacific immigrants: The demographic background. In B. O. Hing & T. Lee (Eds.), *The state of Asian Pacific Americans: Reframing the immigrantion debate* (A Public Policy Report; pp. 35-58; table 7, p. 52). Los Angeles: University of California at Los Angeles, LEAP and UCLA Asian American Studies Center.

Kar, S. B., Campbell, K., Jimenez, A., & Gupta, S. (1995). Invisible Americans: An exploration of Indo-American quality of life. *Amerasia Journal, 21*(3), 25-52.

Kar, S., Jimenez, A., Campbell, K., & Sze, F. (1998). Acculturation and quality of life: A comparative study of Japanese-Americans and Indo-Americans. *Amerasia Journal, 24*(1), 129-142.

Kar, S. B., & Alex, S. (1999). Public health approaches to substance abuse prevention: A multicultural perspective. In S. B. Kar (Ed.), *Substance abuse prevention: A multicultural perspective.* New York: Baywood.

Lecca, P. J., Greenstein, T. N., & McNeil, J. S. (1987). *A profile of Mexican American health: Data from the Hispanic Health and Nutrition Examining Survey 1982-84.* Arlington, TX: Health Services Research.

Lin, K., Masuda, M., & Tazuma, L. (1982). Problems of Vietnamese refugees in the United States. In R. C. Nann (Ed.), *Uprooting and surviving: Adaptation and resettlement of migrant families and children.* Boston: D. Reidel.

Logue, E. E., & Jarjoura D. (1990). Modeling heart disease mortality with census tract rates and social class mixtures. *Social Science & Medicine, 31*(5), 545-550.

Lovejoy, N. C., Jenkins, C., Wu, T., Shankland, S., & Wilson, C. (1989). Developing a breast cancer screening program for Chinese American women. *Oncology Nursing Forum, 16,* 181-187.

McPhee, S. J., Bird, J. A., Ha, N. T., Jenkins, C. N. H., Fordham, D., & Le, B. (1996). Pathways to early cancer detection for Vietnamese women: Suc Khoe La Vang! (Health is Gold!). *Health Education Quarterly, 23*(Supp.), S60-S75.

Muecke, M. A. (1983). Caring for the Southeast Asian refugee patients in the USA. *American Journal of Public Health, 73,* 431-438.

National Center for Health Statistics. (1998). *Health, United States, 1998* (DHHS Publication No. PHS 98-1232). Atlanta, GA: Centers for Disease Control.

National Institutes of Health. (1989). *Making health communication programs work: A planner's guide* (NIH Publication No. 89-1493). Washington, DC: U.S. Department of Health and Human Services.

Orlandi, M. A. (1992). The challenge of evaluating community-based prevention programs: A cross-cultural perspective. In M. A. Orlandi, R. Weston, & L. G. Epstein (Eds.), *Cultural competence for educators* (DHHS Publication No. ADM 92-1884). Washington, DC: U.S. Department of Health and Human Services.

Pasick, R. J., D'Onofrio, C. N., & Hiatt, R. A. (Eds.). (1996). Promoting cancer screening in ethnically diverse and underserved communities: The Pathways report. *Special Issue of Health Education Quarterly, 23*(Supp.).

Pasick, R. J., D'Onofrio, C. N., & Otero-Sabogal, R. (1996). Similarities and differences across cultures: Questions to inform a third generation for health promotion research. *Health Education Quarterly, 23*(Supp.), S142-S161.

Pasick, R. J., Sabogal, F., Bird, J. A., D'Onofrio, C. N., Jenkins, C. N. H., Lee, M., Engelstad, L., & Hiatt, R. A. (1996). Problems and progress in translation of health survey questions: The Pathways experience. *Health Education Quarterly, 23*(Supp.), S28-S40.

Pèrez-Stable, E. J. (1987). Issues in Latino health care medical staff conference. *Western Journal of Medicine, 146,* 213-218.

Pèrez-Stable, E. J., Otero-Sabogal, R., Sabogal, F., & Nápoles-Springer, A. (1996). Pathways to early cancer detection for Latinas: En Acción Contra el Cancer. *Health Education Quarterly, 23*(Supp.), S41-S59.

Pew Health Professions Commission. (1998) *Executive summary: Critical challenges: Revitalizing the health professions for the twenty-first century.* San Francisco: University of California at San Francisco, Center for the Health Professions.

President's Initiative on Race. (1999). *Changing America: Indicators of social and economic well-being by race and Hispanic origin.* Washington, DC: National Center for Health Statistics.

Sabogal, F., Marín, G., Otero-Sabogal, R., Marín, B. V., & Pèrez-Stable, E. J. (1987). Hispanic families and acculturation: What changes and what doesn't? *Hispanic Journal of Behavioral Science, 9,* 397-412.

Shi, L., & Shi, P. (1992). *Experience in treating cancers with traditional Chinese medicine.* Beijing: Shandong Science and Technology Press.

Subervi-Velez, F., & Colsant, S. (1993). The television world of Latino children. In G. Berry & J. K. Asamen (Eds.), *Children and television.* Newbury Park, CA: Sage.

Triandis, H. C. (1972). *The analysis of subjective culture.* New York: Wiley-Interscience.

Triandis, H. C., Marín, G., Lisansky, J., & Betancourt, H. (1984). Simpatía as a cultural script of Hispanic. *Journal of Personality & Social Psychology, 47,* 1363-1375.

United Way of Greater Los Angeles. (1994). *The Los Angeles fact book: 1994, a report on Asian American needs-assessment.* Data obtained from CD-ROM. (Available from the United Way of Greater Los Angeles, 523 W. Sixth Street, Los Angeles, CA 90014)

United Way of Greater Los Angeles. (1999). *State of the county report, Los Angeles 1998-99.* Retrieved June 15, 2000 from the World Wide Web: http://www.unitedwayla.com/pages/uwresources/StateOfCounty/StateofCounty.html

U.S. Bureau of the Census. (1990). *Census of population 1990: Social and economic characteristics.* Washington, DC: U.S. Department of Commerce.

U.S. Bureau of the Census. (1993). *Asians and Pacific Islanders in the United States.* Washington, DC: Government Printing Office.

U.S. Department of Health and Human Services. (1998), *Health, United States, 1998: Socioeconomic Status and Health Chartbook* (DHHS Publication No. PHS 98-1232U). Washington, DC: Author.

Valdes, I., & Seoane, M. H. (1995). Hispanic buying power (marketing power). *American Demographics, 17*(10), S10.

Wong, P., Lai, C. F., Nagasawa, R., & Lin, T. (1998). Asian Americans as a model minority: Self-perceptions and perceptions by other racial groups. *Sociological Perspectives, 41*(1), 95-121.

5

Communicating With Multicultural Populations

A Theoretical Framework

Snehendu B. Kar
Rina Alcalay
with Shana Alex

A Communication Challenge

Communication is a critical aspect during the transition between cultures. When two or more cultures coexist in the same society, there is a greater risk that the receiver belongs in a culture and space that is different from the sender's; this increases the likelihood that the receiver will misinterpret the intended meaning in the message being delivered, even when the translated words are correct. The result is miscommunication. To be effective, communication campaigns must be in synchronicity with the target audience's culture at all message levels: the textual and the visual, the denotative and the connotative, the explicit and the symbolic.

When communicating with members of other cultures, it is necessary to be aware of and to acknowledge the unique way in which recipients have integrated elements from their culture of origin with those of their culture of destination. How do they "make sense" of the world under their new circumstances? The inclusion, in a process of triangulation, of culture of origin, adopted culture, and the syntheses made of both is at the core of designing health promotion messages. People bring unique personal histories, family constellations, socioeconomic status, religious beliefs, and normative systems into their "being in the world." Efforts to use racial or ethnic background only, as simplistic, straightforward predictors of beliefs or behavior, will lead to harmful stereotyping. Both the cultural definitions and the specific configuration of the target group are necessary for designing effective health promotion messages.

It is difficult to reach any population with health promotion messages. It is much more difficult than promoting commercial products that offer instant gratification to those who consume them. Trying to promote healthy behaviors that offer delayed or uncertain benefits and also entail immediate deprivations makes these efforts even more challenging. Health campaigns usually ask people to stop doing things that bring them pleasure, such as smoking, drinking, and eating high-cholesterol or fast foods. When those difficulties are compounded with trying to reach culturally diverse populations who have different countries of origin, hold different beliefs about health, and often speak languages other than English, the challenge is even greater. Structural and systemic constraints often prevent behavioral changes from occurring, even in the presence of the best planned, most culturally sensitive communication campaigns. People's material conditions of life and their life positions in the social structure greatly affect their behavior, which in turn affects their health (Marmot, Kogevinas, & Elston, 1987; Townsend & Davidson, 1988).

The application of theoretical communication principles to the practice of planning and implementing health promotion campaigns is often prevented by factors such as the complexity of the process of communicating through media, the health issues involved, the nature of the audiences, and the lack of adequate resources to design the best possible campaigns. The complex and multidimensional nature of socioeconomic and cultural challenges defies generalization, yet some sort of standard approach to understanding communication dimensions for facilitating, prioritizing, targeting, and tailoring health promotion campaigns is necessary. The treatment goal of campaigns with multicultural populations must succeed in empowering their targets so as to develop "the ability to cope constructively with the forces that undermine and hinder the achievement of reasonable control over one's destiny" (Chung &

Pardeck, 1997). Feeling powerless, isolated, or alienated is often common, particularly among low-acculturated immigrants. Low-acculturated populations must find ways to overcome their lack of power. Thus, strengthening ego functions and reinforcing external supports must be key goals of health promotion campaigns. Any attempt to influence multicultural groups must incorporate individual, family, community, and policy levels of intervention.

A key goal, particularly with multicultural and disadvantaged populations, is empowerment—in other words, to increase people's ability to cope constructively with their environments and control their own destinies. Thus, strengthening ego functioning (individual changes) and reinforcing external and environmental supports (family, community, policy changes) are key components of intervention. Skill building, self-esteem development, and family strengthening must also occur (Kar, Pascual, & Chickering, 1999; Pinderhughes, 1983). Multicultural populations must learn mechanisms to deal with stress, conflict, and contradiction between elements of their culture of origin and their current cultural milieu.

Communication interventions must work with multicultural individuals, families, and communities to obtain empowerment. Simultaneously, no campaign will succeed without making the social system—including health practitioners, health institutions, and other community organizations—sensitive and responsive to specific needs and characteristics of multicultural populations. Social systems must also be empowered by developing appropriate skills to include multicultural populations as effective participants of the health care system.

Theories stemming from public health, social psychology, communication, community organization, and other social sciences serve as essential tools in understanding and designing health communication interventions. These theories are also useful for communicating with multicultural populations. They help us to understand underlying universal principles of social behavior. They also help us to focus on the specific circumstances of a unique group. If carefully used as guidelines, they provide a framework to design culturally appropriate health communication campaigns.

This chapter reviews selected theories and concepts that are the most widely used by multicultural interventions. First, key factors necessary to enhance the effectiveness of health promotion interventions are presented. Second, theories underlying and explaining social behavior are briefly described. Finally, communication theories explaining the role of mass media for health promotion are discussed. Examples of the application of these concepts and theories to multicultural populations are included throughout the chapter.

Key Factors in Multicultural
Health Communication: An Ecological Perspective

The term *ecology* refers to the study of the relationships between organisms and their environment (Stokols, 1996). Social ecology is a framework, a set of theoretical principles for understanding the interrelations between diverse personal and environmental factors in human health and illness. This perspective reflects not only behavioral and environmental change but also the interplay between persons, groups, and their social, physical, and cultural milieu (Stokols, 1996). With this model, people's behaviors affect and are affected by health at the individual, family, and community levels.

The ecological model states that behavior, regardless of ethnicity, is determined by five levels of influence:

1. *Intrapersonal factors*—individual characteristics, such as knowledge, attitudes, self-concept, skills, and developmental history

2. *Interpersonal factors*—relationships with primary social groups, including the family, peer networks, and the workplace

3. *Institutional factors*—social institutions with organizational characteristics, such as management styles, work schedules, and economic and social resources

4. *Community factors*—primary social groups to which an individual belongs, such as families, friendship networks, and neighborhoods, and relationships among social groups and organizations within a defined boundary

5. *Public policy*—local, state, and national laws and regulations that affect individual health

This model postulates that appropriate changes in these levels are necessary for behavior change to occur (Breslow, 1996; Choi, Yep, & Kumekawa, 1998).

The ecological model of health promotion de-emphasizes the importance of the individual on behavior change and the potential concomitant of blaming the victim for lack of effort or failure to change. Also, it considers both individual and environmental factors as possible explanations for unhealthy behaviors. Thus, it encourages the use of environmental approaches in prevention programs, a key factor for multicultural health communication programs (McLeroy, Bibeau, Steckler, & Glanz, 1988). The ecological model enables programs to understand the complexity of the factors influencing health behaviors and to target these factors at three different levels: individual, interpersonal, and community. Hence, from an ecological perspective, multiethnic media campaigns must engage individuals and their environments.

Accordingly, if the target population's cultural environment promotes the unhealthy behavior that the health promotion campaign wants to change, the impact of media messages will probably be negligible. Campaigns need supportive environments to succeed. Campaigns often have limited resources, yet they must compete with commercial advertising that reinforces the unhealthy behavior and, sometimes, with a community that accepts it. For example, the Hispanic Smoking Cessation Project in San Francisco initially had to confront situations in which Latino neighborhoods were covered with billboards promoting cigarettes. Bus cards offered (in Spanish) free packs of Marlboros to anyone who mailed in one of the attached cards. Cigarette companies regularly sponsored community events, and the prevailing attitude was that it was macho for Latino males to smoke. On the other hand, there were no educational materials to prevent smoking, either in Spanish or designed specifically for this population. It took a significant degree of community mobilization to raise the level of awareness, motivate community leaders to question this pro-smoking environment, and try to change it.

Group Attributes

Some basic universal principles of human communication and human behavior are involved in any process of communication, but population-specific attributes, patterns, and modalities will vary according to the circumstances of each cultural group and each individual. To communicate effectively with groups of diverse cultural origins for purposes of health promotion, health professionals must be guided by communication theories, health behavior theories, and cultural models that appeal to the specific sociocultural circumstances of the target group (Hiatt & Pasick, 1996; Pasick, D'Onofrio, & Otero-Sabogal, 1996; Pasick, Sabogal, et al., 1996). The attitudes, norms, and expectancies of group members toward the target behavior must be taken into consideration (Marín, 1990). How is the risk behavior (i.e., smoking) perceived by the group, and what cultural function does it fulfill?

For example, findings from smoking research among Latino men showed that regardless of their high rates of smoking, they did not see themselves as addicted or victimized by the habit. They perceived smoking as a "stupid vice" that they could drop through sheer willpower, showing a high sense of self-efficacy (Marín, Marín, Otero-Sabogal, Sabogal, & Pèrez-Stable, 1989; Sabogal, Otero-Sabogal, Pèrez-Stable, Marín, & Marín, 1989). Smoking is not only acceptable, but it is also desirable among Asian men, who see smoking as fulfilling the important social function of establishing links in social situations. Among Chinese males in particular, "offering someone a cigarette is a courtesy, a greeting" (Valdez, Alcalay, & Stokes, 1991). The same study also showed that Latino women had great trouble identifying themselves as smokers, and if they did so, they usually said they had smoked in the past, but were not doing so anymore. Low-acculturated Latino women in particular felt that women, if they smoked, did so in private, not in public. African American women in the study had no trouble reporting smoking behavior and were most likely to identify themselves as smokers.

Understanding the cultural norms of the target group toward the health risk behavior enables us to accurately conceptualize the health issue and position the communication strategies accordingly. One framework that looks at culturally conditioned factors influencing health behaviors was conceptualized by Kar, Chickering, and Sze (1999, p. 278). The basic principle of this model is that an individual's culturally conditioned beliefs, values, knowledge, attitudes, and practices (BVKAP) influence his or her health-related behavior through five dimensions/processes: (a) belief about disease etiology, (b) preferred modality of treatment, (c) locus of decision/responsibility, (d) communication and social relations, and (e) accessibility of information and services. These forces will influence how health-related decisions are made.

According to Kar, Chickering, and Sze (1999), some cultures may conceptualize disease etiology in terms of cosmic or unitary force and not in terms of specific causal factors (e.g., germs, genes, toxins, and trauma). Consequently, messages recommending Western medicine may not be relevant and may go unheard in these situations. In addition, in some cultures, religion, spirituality, and healing practices are inextricably linked (e.g., as reflected in the Hmong culture). Some cultural groups prefer traditional medical, spiritual, and self-care treatment modalities, augmented by modern medicine. Cultures also vary significantly in terms of expectations about whether important decisions should be made by individuals or collectively by family members. Ethnic groups may also vary in terms of the sources they prefer to use for health-related information and decisions (Kar & Alex, 1999; Ringwalt, Graham, Sanders-Phillips, Browne, & Paschall, 1999; Sanders-Phillips, 1999). Informal communication networks, traditional healers, and alternative medicine should be incorporated in addition to modern media as channels of communication with multicultural groups, particularly low-acculturated groups.

Communication strategies should be specifically tailored to the needs and characteristics of the target population. Consistent with the principle stated in the proceeding section, the materials developed should be appropriate for the target population. Messages should be comprehensible—that is, expressed in the target group's own words and at the appropriate level of complexity. They should be relevant; that is, the situation should be familiar and should reflect the group's reality. Messages should be believable; that is, the sources or spokepersons should be credible and likable to the target population, or messages should be attractive and well executed technically (National Institutes of Health [NIH], 1989). Channels of communication chosen should be those most widely used and most credible for disseminating health information among the audience. More specifically, designers of a health promotion campaign should select mechanisms that increase the appeal and effectiveness of messages by (a) providing models of desired behaviors, (b) using characters and testimonials that are highly credible and attractive to the target group, (c) portraying situations that reflect cultural themes central to the target population, (d) using plenty of visuals, and (e) using simple, clear, and direct language (Otero-Sabogal, 1990).

Simple translation of available materials has proven not to be an effective mechanism for developing messages. Studies and interventions with minority populations show that there is also a shortage of materials for monolingual, non-English-speaking Asians and Latinos (Valdez et al., 1991). Pretesting is an essential tool during communication strategies and message development processes. Effective communication planners ought to budget a significant part of their resources and time to pretesting. The *Guia Para Dejar de Fumar,* for example, designed by the San Francisco Hispanic Smoking Cessation Project, went through numerous versions of the text in addition to numerous pretests of color photographs, figures, and format (NIH, 1989).

Community Involvement

Ideally, requests for communication interventions should arise from the communities themselves; the community should design communication strategies. These interventions should remain with the community for as long as the health issues require. This ideal situation is rare because of the disadvantaged status of many multicultural communities. The struggle for survival often obscures the possibility of community reflection and analysis of health issues. Thus, the role of change agents—that is, communication planners—can be key to raising awareness and mobilizing community participation.

Communication planners can maximize community participation, representation, and empowerment. Communication planners must work with community leaders and organizations to build support and trust. They must offer communication approaches that are valuable to the community, even if they do not fit with the planners' agenda. And they must act primarily as facilitators with the community leaders and organizations taking the lead for the implementation, acceptance, and maintenance of the intervention. Brenda Dervin (1989) examines this perspective in her discussion about communication as dialogue versus communication as information. Communication as dialogue emphasizes the importance of involving the audience in the planning process, of respecting the unique strengths that the audience brings to the health communication process, and of redefining communication as an active exchange between participants (Dervin, 1989; Freimuth & Mettger, 1990). Community involvement and dialogue proved essential for the success of the Hispanic Smoking Cessation Project in San Francisco. Following the National Cancer Institute guidelines for the proposal, a project was conceived with the goal of designing a culturally appropriate smoking cessation group curriculum that would work with Latino smokers. The communication planners' initial objective was to develop a version of smoking cessation classes that would truly represent the needs and characteristics of the Latino target population. After a systematic community consultation (which involved an ethnographic study, a community survey, and group discussions with community and health leaders), the research team realized that a community intervention using media, interpersonal communication, community events, and the design of a self-help smoking cessation guide was more appropriate for the needs and cultural values of the community.

Thus, formative research helped change the original communication strategies to achieve the project goals. The idea of cessation groups, requiring smokers to make a commitment to go for several sessions and disclose many personal things in front of strangers, seemed alien to this target group, which had neither the time nor the inclination for such activity. By contrast, an intervention that appealed to the family members of the smokers via the mass media to support and encourage the smoker to stop smoking, accompanied by a culturally appropriate manual, to be used in the intimacy of the home and at the smoker's pace, was considered a culturally appropriate and effective communication strategy. Thus, the campaign objectives were modified with positive campaign outcomes (Marín, 1990).

Reinforcement of
Target Group's Positive Health Behaviors

Frequently, positive health behaviors of an ethnic group get lost with accul-turation. It is essential to understand and reinforce the positive health behav-iors of the ethnic group and encourage the group not to loose them through the process of acculturation. Because people belong to minority groups does not mean they are altogether disadvantaged. Culturally diverse populations have much to offer to the rest of society in terms of health behaviors and lifestyles. Health promotion campaign designers must understand and reinforce existing positive behaviors of the minority group regarding the desired behavior, not assume an all-negative approach. This will enable the production of messages emphasizing differences rather than deficits in the health behaviors of the tar-get group (Dervin, 1989; Freimuth & Mettger, 1990).

For example, rates of smoking, drinking, and use of nonprescribed drugs are significantly lower in some segments of minority groups. Social support sys-tems, care and concern for the elderly, and family values are generally much stronger among certain minority groups. Nutrition patterns are also healthier and more balanced in some of these groups. These positive behaviors have been shown to protect the group's health; that is, research has shown that regardless of the fact that low-acculturated Latinas have less access to prenatal care ser-vices and are less likely to avail themselves to these services, the rates of low-birth-weight babies are no worse than among non-Latino white women. Latinas smoke less, drink less, use fewer nonprescribed drugs, and have stron-ger social support networks during pregnancy than do non-Latina whites (Alcalay, 1992/1993). It is important to reinforce these positive health behav-iors, particularly because these advantages diminish with acculturation. It is also important because understanding and disseminating information about alternative, positive ways to deal with health risks can benefit not only minori-ties but society at large.

Multicultural Health Campaigns'
Foundation in Social Behavior Theories

Health communication interventions with multicultural populations must (a) make use of available descriptive and explanatory models for planning campaigns, (b) have a realistic understanding of the possibilities and constraints of using mass media, and (c) incorporate specific cultural considerations in the design and implementation of interventions. They need to evaluate the role of structural constraints, consider the possibility of making a difference with communication strategies, and advocate policies, beyond just communication interventions, that will eliminate structural barriers that prevent good health status among multicultural groups.

A communication intervention/campaign is the process of crafting and delivering messages and strategies, based on consumer research, to promote social change at the individual, community, and policy level. Theories of behavior and environmental change guide communication interventions/campaigns. They help health practitioners and planners ask the right questions and develop effective plans to address the issues at stake. Multilevel intervention, encompassing individual and environmental levels, are more powerful and appropriate for long-term, durable changes. Theories introduce understanding and systematization to the various stages of planning, implementing, and evaluating interventions. Familiarity with these key theories will assist in answering questions about (a) how and why people behave or fail to behave in certain ways regarding a health behavior, (b) what we need to know before designing an intervention, (c) how to shape programs to achieve certain goals, and (d) what we can expect from different communication interventions.

Various social behavior theories have guided multicultural communication interventions. These theories address different levels of intervention. Social learning theory, stages of change, and the theory of planned behavior explore how changes occur at the individual level. Diffusion of innovations helps to explain how changes occur at the community level. Social marketing provides a macrosocial, systemic planning approach to communication interventions. And media advocacy presents possibilities for empowering communities to achieve desired policy changes via communication as a strategy for achieving social change.

Individual-Level Theories

Social Learning Theory. This theory has been useful with multicultural populations both in the United States and abroad. It is particularly useful because it includes modeling and the increase of self-efficacy among its key concepts. Low-literacy and low-acculturated individuals benefit particularly with the presentation of visual models to imitate and with the enhancement of their skills to enact healthy behaviors. In social learning theory, human behavior is explained as an interaction between individual characteristics, environmental influences, and behaviors. A basic premise is that people learn not only from their own experiences but also by observing the actions of others and the results of those actions (Glanz & Rimer, 1997). Thus, this theory explains both human behavior and strategies to promote behavioral change.

In fact, social learning theory has great value for planning and explaining how media interventions work. It supports the notion that media can have an effect by showing characters modeling desired and undesired behaviors and by showing the positive consequences that result from the adoption of the desired behaviors. Modeling the new desired behaviors to those people who are the target population is an effective strategy of media use for health promotion. By modeling desired new behaviors and showing positive consequences of adopting such new behaviors, people are persuaded, according to social learning theory (Bandura, 1977). Thus, people learn by observing how to perform the desired health behavior; ideally, they then adopt it.

In addition, by being exposed to media messages, people may learn the necessary skills to perform desired behavior. In other words, people will increase their sense of self-efficacy, a characteristic considered essential for successful behavior change. Multicultural populations, particularly low-acculturated populations, often have low levels of self-efficacy and a high sense of powerlessness. Thus, education, empowerment, skills development, enhancement of support groups (e.g., churches, schools, friends, and service groups, such as Big Brothers) should be a priority. Communication interventions can help individuals and families adapt to their new environment in a fundamental way by enabling them to increase their self-efficacy. One positive consequence of empowerment is the ability to manage conflict, negotiation, and compromise. Campaigns can help target audiences develop such capacities by modeling the sharing of differing perceptions without blaming, withdrawing, or denying (Pinderhughes, 1983). Entertainment formats such as soap operas and/or music videos throughout the world, used for promoting healthy behaviors, have frequently based their communication strategies on social learning theory (Singhal & Rogers, 1989).

Stages of Change Model. This model concerns an individual's readiness to change or attempt to change toward the desired healthy behavior (Prochaska & DiClemente, 1983). It helps determine, prior to designing a campaign, where the target audience is in relation to the desired health promotion outcome. Five distinct stages are identified in the stages of change model: (a) precontemplation (person/population is unaware of problem and has not thought about change), (b) contemplation (thinking about changing behavior in the future), (c) decision/determination (deciding to act and making a plan to change), (d) action (implementing specific action plans), and (e) maintenance (continuing of desired changes) (Prochaska & DiClemente, 1983, 1984a, 1984b; Prochaska, DiClemente, Velicer, Ginpil, & Norcross, 1985). Is the audience already aware of the health risks of a certain behavior? Is it already favorably predisposed to change? Does the target group already have the skills to actually change its behavior? The answer to these questions will help focus campaign efforts on the appropriate level of intervention (Solomon, 1984). For example, if the target audience is aware of the risks of smoking and is motivated to quit, then a culturally appropriate cessation intervention may be in order. If, on the other hand, there is still a low level of awareness about those risks or those risks are minimized, as was found, for example, among low-acculturated Asian men, then an awareness-raising campaign is necessary (Valdez et al., 1991).

The stages of change model enables us to understand and place audiences at the appropriate level of intervention. Multicultural populations may be at different stages of readiness for change regarding various health behaviors. Sometimes they already have healthier behaviors than other groups, such as many nutrition habits among Asian populations or the low level of smoking and drinking among low-acculturated Latino women. Sometimes they are not even aware of health risks that other groups already take for granted, such as the importance of exercise to prevent heart disease or the need to alter nutrition patterns to prevent diabetes among Latinos. Stages of change is a useful framework to place a cultural group and thus to tailor the specific health promotion intervention to make it relevant and appropriate for that group.

The Model of Planned Behavior (Ajzen, 1985; Ajzen & Fishbein, 1980). This model also looks at the individual as the unit of analysis, enables the understanding of how the psychological process of change occurs in the individual, and helps identify the variables involved. As a result of this understanding, the health promotion campaign can develop components that modify all the necessary levels. The theory defines *behavior* as a result of people's attitudes toward such behavior, plus the individual's subjective norms about it (Ajzen, 1985; Ajzen & Fishbein, 1980). For example, a person's intention to exercise will depend on his or her own personal beliefs about the relative costs and benefits of engaging in such behavior, plus the individual's perception of how others in his or her community of reference feel about exercising.

This theory is useful to understand and place individuals within their own cultural norms and values systems. If, for example, there is a perception that smoking is the socially desirable thing to do among the people that matter to the target audience, it will be a lot harder to affect individual change unless the subjective norm can be modified. A smoking prevention campaign for teenagers should stress the message that most teenagers do not smoke, that smoking is not the norm among their peers, and that it is far from being universally accepted. If the campaign succeeds in having teenagers accept nonsmoking as their subjective norm, they will feel less pressure to smoke (Syme & Alcalay, 1982). The combination of both the individual's own attitude plus his or her perception of the subjective norm will determine the person's intention to behave in a certain manner. In addition, for the behavioral change to occur, the individual needs to feel confident that he or she has the necessary skills to implement the new behavior. Thus, self-efficacy is a necessary mediating step conducive to behavioral change.

Community-Level Theories

Diffusion of Innovations. Diffusion of innovations theory (Rogers, 1983) attempts to explain change at the community level. This theory describes and explains how the process of dissemination of a new health promotion idea occurs and how the advocated health behavior gets adopted by various segments of a community, until all the members of the community have done so. Diffusion of innovations is based on the assumption that a minority's current behavior is poorly adapted to environment. Due, in part, to lack of knowledge, people do not act optimally. Diffusion derives from the theory of modernization, a perspective that assumes the benefit of change toward the mainstream and away from the traditions in the cultures of origin. In this perspective, media can accelerate this process of change by spreading knowledge, which equals power to improve life and better use resources (Rogers, 1983).

Hence, diffusion of innovations focuses the attention on the following components: (a) the dissemination of the innovation (a new idea, practice, or technology), (b) the communication channels, and (c) the various stages of adoption (a time element) among the members of a social system (types of communities). Examples of innovations disseminated include annual cancer prevention screenings among Asian or Hispanic women, exercise as a health promotion lifestyle change among multicultural groups, and the use of condoms for AIDS prevention. Change is brought to the community via a partnership of change agents (outside professionals) with community opinion leaders (from inside the community). The latter can be health professionals and community leaders from the target community. According to diffusion of innovations theory, community leaders serve as an intermediate channel, in a two-step flow of communication, between the media and the community at large. Rates of adoption, another important concept in diffusion of innovations theory, acknowledges that change will reach different members of the target group at different times, depending on their readiness for change and the speed with which they will adopt.

This theory is useful to identify which actors in the specific cultural group are trusted and imitated by the specific community and thus can serve as opinion leaders for the communication intervention. It also helps predict how and if the innovation will be disseminated in the community.

Social Marketing Model. The social marketing model (Solomon, 1989) refers to the use of marketing principles and techniques for designing, implementing, and evaluating programs seeking to increase the acceptability of a health behavior. "Social marketing is the application of concepts and techniques drawn from the private sector to problems of influencing socially important voluntary behaviors such as drug use, smoking, safe sex, family planning, and child care" (Andreasen, 1994, p. 7). Its main purpose is to tailor interventions to best serve a defined target group. It borrows the concept of market segmentation to understand and organize potential target audiences. Key characteristics of social marketing are (a) a consumer orientation, (b) a behavior change orientation, and (c) a research basis (i.e., audience analysis, whereby efforts are centered on identifying and responding to consumers' needs and identifying resistance points).

A social marketing-based intervention will include at least the following six stages: analysis, planning, development of plan elements, implementation, assessment of effectiveness, and feedback. There is constant research-based feedback and planning within each stage as well (Glanz & Rimer, 1997). A social marketing intervention is concerned not only with the production of advantageous health promotion products (ideas, behaviors, or actual artifacts) for the target audience but also with the place (easy distribution system or point for the product), pricing (a health behavior must be associated with minimum effort and psychological, social, or monetary cost), promotion (media-based and interpersonal communication strategies that inform, persuade, and influence beliefs and behaviors relevant to the product), and positioning (identification of the special niche the product or behavior seeks to fill) of those social marketing products (Kotler & Roberto, 1989; Winett, 1995). Social marketing is used by communication planners in different world regions for the promotion of healthy lifestyles.

Policy-Level Theories

Media advocacy is the strategic use of mass media for advancing a social or public policy initiative (NIH, 1988). It criticizes the emphasis of social marketing on changing people's behaviors and advocates the use of media to change policies (Wallack, 1990). Media advocacy, by means of communication strategies, attempts to mobilize communities and their representatives to change policies that favor unhealthy behaviors such as smoking, drinking, and polluting the air. According to media advocacy, it is not by asking individuals to change their behaviors but by supporting policies that encourage healthy behaviors that real and effective changes occur. Thus, a main focus of this approach is to reframe the way the issues are perceived and to promote public debate via the mass media, encouraging a "system blame" instead of an "individual blame" perspective on the public health issue.

Reframing is a key strategy for media advocacy that promotes the use of "creative epidemiology." The latter is the use of new scientific evidence and existing data to gain media attention and convey the importance of a public health issue. This point is exemplified by an American Cancer Society videotape that explains that 1,000 people quit smoking every day by dying, and equates this number to 2 fully loaded jumbo jets crashing every day with no survivors (Wallack, 1990). Thus, creative epidemiology is not a misleading use of epidemiological data; it is a reframing of data to encourage social action.

Proponents of this approach support the notion that media advocacy "empowers the public to participate more fully in defining the social and political environment in which decisions affecting health are made" (Wallack, 1990, p. 159). For example, the smoking control movement in this country has used this approach with quite successful results. The tobacco industry has crafted an image of itself as an advocate of civil rights, protector of free speech, and good community citizen. Antismoking groups were characterized as dictatorial zealots and health nuts. These strategies had been successful until recently when the antismoking movement, with government support, succeeded in reframing the issues by presenting tobacco producers as exploiters of youth, women, and minorities. The movement continually makes the link between death and tobacco explicit, thus stripping the industry of its positive symbols. In sum, media advocacy requires a more confrontational, political, system blame, and policy change orientation from media interventions.

Multicultural Health Promotions'
Foundation in Mass Communication Theories

According to communication scholars, DeFleur and Dennis (1998), "Mass communication is a process in which professional communicators use media to disseminate messages widely, rapidly, and continuously to arouse intended meanings in large and diverse audiences in attempts to influence them in a variety of ways" (p. 24). Mass media is used in health promotion interventions for many reasons, such as speed, attractiveness, and lower cost for reaching larger audiences. The term *mass media* includes a wide spectrum of technologies, from network television and national newspapers to specialized cable television, magazines, and local newspapers. Public communication campaigns are a common mechanism to use mass media to reach diverse populations with health promotion messages.

Communicating with multicultural populations brings the additional challenge of trying to reach diverse target audiences who come from a multiplicity of backgrounds, speak multiple languages, and have culturally diverse perspectives. Rogers and Storey (1987) define public communication campaigns as deliberate attempts to inform, persuade, or motivate behavior changes in a relatively well-defined, large audience, for noncommercial benefits to the individual and/or society at large, typically within a given time period, by means of organized communication activities involving the mass media and often complemented by interpersonal support. Health campaigns deal with a variety of issues, such as family planning, smoking prevention, nutrition education, and AIDS prevention. Target populations often originate from a variety of ethnic or socioeconomic backgrounds, and the level of intervention varies from campaigns targeted to individuals, through families, organizations, community, and policy. Campaigns often show a lack of realistic expectations of the capabilities or constraints of the media. This chapter will discuss research and theories of media effects to provide a better understanding of the possibilities and the limitations of using mass media, particularly in the context of multicultural communication. The clarification of how media effects occur should facilitate the design of carefully tailored, sensible, and realistic health communication campaigns. These theories are universal and not culturally specific. They are based on research done over several decades, in many cultures and countries. In other words, they seem to reflect intrinsic qualities of the interactions between human beings and media, yet their application is culturally specific.

Media Can Have Powerful Effects

The media have powerful effects on their audience. However, those influences seldom occur directly and as an immediate response to a single campaign. Planners often assume that communication effects are direct and become disappointed when people's behaviors are not changed as a result of the campaign. Research shows that it takes cumulative interventions introduced over an extended period of time to achieve the desired impact (Lowery & DeFleur, 1995).

Cultivation of Beliefs Model. This phenomenon, whereby media messages that repeat certain worldviews, end up having powerful effects on people's definition of reality, has been called the cultivation of beliefs (Gerbner, Gross, Morgan, & Signorelli, 1986). According to Gerbner et al., "Television cultivates from infancy the predispositions and preferences that used to be acquired from other primary sources. The repetitive pattern of television mass-produced messages and images forms the mainstream of a common symbolic environment" (p. 18). From the point of view of the cultivation of relatively stable and common images, the pattern that counts is that of the total pattern of programming to which communities are regularly exposed over periods of time.

Gerbner's research showed that heavy viewers (people who watched over 4 hours of television daily) shared more similar beliefs among themselves on a variety of issues compared with light viewers (those individuals who watched less than 4 hours of television per day). This capacity of media helps to explain the differences within cultural groups that occur in the course of one generation. For example, Latinos or Asians who have been raised in other countries and continue to expose themselves to foreign language and foreign-produced programs will shield themselves from acculturation and assimilation to this country's values. On the other hand, those members from other cultural groups whose frame of reference becomes increasingly the "majority media," will become more acculturated and will tend to at least become bicultural.

The cultivation of beliefs principle has been a useful tool to explain why multicultural communities hold on to certain patterns of health behavior and what role the media can play to either maintain or change some of those patterns. For example, when the Latino Smoking Cessation Project introduced its smoking cessation campaign in San Francisco, it found a media environment that supported smoking and portrayed smoking behavior as a socially desirable behavior for Latinos. It took several years of communicating antismoking messages via those same media to have a significant impact and to change favorable cultural patterns toward smoking to more critical ones. The effect of this effort was cumulative and long-term, and in no way did it result from one single message communicated over one single medium.

Multilanguage Media in the United States. Little research has been done to analyze or use programming targeted at minority populations. Yet large cultural groups in this country routinely consume mass media in a language other than English, with a significant percentage of the programming produced abroad. One example is the Hispanic media world in the United States, a powerful force and resource often neglected and poorly understood by communication planners. An example of a culturally different media reality in the United States is represented by the Spanish language media. Telemundo and Univisiòn, Spanish-language television networks, reach 21 million people in this country alone (Subervi-Velez & Colsant, 1993). Univisiòn is the largest Spanish language network in the United States. Thus, Spanish language media can be a powerful tool to cultivate positive health beliefs among Latinos. Asian television stations and Asian newspapers are also an important source of information and influence (Delener & Neelankavil, 1990).

According to the 1990 U.S. census, Spanish is the most commonly spoken language in the United States after English. For more than 15 million people aged 5 and older, Spanish was the primary language spoken at home in four states (California, Texas, New York, and Florida), which account for 70% of U.S. Spanish-speaking population. About 34 million people speak Spanish at home (U.S. Bureau of the Census, 1995). The U.S. Spanish language media has become a principal source of information for events taking place in the Spanish-speaking areas of the world and the main vehicle to keep Hispanics abreast of local and national events.

In 1961, Spanish International Communication Corporation (SICC) and its sister company, Spanish International Network (SIN) were formed. Later, they became the Univisiòn Group (Valdes & Seoane, 1995). Currently, the three major Spanish television networks, Univisiòn, Telemundo, and Galavision, transmit to 64 cities across the country via 95 stations (Nielsen Media Research, 1993a, 1993b). Together, the two leading Spanish networks reach an average of 6 million households, or 89% of the total Hispanic market. Galavision, the third Spanish network, serves California, Texas, and Arizona, reaching more than 3 million households, up from 160,000 in 1988. They transmit to 64 cities across the country via 95 stations (Valdes & Seoane, 1995). In 1992, Nielsen Media Research introduced a service, the Nielsen's Hispanic Television Index, designed to measure specifically Hispanic households. It gathers its data from a sample of more than 800 Hispanic households representing approximately 3,000 people. According to the Nielsen Hispanic Television Index (1993a), Hispanic viewers vastly prefer Spanish language television. During prime-time, for example, the average rating of English language television networks for all Hispanic viewers averages 43% lower—and, for Spanish dominants, 75% lower—than for the general population.

Spanish language radio includes news, talk shows, sports, and music, mainly from and about Latin America, other Hispanic countries, and to a lesser extent, the United States. Hispanics prefer Spanish language over English language radio not only because they can understand the language but because radio offers a unique cultural forum with which Hispanic groups can identify. In less than a decade, the number of AM and FM stations owned or represented by the Spanish Katz Radio Group more than doubled in the eastern United States and quadrupled in the West. In Los Angeles, KLAX-FM radio reported that during an average week, about 850,000 people 12 years of age and over tune in, making KLAX a star in the national radio industry, regardless of language of broadcasting. In 1993, the station held number-one status in Los Angeles. Population density, size, language, and cultural sensitivity were all factors included in the marketing plan of this radio station. According to Arbitron (1993), Spanish-language radio is the preferred medium of Hispanics aged 12 and over.

Also, Hispanics have unique listening habits. For example, they prefer the Top 40 music program significantly more than the rest of the population. Urban music, a combination of hip-hop, rhythm, blues, and rap, a big favorite among African Americans (54.5%), is not popular among Hispanics (4.2%) (Arbitron, 1993, p. 7). Another interesting factor is the lack of seasonality, or time of day, preference among Hispanics. According to Arbitron, large segments of the Hispanic market will have the radio on all day long, all year round, particularly those Hispanics ages 25 to 64 (Arbitron, 1987, p. 22). Research also shows that although proportionally fewer Hispanics than general market consumers read, those who do read spend as much time as Anglos in a given day reading the newspaper (Greenberg, Burgoon, Burgoon, & Korsenny, 1983). Outdoor advertising, including billboards and public transportation, are particularly appropriate for reaching those Hispanics with lower readership skills and limited knowledge of English.

On the other hand, studies show that in English language media, particularly television, characters from other cultural groups are greatly underrepresented. This is particularly true for Latino character representation, which is almost completely absent from commercial television according to a 1990 study by Subervi-Velez (Subervi-Velez & Colsant, 1993). Although television and radio can have a large impact on the Hispanic population, this impact can be ephemeral and not always the most effective for campaigns. Given the immigrant status of large segments of populations, this can be a handicap. These populations need substantially more time to understand and get oriented to the messages conveyed by the media. In this sense, a piece of paper in their hands is a greatly valued and effective communicative device. It provides visual repetition and reinforcement. The significant success of the California *Wellness Guide* with multicultural populations attests to this issue (Alcalay & Bell, 1996).

Agenda-Setting. This widely used communication theory states that another effect of the media is its capacity to set the public's agenda. In other words, the media tends to affect what people will think about and perceive as important. This effect is generally associated with news media (McCombs & Shaw, 1991). The agenda-setting hypothesis maintains that the more importance the media gives to an issue, the more importance the public will attach to it as well. Conversely, the less exposure an issue has on the media, the less it will be perceived as important. This latter effect, called "the spiral of silence," assumes that those opinions that are not aired are eventually silenced (Noelle-Newmann, 1974).

This consequence is particularly serious with minority groups whose opinions, perceptions, and values are seldom portrayed in mainstream media. Different cultures bring different definitions of health, treatment, and health procedures, such as childbirth customs. Anne Fadiman (1998) in her book *The Spirit Catches You and You Fall Down* illustrates the different agendas that the Hmong culture and American doctors bring to the process of communication and how these cultures collide. Deeply meaningful symbols, like the need to bury a newborn's placenta so that when the moment of death comes, the person will find its original home and thus the soul will find peace, are completely ignored by the medical system. Multicultural groups' agendas are unfamiliar or ignored by the system. Also, these groups are not familiar with the premises of Western medical care. Health promotion professionals, who want to get a particular health issue on the agenda, should consider using the media and public relations activities to reach their target population. In the case of advancing an agenda on health issues, the target may be journalists or policymakers as opposed to the general public. The agenda-setting function also points to the difficulty that communication planners face in having to compete with many other issues for the public's attention.

Knowledge Gap. One of the unwelcome effects of disseminating health messages is that they sometimes widen the knowledge gap. According to Tichenor,

Donohue, and Olien (1970), a knowledge gap occurs when, as a result of increased infusion of mass media information into a social system, segments of the population with higher socioeconomic status acquire this information at a faster rate than do lower-status segments. As a result, the gap in knowledge between these segments tends to increase rather than decrease. In other words, those who initially have more resources will gain knowledge faster than those who have fewer resources. If the purpose of the campaign is to reach those who need it the most, then the messages and communication strategies must be carefully tailored to those groups. Poorer people have less access not only to services but also to valuable information about health. Therefore, the notion that mass media information can increase inequalities in a social system deserves serious consideration.

An example of the knowledge gap was revealed by the evaluation of the California Smoking Control Programs for Targeted Populations (Valdez et al., 1991). Several organizations participating in the evaluation reported that when the state made funding available to community organizations for the development of cessation and prevention strategies for minority groups, it was the more visible and more resourceful organizations that found out about the availability of funds, presented proposals, and got funded. In many instances, grassroots organizations that were more representative and worked closely with minority groups in the community were either not notified about the availability of funds, or if they were, they were unable to submit a competitive proposal because of a lack of material and human resources. This fact helped reinforce the feeling that those organizations that were better off, not necessarily those that were more representative of minorities, got stronger and that many of the community organizations that truly served and represented minorities groups got weaker by comparison.

Uses and Gratifications and/or Media Dependencies. This approach looks at the ways the media offer gratifications to the people. In other words, it describes the functions that media perform for people. Some of the functions that have been identified are entertainment (e.g., relaxation, fantasy), orientation (e.g., how to conduct oneself in a certain situation, role modeling), and information (e.g., how to apply to citizenship, where to get health care services) (Berger, 1991; Blumler & Katz, 1974; Grant, Guthrie, & Ball-Rokeach, 1991). Although much research has been done on this topic, little is known about the uses and gratifications of various media and media formats among diverse populations and even less among low-acculturated populations. What are the functions that media fulfill for ethnically diverse populations? Research on this topic should help health communication planners to use more appropriate formats and appeals for reaching multicultural populations. For example, much has been said about the use of fotonovelas (picture magazines with some text) either working or not working to reach Latino women. Advocates encourage the use of fotonovelas as a popular format among this segment of the population group. Others reject the value of this format for health promotion because of the association of fotonovela with entertainment and not with a format or channel more appropriate for conveying public health-type information. Although fotonovelas can work, it cannot be assumed that because they fulfill an entertainment function, they will also work as an information tool.

Beyond Communication: Community Partnership and Empowerment

Advocacy for and empowerment of the underserved has emerged as a major goal of health promotion ("Ottawa Charter," 1996; U.S. Department of Health and Human Services, 1991). We have much to learn from successful grassroots movements in diverse cultures around the world about how these initiatives have successfully mobilized communities for collective action. In the political literature, there are many examples of massive nonviolent grassroots movements that have fundamentally transformed disadvantaged and oppressed societies. Notable examples include the Gandhian "Sarvodaya," or nonviolent civil disobedience movement, which helped liberate India from centuries of British colonial rule, and Martin Luther King, Jr.'s nonviolent civil rights movement, modeled after the Gandhian movement, which had a profound influence on the quality of life of African Americans and others. More recently, Nelson Mandela's mass movement has brought an end to apartheid in South Africa. But most American psychologists and sociologists involved with health-related theory development and research have been preoccupied with individuals and microsystems, neglecting the valuable lessons that can be learned from disadvantaged and disenfranchised communities that have undertaken nonviolent social actions to enhance their health and quality of life.

Social activists and community organizers, on the other hand, have carefully studied and applied the lessons learned from successful grassroots movements; unfortunately, activists do not generally produce scholarly writings, and as a consequence, most of their experiences are not reflected in the literature. There are notable exceptions—namely, Alinsky (1969, 1971), Freire (1970, 1973), McKnight (1978, 1997), and Tropman, Erlich, and Rothman (1995), who have articulated the basic precepts and processes of empowerment and social action movements through their actions and writings. Due to space constraints, we extract here only the essence of their contributions that are relevant to this discussion. The basic premise of the social action model is that disadvantaged people must be empowered, organized, and educated if they are to summon up the psychological will, skills, and organized group support (group efficacy and power as distinct from psychological self-efficacy) requisite for social action in a common cause. The strategies advocated by Alinsky, Freire, and McKnight, however, vary to some extent. Alinsky (1969, 1971) advocates *winnable confrontations* to enhance the *social power* of the disadvantaged, which is a requisite for social action. He holds that have-nots have limited confidence in their own judgment and abilities and that the community organizer must represent a powerful force and must present have-nots with a reasonable prospect for success (Alinsky 1969, 1971).

Freire (1973) advocates the necessity of *education for a critical consciousness* so that the disadvantaged will be able to define the problem, evaluate their options, and mobilize themselves to achieve the preferred solution. Empowerment education is critical if the disadvantaged are to gain and internalize the new knowledge, confidence, and competencies that will enable them to overcome their powerlessness. McKnight (1997) advocates a *resource mobilization* strategy; he holds that communities have untapped resources for social action that must be mobilized for the solution of local problems. Coleman (1988) and others echo this approach by proposing the mobilization of *social capital* in dealing with local problems. Social capital is defined as using resources within social structure and social organization (including cultural capitals) by which individuals can achieve their needs and interests (Korbin & Coulton, 1996, p. 165). An example of this approach is the community organization for care of the elderly in a highly distressed neighborhood of San Francisco (Minkler, 1992); among other services, the program provided the elderly with volunteer escorts who enabled them to go about their daily business without the fear of becoming crime victims. In this case, the community escorts represented the social capital. Another example is the program to combat child maltreatment in the Cleveland Metropolitan Area; in this case, the social capital consists of the neighbors' willingness to report child abuse, offer material help to abused children, and volunteer to watch neighbors' children (Korbin & Coulton, 1996). Our study shows that successful social action movements depend on effective mobilization of social capital to meet a just and pressing human need (Kar, Pascual, et al., 1999). Analysis identified seven methods that make up the EMPOWER model:

1. *E*mpowerment education and training
2. *M*edia use and advocacy
3. *P*ublic education and participation
4. *O*rganizing associations and unions
5. *W*ork training and microenterprise
6. *E*nabling services and support
7. *R*ights protection and promotion (Kar, Pascual, & Chickering, 1999)

Conclusions

This chapter reflected on some of the special challenges underlying communication processes with multicultural populations living in the United States. It presented some of the key considerations that can render these processes more effective; it reviewed selected theories of social behavior and their application to influencing multicultural population; and it discussed key communication theories within a framework of multicultural communication. This chapter presented a selection of theoretical concepts from a variety of social sciences that are commonly used by multicultural health campaigns. Although many of these theories and principles were not developed specifically for addressing multicultural communication, they are nevertheless useful tools to guide the process of multicultural campaign planning, design, and evaluation. They can guide a process in which the specific contents must be filled by carefully working with the diverse cultural groups.

References

Ajzen, I. (1985). From intentions to actions: A theory of planned behavior. In J. Kuhl & J. Beckman (Eds.), *Action control: From cognition to behavior.* Berlin: Springer-Verlag.

Ajzen, I., & Fishbein, M. (1980). *Understanding attitudes and predicting social behavior.* Englewood Cliffs, NJ: Prentice Hall.

Alcalay, R. (1992/1993). Perceptions about prenatal care among health providers and Mexican-American community women: An exploratory study. *International Quarterly of Community Health Education, 13*(2), 107-118.

Alcalay, R., & Bell, R. A. (1996). Ethnicity and health knowledge gaps: Impact of the California Wellness Guide on poor African-American, Hispanic, and non-Hispanic white women. *Health Communication, 8*(4), 303-329.

Alinsky, S. D. (1969). *Reveille for radicals.* New York: Vintage.

Alinsky, S. D. (1971). *Rules for radicals: A practical primer for realistic radicals.* New York: Vintage.

Andreasen, A. R. (1994). Social marketing: Its definition and domain. *Journal of Public Policy and Marketing, 13*(1), 108-114.

Arbitron. (1987). Arbitron ratings: Radio year round. In *The medium of all seasons.* New York: Author.

Arbitron. (1993). How Hispanics listen to radio. In *Beyond the ratings.* Beltsville, MD: Author.

Bandura, A. (1977). *Social learning theory.* Englewood Cliffs, NJ: Prentice Hall.

Berger, A. A. (1991). *Media analysis techniques.* Newbury Park, CA: Sage.

Blumler, J. G., & Katz, E. (Eds.). (1974). *The uses of mass communications: Current perspectives on gratifications research.* Beverly Hills, CA: Sage.

Breslow, L. (1996). Social ecological strategies for promoting healthy lifestyles. *American Journal of Health Promotion, 10*(4), 253-257.

Choi, K. H., Yep, G. A., & Kumekawa, E. (1998). HIV prevention among Asian and Pacific Islander American men who have sex with men: A critical review of theoretical models and directions for future research. *AIDS Education and Prevention, 10*(Suppl. A), 19-30.

Chung, W. S., & Pardeck, J. T. (1997). Treating powerless minorities through an ecosystem approach. *Adolescence, 32*(127), 626-634.

Coleman, W. D. (1988). *Business and politics: A study of collective action.* Kingston, Ontario, Canada: McGill-Queen's University Press.

DeFleur, M. L., & Dennis, E. E. (1998). *Understanding mass communication: A liberal arts perspective* (6th ed.). Boston: Houghton Mifflin.

Delener, N., & Neelankavil, J. (1990, June-July). Informational sources and media usage: A comparison between Asian and Hispanic subcultures. *Journal of Advertising Research,* pp. 45-52.

Dervin, B. (1989). Audience as listener and learner, teacher and confidante: The sense-making approach. In R. Rice & B. Paisley (Eds.), *Public communication campaigns.* Newbury Park, CA: Sage.

Fadiman, A. (1998). *The spirit catches you and you fall down: A Hmong child, her American doctors, and the collision of two cultures.* New York: Farrar Straus & Giroux.

Freimuth, V., & Mettger, W. (1990). Is there a hard-to-reach audience? *Public Health Reports, 105*(3), 232-238.

Freire, P. (1970). *Cultural action for freedom.* Cambridge, MA: Harvard Educational Review.

Freire, P. (1973). *Education for critical consciousness.* New York: Continuum.

Gerbner, G., Gross, L., Morgan, M., & Signorelli, N. (1986). Living with television: The dynamics of the cultivation process. In J. Bryant & D. Zillman (Eds.), *Perspectives on media effects.* Hillsdale, NJ: Lawrence Erlbaum.

Glanz, K., & Rimer, B. K. (1997). *Theory at a glance: A guide for health promotion practice.* Bethesda, MD: U.S. Department. of Health and Human Services, Public Health Service, National Institutes of Health, National Cancer Institute.

Grant, A. E., Guthrie, K. K., & Ball-Rokeach, S. J. (1991). Television shopping: A media system dependency perspective. *Communication Research, 18*(6), 773-798.

Greenberg, B. S., Burgoon, M., Burgoon, J., & Korsenny, K. (1983). *Mexican Americans and the mass media.* Norwood, NJ: Ablex.

Hiatt, R. A., & Pasick, R. J. (1996). Unsolved problems in early breast cancer detection: Focus on the underserved. *Breast Cancer Research Treatment, 40,* 37-51.

Kar, S. B., & Alex, S. B. (1999). Public health approaches to substance abuse prevention: A multicultural perspective. In S. B. Kar (Ed.), *Substance abuse prevention in multicultural communities.* Amityville, NY: Baywood.

Kar, S. B., Chickering, K. C., & Sze, F. (1999). Summary and implications. In S. B. Kar (Ed.), *Substance abuse prevention in multicultural communities.* Amityville, NY: Baywood.

Kar, S. B., Pascual, C. A., & Chickering, K. L. (1999). Empowerment of women for health promotion: A meta-analysis. *Social Science and Medicine, 49* 1431-1460.

Korbin, J. E., & Coulton, C. J. (1996). The role of neighbors and the government in neighborhood-based child protection. *Journal of Social Issues, 52*(3), 163-176.

Kotler, P., & Roberto, E. L. (1989). *Social marketing: Strategies for changing public behavior.* New York: Free Press.

Lowery, S., & DeFleur, M. L. (1995). *Milestones in mass communication research: Media effects* (3rd ed.). White Plains, NY: Longman.

Marín, G. (1990, December). *Culturally appropriate interventions in health promotion: Why and how.* Paper presented at the First International Workshop of Experts on Drug Abuse Prevention, Santa Pola, Alicante, Spain.

Marín, G., Marín, B., Otero-Sabogal, R., Sabogal, F., & Pèrez-Stable, E. (1989). The role of acculturation on the attitudes, norms and expectancies of Hispanic smokers. *Journal of Cross-Cultural Psychology, 20,* 399-415.

Marmot, M. G., Kogevinas, M., & Elston, M. A. (1987). Social/economic status and disease. *Annual Review of Public Health, 8,* 111-135.

McCombs, M., & Shaw, D. (1991). The agenda-setting function of mass media. In D. Protess & M. McCombs (Eds.), *Agenda-setting: Readings on media, public opinion, and policymaking.* Hillsdale, NJ: Lawrence Erlbaum.

McKnight J. (1978). Community health in a Chicago slum. *Development Dialogue, 1,* 62-68.

McKnight, J. L. (1997). A 21st-century map for healthy communities and families. *Families in Society: The Journal of Contemporary Human Services, 78*(2), 117-128.

McLeroy, K., Bibeau, D., Steckler, A., & Glanz K. (1988). An ecological perspective on health promotion programs. *Health Education Quarterly, 15,* 351-377.

Minkler, M. (1992). Community organizing among the elderly poor in the United States—A case study. *International Journal of Health Services, 22*(2), 303-316.

National Institutes of Health. (1988). *Smoking control media advocacy guidelines.* Washington, DC: Advocacy Institute for the National Cancer Institute.

National Institutes of Health. (1989). *Making health communication programs work: A planner's guide* (NIH Publication No. 89-1493). Washington, DC: U.S. Department. of Health and Human Services.

Nielsen Media Research. (1993a). *National Hispanic television index newsletter* (Vol. 3.). New York: A. C. Nielsen Co., Media Research Division.

Nielsen Media Research. (1993b). *National Nielsen television index* (p. 20). New York: A. C. Nielsen Co., Media Research Division.

Noelle-Newmann, E. (1974, Spring). The spiral of silence: A theory of public opinion. *Journal of Communication,* pp. 43-51.

Otero-Sabogal, R. (1990, January). *Diversity and similarities among Hispanics.* Paper presented at the American Cancer Society Communication Conference, Washington, DC.

The Ottawa Charter for Health Promotion (17-21 November 1986). (1996). In *Health promotion anthology* (Scientific Publication No. 557). Washington, DC: World Health Organization, Pan American Health Organization.

Pasick, R. J., D'Onofrio, C. N., & Otero-Sabogal, R. (1996). Similarities and differences across cultures: Questions to inform a third generation for health promotion research. *Health Education Quarterly, 23*(Supp.), S142-S161.

Pasick, R. J., Sabogal, F., Bird, J. A., D'Onofrio, C. N., Jenkins, C. N. H., Lee, M., Engelstad, L., & Hiatt, R. A. (1996). Problems and progress in translation of health survey questions: The Pathways experience. *Health Education Quarterly, 23*(Supp.), S28-S40.

Pinderhughes, E. (1983). Empowerment for our clients and for ourselves. *Journal of Contemporary Social Work, 4*(6), 331-338.

Prochaska, J. O., & DiClemente, C. C. (1983). Stages and processes of self-change of smoking: Toward an integrative model of change. *Journal of Consulting and Clinical Psychology, 51*(3), 390-395.

Prochaska, J. O., & DiClemente, C. C. (1984a). Self-change processes, self-efficacy and decisional balance across five stages of smoking cessation. *Progress in Clinical and Biological Research, 156,* 131-140.

Prochaska, J. O., & DiClemente, C. C. (1984b). *The transtheoretical approach: Crossing traditional boundaries of therapy.* Homewood, IL: Dow Jones-Irwin.

Prochaska, J. O., DiClemente, C. C., Velicer, W. F., Ginpil, S., & Norcross, J. C. (1985). Predicting change in smoking status for self-changers. *Addictive Behaviors, 10*(4), 395-406.

Ringwalt, C., Graham, P., Sanders-Phillips, K., Browne, D., & Paschall, M. (1999). Ethnic identity as a protective factor in the health behaviors of African-American male adolescents. In S. B. Kar (Ed.), *Substance abuse prevention in multicultural communities.* Amityville, NY: Baywood.

Rogers, E. (1983). *Diffusion of innovations* (3rd ed.). New York: Free Press.

Rogers, E. M., & Storey, D. (1987). Communication campaigns. In C. Berger & S. Chaffee (Eds.), *Handbook of communication science.* Newbury Park, CA: Sage.

Sabogal, F., Otero-Sabogal, R., Pèrez-Stable, E., Marín, B., & Marín, G. (1989). Perceived self-efficacy to avoid cigarette smoking and addiction: Differences between Hispanics and non-Hispanics. *Hispanic Journal of Behavioral Sciences, 11*(2), 136-147.

Sanders-Phillips, K. (1999). Psychosocial factors influencing substance abuse in Black Women and Latinas. In S. B. Kar (Ed.), *Substance abuse prevention in multicultural communities.* Amityville, NY: Baywood.

Singhal, A., & Rogers, E. (1989). Prosocial television for development in India. In R. Rice & C. Atkin (Eds.), *Public communication campaigns.* Newbury Park, CA: Sage.

Solomon, D. (1984). Social marketing and community health promotion: The Stanford heart disease prevention program. In L. Frederiksen, L. Solomon, & K. Brehony (Eds.), *Marketing health behavior.* New York: Plenum.

Solomon, D. (1989). A social marketing perspective on communication campaigns. In R. Rice & B. Paisley (Eds.), *Public communication campaigns.* Newbury Park, CA: Sage.

Stokols, D. (1996). Translating social ecological theory into guidelines for community health promotion. *American Journal of Health Promotion, 10*(4), 282-298.

Subervi-Velez, F., & Colsant, S. (1993). The television world of Latino children. In G. Berry & J. K. Asamen (Eds.), *Children and television.* Newbury Park, CA: Sage.

Syme, L., & Alcalay, R. (1982). Control of cigarette smoking from a social perspective. *Annual review of Public Health, 3,* 179-99.

Tichenor, P., Donohue, G., & Olien, C. (1970). Mass media flow and differential growth in knowledge. *Public Opinion Quarterly, 34*(2), 159-170.

Townsend, P., & Davidson, N. (Eds.). (1988). *Inequalities in health: The Black report.* London: Penguin.

Tropman, J. E., Erlich, J. L., & Rothman, J. (Eds.). (1995). *Tactics and techniques of community intervention* (3rd ed.). Itasca, IL: F. E. Peacock.

U.S. Bureau of the Census. (1995). *1995 statistical abstract of the United States.* Washington, DC: Author.

U.S. Department of Health and Human Services. (1991). *Healthy people 2000: National Health promotion and disease prevention objectives* (DHHS Publication No. PHS 91-50212). Washington, DC: Government Printing Office.

Valdez, R., Alcalay, R., & Stokes, M. (1991). *Asian, Black and Latino concerns and recommendations regarding California's antitobacco campaign effort.* Sacramento: California Department of Health Services, Tobacco Control Section.

Valdes, I., & Seoane, M. H. (1995). Hispanic buying power (marketing power). *American Demographics, 17*(10), S10.

Wallack, L. (1990). Improving health promotion: Media advocacy and social marketing approaches. In C. Atkin & L. Wallack (Eds.), *Mass communication and public health.* Newbury Park, CA: Sage.

World Health Organization/United Nations International Children's Emergency Fund. (1978). *ALMA-ATA 1978 primary health care: Report of the International Conference on Primary Health Care.* Geneva, Switzerland: Author.

Winett, R. (1995). A framework for health promotion and disease prevention programs. American Psychologist, 50 (5), 341-350.

PART II

HEALTH COMMUNICATION IN HIGH–RISK MULTICULTURAL POPULATIONS

6

Childhood Unintentional Injury Prevention
Multicultural Perspectives

Deborah Glik
Angela Mickalide

In developed countries today, unintentional injuries are the leading cause of death and disability among children 14 years of age and under. In this chapter, we frame this issue to take account of the increasing cultural diversity in American communities, exploring how beliefs and behaviors embedded within specific cultural contexts play a role in the causes and prevention of injuries. The chapter is organized into the following six sections: First, we will (a) describe the scope of the unintentional injury problem, (b) outline the major risk factors, and (c) show how ethnic group membership is related to increased incidence of specific types of injuries. Then we will (d) discuss how "cultural factors" can be better conceptualized and measured in injury research, (e) present in summary fashion results from studies we have participated in that take these factors into account, and (f) conclude by describing some elements of culturally informed injury prevention programs.

The Childhood Injury Problem

Over the past decade, the childhood unintentional injury death rate has declined by 26% (O'Donnell & Mickalide, 1998). Yet injury remains the leading health threat to America's children. In 1995 in the United States, more than 6,600 children ages 14 and under died from unintentional injuries and nearly 120,000 were permanently disabled (National Center for Health Statistics [NCHS], 1995). One of every four children, or more than 14 million children aged 14 and under, sustain injuries serious enough to require medical attention each year (Scheidt et al., 1995). Each year, injuries to children ages 14 and under result in 246,000 hospitalizations (Graves & Gillum, 1996), nearly 8.7 million emergency room visits (Stussman, 1997), and more than 11 million visits to physicians' offices (Woodwell & Schappert, 1997). These injuries have enormous financial, emotional, and social effects, not only for the child and the family but for the community and society as a whole (Kogan, Overpeck, & Fingerhut, 1995; Miller, 1993, 1996). Yet we know that injuries are not random events: They can be linked to specific environmental, social, and individual risk factors, and many unintentional childhood injuries can be prevented (Baker, O'Neill, Ginsburg, & Li, 1991; Miller, 1993, 1996).

In general, children are primarily at risk for unintentional injury-related death from motor vehicle injuries that include children as occupants, pedestrians, and bicyclists (see Figure 6.1) (Division of Injury Control [DIC], 1990; see also NCHS, 1995). They are also at risk for drowning in swimming pools, bathtubs, lakes, ponds, and streams (Baker et al., 1991). House fires, burns from household appliances, and scalds from hot water also take their toll on young children (McLouglin & McGuire, 1990). Suffocation is the leading cause of death for children under 1 year of age, whereas choking on small objects and poisoning from household products are serious risks for 1- to 4-year-olds (NCHS, 1995). Finally, unintentional injuries from firearms, falls, and sports are categories of injuries that pose risks for children (NCHS, 1995).

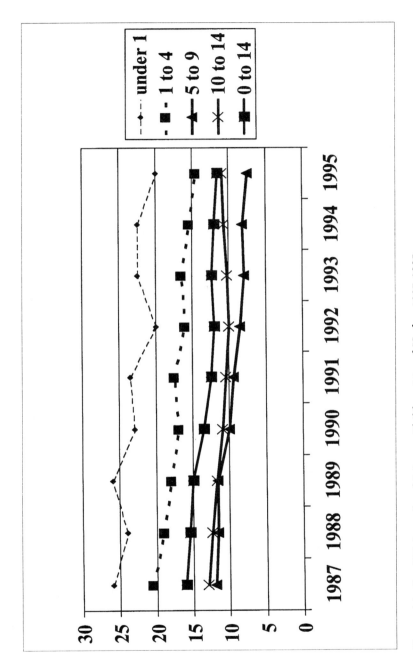

Figure 6.1. Fatal Unintentional Injury—Children 14 and Under, 1987-1995

SOURCE: Fingerhut and Warner (1997).

143

Children at Risk

A number of sets of risk factors for childhood injury have been identified. For example, injury rates vary with a child's age, gender, race, and socioeconomic status (SES) (NCHS, 1995). Thus, younger children, males, minorities, and poor children suffer disproportionately (Singh & Yu, 1996). Risk factors for childhood injury can be categorized into four general areas: (a) the physical environment and exposure to hazards, (b) the social environment, (c) child development and behavior, and (d) parenting practices and protective behaviors.

The Physical Environment and Exposure to Hazards. Children are exposed to numerous hazards linked to injury in residential, school, playground, and outdoors environments. For the young child, encounters with residential hazards such as poisons, electrical outlets, scalding tap water, automatic garage doors, swimming pools, stairs, carbon monoxide, fires, baby walkers, pets, or sharp objects can lead to injury. Older children are exposed to hazards such as traffic, playground equipment, sports activities, bicycles, rollerblades, skateboards, tools, and firearms (DIC, 1990). Children are more likely to be injured during the summer months when the longer days permit more recreation and unsupervised activity and also at night when visibility is lower (Mazurek, 1994). Children living in rural areas are at greater risk from unintentional injury-related death than are children living in urban areas (Fingerhut & Warner, 1997) and are often exposed to farm equipment, lakes, rivers and streams, car crashes, firearms, and house fires. Injuries in rural settings occur in remote, sparsely populated areas that tend to lack organized systems of trauma care, resulting in prolonged response and transport times, thereby increasing the threat of mortality (Kogan et al., 1995).

The Social Environment. Unintentional injuries disproportionately affect poor children and result in more fatalities than among children with greater economic resources (Baker et al., 1991; DIC, 1990; Scheidt et al., 1995; Singh & Yu, 1996). Children from low-income families are twice as likely to die in motor vehicle crashes, four times more likely to drown, and five times more likely to die in a house fire (DIC, 1990; Rivara, 1990). Several factors common to low-income families may increase a child's risk of injury, including living in single-parent households, lack of education, young maternal age, and multiple siblings (NCHS, 1995; Rivara, 1995). Children from low-income families live in more hazardous environments (Durkin, Davidson, Kuhn, O'Conner, & Barlow, 1994), including substandard and overcrowded housing, lack of safe recreational facilities, proximity of housing to busy streets, inadequate day care and/or supervision, increased exposure to physical hazards, and limited access to health care, all of which may increase their risk of injury (Santer & Stocking, 1991). Low-income families are less likely to use safety devices due to a lack of money, a lack of transportation to obtain safety devices, a lack of control over housing conditions, or any combination of these factors (Glik, Greaves, Kronenfeld, & Jackson, 1993; Glik, Kronenfeld, & Jackson, 1993; Greaves, Glik, Kronenfeld, & Jackson, 1994; Hsu & Williams, 1991; Mickalide, 1993).

Child Development and Behavior. Leading causes of unintentional injury-related death vary throughout childhood and depend on a child's developmental abilities, behaviors, and exposure to potential hazards (Guyer, Talbot, & Pless, 1985; Pless, Peckham, & Power, 1989; Rivara, 1995). As Agran (1987) points out, the risk of injury for children is inextricably bound to developmental stages of the child, which cannot be sequentially altered. Although there is little evidence that there are "injury-prone children," injuries tend to occur when the demands of a task exceed the abilities of the child to safely complete the task. Infants have higher rates of unintentional injury-related death and are more likely to die or sustain nonfatal injuries from fires and burns, suffocation, drowning, motor vehicle crashes, and falls (NCHS, 1995). Preschoolers are developing better motor skills but have poor impulse control and judgment (Christoffel, Christoffel, & Tanz, 1988; Rivara, 1995). Their natural curiosity and lack of fear lead them into potentially dangerous situations. These children are more likely to die from fires and burns, drowning, motor vehicle occupant crashes, pedestrian injuries, poisoning, and choking (NCHS, 1995). School-age children believe they have better skills and abilities than they actually do and are more likely to participate in high-risk behaviors. These children have higher fatality rates from motor vehicle crashes, pedestrian injuries, bicycle injuries, drowning, and unintentional firearm injuries.

For virtually all ages, and all causes of injury, males are at greater risk of unintentional death and injury than are females. Higher male risk is primarily due to greater exposure to activities that result in injury and patterns of risk taking and rougher play activities that result in injury (Kogan et al., 1995). Children with emotional or behavioral problems, with developmental delay, or who are inattentive or easily distracted tend to sustain more unintentional injuries than do other children (Bussing, Menvielle, & Zima, 1996; Jacquess & Finney, 1994). Thus, the causes and consequences of injuries vary considerably by age and developmental level, reflecting differences in children's cognitive, perceptual, and motor/language abilities.

Parenting Practices and Protective Behaviors. A final set of risk factors is that of parental patterns of supervision, safety behaviors, and management of the home environment, in addition to the accuracy of parents' perceptions of the child's abilities and injury risk. Although we do have evidence that increased use of certain devices (e.g., child safety seats, smoke alarms, window guards) reduce injury morbidity and mortality, we do not have direct evidence yet that overall parental safety proofing and supervisory behaviors as defined alter substantially the risk of injury to young children. On the other hand, there are some indications that lower income, ethnic minority parents demonstrate more limited understanding of child safety (Eichelberger, Gotschall, Feely, Harstad, & Bowman, 1990; Hoffman, 1986; Glik, Greaves et al., 1993; Glik, Kronenfeld, & Jackson, 1991; Glik, Kronenfeld et al., 1993) and are less likely to use or be aware of child injury prevention measures (Hoffman, 1986). National SAFE KIDS Campaign surveys have indicated that parents underestimate the threat posed by unintentional injury to their children and that this trend is worsening over time. In 1997, only 20% of parents identified injury as a leading health risk to children compared with 24% in 1992 and 32% in 1987. Conversely, parents overestimate the threat of violence and drugs relative to the threat of unintentional injury (Mickalide, 1993).

Ethnic Differences in Injury Rates

A great deal of descriptive epidemiological data suggest that cultural and ethnic differences do play a role in injury causation. African American and Native American children have higher rates of death and injury rates compared with white children (Kogan et al., 1995; NCHS, 1995). The argument is often made that ethnic disparities in unintentional injury rates appear to have more to do with living in impoverished, risky environments; lower levels of parental education, employment, and income; and safety behaviors than with ethnicity per se (DIC, 1990; National SAFE KIDS Campaign [NSKC], 1997). Yet children in specific ethnic groups are more likely to lack health insurance, have more difficulty obtaining appropriate and necessary medical care, and have lower incomes, creating significant financial barriers to receiving care. They are also more likely to receive care in hospital emergency rooms and are less likely to receive lifesaving preventive services (DiSorbo, 1995; Elders, 1995). Although poverty does have a strong direct effect on injury rates, typically not teased out of injury research is how cultural factors may have unique effects on injury outcomes.

Most injury prevention research treats race/ethnicity as either an ordinal independent or a risk factor variable, or as a confounder, without a great deal of explication other than "culture of poverty" arguments as to why being a member of a specific ethnic group would increase or lessen risk. Many articles, moreover, equate ethnicity with minority status, often correlated with economic disadvantage, which, as shown above, is an important risk factor in child injury. Nor has the literature typically assessed the impact of acculturation on risk, a factor particularly important among newer immigrant groups. Another aspect of cultural life is the impact of living in multicultural communities with many different norms and practices that could also affect child injury rates in the same geographic area. Also, until the late 1980s, most data sets did not differentiate Hispanic or Native American children from white children. Notwithstanding these deficiencies in the child injury literature, it is interesting to look at the evidence that does exist concerning multicultural contributors to childhood injury.

If we look at overall (unadjusted for SES) rates of injury death from all causes for children in the four traditional ages ranges for injury research—under the age of 1, 1 to 4, 5 to 9, and 10 to 14—and break it down by four ethnic groups of white, African American, Native American, and Asian American, it is clear that African American and Native American children have much higher injury mortality rates than do white and Asian populations, especially in the under 1 year and 1 to 4 age groups (Baker & Waller, 1989; James, 1994-1995). Although many data are limited to white and African American comparisons, overall, Native American children have the highest rates of injury of any ethnic group for most categories of injury (Baker et al., 1991; U.S. Department of Health and Human Services [DHHS], 1995). In a 1990 report from the Centers for Disease Control, African American children had death rates 1.3 to 2 times higher than white children for all age groups 0 to 14 (DIC, 1990), rates consistent with more recent data (NCHS, 1994-1995). The Baker et al. (1991) report, which had more extensive ethnic breakdown, shows that Native American injury rates are slightly higher than African American rates. These rates are, of course, confounded by poverty and rural residency, both risk factors for injury in their own right (Baker et al., 1991).

Data for Hispanic children present a slightly different picture, however. Even though poverty rates are three times those of white children and one third of Hispanic children live in single-parent households, overall injury rates for Hispanic children are comparable to white children (Fingerhut, 1991-1992). For example, in 1995, unintentional injury death rates (per 100,000 children) were 12.8 for Hispanic and 13.0 for white children ages 1 to 4, and for ages 5 to 14 they were 7.5 and 8.7, respectively (Anderson, Kochanek, & Murphy, 1997). These types of data suggest that the poverty argument may gloss over differences in risk attributable to culture, such as family structure, living arrangements, patterns of child rearing, or exposure to hazards.

Rates for ethnic differences in injury rates are confirmed by more regional, state, and local data sets. When Hispanic children are considered as a group separate from non-Hispanic whites, they have rates of childhood injury lower than Native Americans and African Americans and comparable to those for white and Asian American rates for some but not all types of injuries (Fingerhut, 1991-1992; Lyman, Acee, Kelter, & Trent, 1992). A study in a low-income community in Northern Manhattan found that within this context, African American children had higher rates of unintentional injuries than did Hispanic children and speculated that crowded housing conditions can possibly have a protective effect for Hispanic children, because there would be more adult supervision (Durkin et al., 1994).

When specific categories of unintentional childhood injury are examined, a more complex pattern of ethnic differences emerge. For motor vehicle passenger injuries, an injury that is a leading cause of injury-related death for young children, national data suggest that Native American children have almost 2 times the mortality rate of Asian American and white children, with rates for African American children in between. However, there are also regional differences. California data show that, overall, white children 14 and under have motor vehicle occupant death rates similar to Hispanic and Asian American children, with African American children having the highest rates overall. Looking even more locally, Los Angeles County data suggest a similar pattern. Lack of great differentiation between ethnic groups, even when taking poverty into account, may have to do with a culture of driving, with white children experiencing more exposure to risk due to more time spent in the car, whereas ethnic minority children may have lower overall time spent in a car but higher risk exposure due to older more dangerous vehicles and less use of safety devices.

Another category of motor vehicle injury, pedestrian-motor vehicle injuries, also shows different patterns depending on ethnicity. On the basis of national data, Rivara (1990) reports that nonwhite children had pedestrian injury rates 1.5 times higher than are white children. A study in New Mexico showed that Native American children are 2.5 times as likely to be killed in pedestrian incidents than children in other ethnic groups (Olson, Sklar, Cobb, Sapien, & Zumwat, 1993). California statewide data show that African American and Hispanic children are both 2 times as likely as white or Asian American children to be killed in these situations (Lyman et al., 1992). This can vary by region as well. A study in Long Beach showed that all the nonwhite ethnic groups had pedestrian injury rates 2 times higher than those of white children. Higher Asian American rates may be due to a large, less acculturated immigrant population in Long Beach (Kraus et al., 1996). Similar trends are found for bicycle versus motor vehicle injury rates in these populations.

For some types of injuries—namely, sports injuries and swimming pool drownings among younger children—white children have higher rates due to higher exposure to sports activities and to swimming pools (Baker et al., 1991; Ellis & Trent, 1997). However, for non-pool-related drowning among older age groups in lakes, streams, and ponds, Native American and African American drowning rates are higher than either Hispanic or white rates, related also to rural areas where rates are higher. This is confirmed as well by data from Texas where rates of drowning in one metropolitan county were 56% higher among African Americans compared with whites and 19% higher among Hispanic children (Warnecke & Cooper, 1994). In this study, drowning rates were higher for white children in private swimming pools and hot tubs, whereas African American and Hispanic children drowned mainly in apartment pools. For bathtub drownings, rates were twice as high among Hispanic children than for either African American or white children, whereas for drowning in other bodies of water, rates were highest for African American children (Warnecke & Cooper, 1994)

Death from falls are higher for African American children than for whites, and for Native American children, death from falls is highest under the age of one year. Asian American children also experience an elevated rate of falls between ages 1 and 4 (Baker et al., 1991; DIC, 1990). Childhood poisoning, a type of injury death that has fallen dramatically over past decades is still substantially higher among African American and Native American children (Baker et al., 1991; DIC, 1990). Unintentional firearm-related deaths are highest among Native Americans, with similar lower rates among whites and African Americans and very low rates among Asian Americans. Native American children are at the highest risk for death due to house fires (McLouglin & McGuire, 1990).

Culture Reconsidered

Increased recognition of multiculturalism in U.S. society over the past decade has not been well assimilated into the injury research field, traditionally dominated by researchers with epidemiological or interventionist orientations. Behavioral approaches have tended to draw on developmental and social psychological research frameworks, often glossing over cultural explanations for differences in injury rates between members of different social or ethnic groups. Yet as Margaret Mead pointed out over 70 years ago, cultural variation in child rearing is a key to understanding human development (Mead, 1930). In addition, exposure to different types of risks throughout childhood may be culturally mediated (Valsiner, 1997). Thus, many of the factors that create excess injury-related morbidity and mortality among children may be determined in part by the cultural context in which the child lives.

How is culture related to injury among children? Population differences in environmental adaptation are mediated by normative models of behavior that are socioculturally scripted (Levine, 1988). Taking a structural functional viewpoint, social adaptation can be seen to be driven by four basic needs of population groups: survival, reproduction, communication, and self-regulation—all considered to be universal. How children are reared and what level of risk they are exposed to conforms to those needs and varies by cultural group, which in turn are linked to biological, economic, historical, and demographic patterns of culture that include housing, work, education, family structure, and social structure (Levine et al., 1994).

From a developmental perspective, the process of child development can be understood to be embedded within a structurally organized environment that is interconnected with the system of cultural meanings of the society the child is born into, which itself is dynamic and changing (Valsiner, 1997). Environmental changes, whether caused by the child himself or herself, the family, larger social groups, or through unanticipated events creates uncertainty and to some degree risk. *Cultural variation* can be seen in the degree to which parents allow freedom of action to a child versus directing the child's action. Other terms for this could be *promoting autonomy* or *dependence for self-directed action*. These ideas supersede the notion of parenting style, permissive or strict, as a function of parental personality. Rather, these parent-child-environment interactions are seen to be the outcome of cultural norms (Valsiner, 1997).

Specifically, culture has ideational, relational, and material attributes that can influence cognitions, environment, child development, and social behavior (Geertz, 1973; Mead, 1930)—all factors implicated in childhood injuries. Ideationally, culture can influence risk perceptions, belief systems in regard to the etiology of injuries, or responses to injuries once they occur. Explanatory models for illness and disease can also be constructed for risk perceptions and prevention beliefs (Kleinman, 1980; Kronenfeld & Glik, 1990). Relational elements have to do with family structure, kinship and reproductive patterns, living arrangements, and who cares for children. Material culture has to do with the nature of physical elements in and outside of households, including housing stock, transportation, cultural artifacts, foods, tools, and so on.

"Cultural scripts" serve to mediate child-rearing practices, which can include parenting styles, child care and supervision, family structures, and kinship relations (Levine et al., 1994; Valsiner, 1997). Such scripts have been studied in diverse cultures and show both inter- and intracultural variation (Levine et al., 1994). For example, among the highly fertile Gusii of Kenya, where women work in the fields by day, once the child is a toddler, older children are caretakers. This is in contrast with certain low-fertility cultures where women do not work out of the household and hence older women whose children are grown participate more fully in others' child care and supervision. In developed countries, cultural differences are seen in the level at which women participate in the workforce outside of home, which, of course, has implications for child development and supervision.

In the United States, numerous scripts dictate who takes care of children and in what settings. In addition, attributes of material culture, such as how homes are built or lived in, may vary by region and by cultural group. Still, there may be cultural distinctions in regard to the way homes are arranged or used (fenced, open, crowded, well lit), elements in homes that may be risky (hazards such as poisons, plants, foods, pets, toys, tools), the acquisition of cultural artifacts (e.g., cars, bicycles, rollerblades, swimming pools), or even how children are supervised—all of which may pose risks. For example, low-income Hispanic families may acquire trucks for transport, which in turn are risky because children often ride in the truck bed, not in the cabin, putting them at greater risk for injury (Agran, Winn, & Castillo, 1991). Or cultural practices in households with many children may be to have older children supervise younger children, a risk if older children are not familiar with injury prevention guidelines or are themselves children. In some households of Middle Eastern origin, babies are always put on their backs to sleep so that the child "can face Allah," which may decrease the risk of SIDS (sudden infant death syndrome) in these children. Among Mexican Americans, botanicals with a lead base have been implicated in lead poisoning among children (personal communication,

A. Martinez, Los Angeles County Department of Health Services, December, 1991). Among some immigrants from Latin America, mercury vapors used in religious rituals have been linked to slow poisoning of household members, and overdoses from herbal remedies have been noted among children from Asian American families.

Culturally Informed Child Injury Research

Rather than just assessing the degree to which the variable of ethnicity predicts some outcome, be it injury rates or behavior, the research issue can be reframed to asked how members of different ethnic groups within a community or larger social system assess and respond to injury risks. One research orientation that may give valuable insight into the reasons for sociocultural variations in childhood injury is to study parental beliefs, behaviors, knowledge, and risk perceptions and to link these elements theoretically and analytically.

Accurate information and positive beliefs and behaviors about injury control are predictive of parental safety behaviors (Garling & Garling, 1993; Garling, Garling, Mauritzon-Sandberg, & Bjornstig, 1989; Glik, Greaves, et al., 1993; Glik, Kronenfeld, & Jackson, 1993; Langley & Silva, 1982). At the same time, studies have shown that many parents and caretakers have unrealistic expectations of their children's risk negotiation skills or may not fully subscribe to certain safety measures (DiGuiseppi, Rivara, Koepsell, & Polissar, 1989; Dunne, Asher, & Rivara, 1992; Rivara, Bergman, & Drake, 1989). However, in general, detailed studies looking at parental risk perceptions and behaviors have not taken ethnicity into account. Three studies that do look at ethnic differences in parental responses to injury risks that the authors have participated in will be summarized here.

South Carolina Study. Research carried out by Glik and colleagues in a southeastern state in 1986 to 1989, used survey research methods with a large sample of parents of young children ($N = 1,247$) to assess sociocultural correlates of injury control (Glik et al., 1991; Kronenfeld, Reiser, Glik, Allatore, & Jackson, 1997). In this study, responses to childhood injury risk were conceptualized as risk perceptions with dimensions of seriousness and likelihood of injury and seriousness and likelihood of hazards. Safety behaviors were measured using a modified version of the American Academy of Pediatrics TIPP scale (Bass, Mehta, & Ostrovsky, 1985). The data set included a substantial number of low-income African American respondents. Thus, one analytic strategy was to compare ethnic differences on some of the subscales as well as to analyze theoretical models within subsamples of the data set. Findings showed that on the risk perceptions measures, African American respondents had consistently higher scores than did white respondents, indicating that they perceived specific injuries, and hazards linked with injuries, as more serious and more likely to affect their children (Glik, Kronenfeld, & Jackson, 1993). In regard to safety behaviors conceptualized as using smoke detectors, child safety seats, safe product storage, knowing the Heimlich maneuver, keeping Ipecac syrup in the house, and supervising children in the bathtub, African Americans relied more on supervisory practices to control children than on using certain passive strategies such as car seats or other devices promoted for this purpose. Thus, although perceptions of danger and risk were greater and African American parents supervised their children as effectively as white parents, African Americans used fewer costly countermeasures, and those they did use were less effective (Glik et al., 1991; Glik, Kronenfeld, & Jackson, 1993)

When data were analyzed using structural equation models, there were some differences for African Americans and whites (Kronenfeld et al., 1997). Specifically for both groups, higher risk perceptions were related to stress, which mediated the relationship between risk perceptions and safety behaviors. Coping was also an important mediating factor. For African American mothers, the role of education was much more important than for white mothers in predicting the degree to which they practiced injury control (Kronenfeld et al., 1997).

National SAFE KIDS Campaign (NSKC) Survey. In 1997, the National SAFE KIDS Campaign commissioned a national telephone survey of parents to determine parental knowledge, attitudes, and self-reported behaviors concerning unintentional childhood injury (NSKC, 1997). The unweighted sample consisted of 968 whites (62%), 265 African Americans (17%), and 217 Hispanics (14%). Through analysis, statistically significant differences in safety practice among the three ethnic groups emerged, as presented in Table 6.1.

White parents (37%) were more likely to report that they knew almost everything about child safety devices and precautions prior to the telephone interview compared with lower knowledge rates among African Americans (24%) and Hispanics 24%. On most of the items, white parents had higher levels of compliance with child safety recommendations. On three items—child rides in back seat of car, toys removed from crib, and child wears pads for sports—Hispanic parents scored better than white parents. Perhaps the most interest-

Table 6.1   National SAFE KIDS Survey Data, 1997 (in percentages)

Item	White	African American	Hispanic	Chi-Square Tests
Child always follows safety rules	73	62	67	$p < .009$
Have smoke detector	99	98	94	$p < .001$
Have first aid kit	92	78	88	$p < .000$
Have fire extinguisher	81	60	59	$p < .000$
Have Ipecac syrup	55	34	25	$p < .000$
Have carbon monoxide detector	32	20	19	$p < .000$
Have window guards	27	44	46	$p < .000$
Child wears life vests in boats	94	84	92	$p < .000$
Child rides only in back seat of car	59	59	72	$p < .008$
Water heaters set at < 120 degrees	68	59	62	$p < .034$
Pillows/toys removed from crib	68	77	86	$p < .030$
Child wears pads while skating	62	62	77	$p < .017$

SOURCE: National SAFE KIDS Campaign (1997).

ing finding of all is that ethnically diverse parents were less likely than whites to own safety devices, but they were no less likely to use them once they had them. This bolsters the need to distribute child safety products (e.g., smoke alarms, bike helmets, child safety seats) to families in need and to develop culturally sensitive educational materials to promote their use (NSKC, 1997).

California Study of Parents of Elementary School Children. Survey data ($N = 113$) were collected by telephone in Los Angeles County to compare differences between recently immigrated Mexican Americans ($n = 59$) and middle-class white parents ($n = 54$) on their cognitive beliefs and protective behaviors related to injury risks for their elementary school-age child (aged 5-9 years). Questions comprised measures of parents' injury risk perceptions, perceptions of control and efficacy, risk control behaviors, estimates of children's exposure to injury risks, child attributes, and injury experiences. The basic aim of this study was to create a viable model of parents' behavioral responses to their children's injury risk, with measures developed derived from epidemiological findings on injury. We were interested in whether parents' perceptions and behaviors were linked to cultural or ethnic differences.

Contrasts in educational level, employment, Spanish language versus English language fluency, and income were clearly different between groups. Child injury experience and age of the child were not different (see Table 6.2).

Mexican American parents perceived their children to have a higher likelihood of injury. For perceived seriousness of injury, there was a less clear-cut trend between white and Mexican American subjects. In general, Mexican American parents did not differentiate between serious and less serious injury. Mexican American parents had significantly higher injury hazard perceptions, in regard to both chance and dangerousness. The degree to which a child was exposed to risks was not significantly different between groups. However, based on item analyses, Mexican American children were more exposed to busy streets, using stoves by themselves, bicycling on streets, using rollerblades and skateboards on streets, team sports, and storing guns in the home. White parents saw their children as more exposed to risks associated with riding in a car as a passenger, living in areas of high-density traffic, and using swimming pools and playground equipment.

White parents report more hazard control and had a greater sense of self-efficacy in obtaining their child's cooperation in risk reduction efforts than did Mexican American parents. White parents were more likely to report that their 5- to 9-year-old child could do a variety of unsupervised activities (e.g., cross busy streets, walk around the neighborhood alone) and were more likely to teach their children safe practices for a variety of activities, such as crossing the street, using the stove, swimming, cycling, skating, and using the playground. Both groups claimed they teach their children about gun safety. In regard to safety devices, Mexican American parents were less likely to use seat belts for their children and more likely to keep a locked gun at home. Both groups reported similar low levels of bicycle helmet use and use of protective gear when their children were rollerblading or skateboarding. White parents had significantly greater knowledge about safety practices than did Mexican American parents.

Further analyses using multiple regression models show that Mexican Americans had a higher level of risk perception but that those levels were not

Table 6.2   One-Way Analysis of Variance: Summed Variables, by
Ethnicity—California Data

Variables	ANG-AM/MSES $(n = 54)$[a]	MEX-AM/LSES $(n = 59)$[a]	F (df)	Probability
		Ethnicity		
Perceived risk items				
Perceived chance of injury (18 items)	46.07 (9.2)	51.11 (14.2)	4.72 (1,110)	.03
Perceived seriousness of injury (18 items)	62.53 (13.2)	67.91 (15.0)	3.95 (1,110)	.04
Perceived chance of hazards (17 items)	53.06 (12.3)	65.76 (10.7)	33.12 (1,107)	.0001
Perceived dangerousness of hazards (17 items)	55.16 (10.3)	68.76 (9.6)	51.75 (1,108)	.0001
Response to risk items				
Hazard exposure (10 items)	21.05 (4.2)	22.47 (4.0)	3.32 (1,110)	ns[b]
Hazard control (14 items)	47.50 (6.3)	42.19 (6.2)	20.04 (1,110)	.0001
Outcome expectations (10 items)	36.59 (6.3)	34.94 (4.4)	2.66 (1,110)	ns[b]
Self-efficacy (10 items)	42.43 (4.7)	39.36 (4.7)	11.73 (1,110)	.001
Knowledge of safety (6 items)	3.19 (1.2)	.98 (.95)	114.27 (1,110)	.0001

NOTE: ANG-AM data are for middle-class white parents; MEX-AM data are for recently immigrated Mexican American parents.
a. Numbers in this column represent mean (standard deviation).
b. Nonsignificant.

significantly associated with increased hazard control behaviors. In contrast, white parents had lower levels of risk perception but reported more safety promotion with their children, specifically giving their children more autonomy to negotiate risk. In both groups, injury risk control is strongly mediated by attitudes and perceptions.

Findings suggest that white parents were both more permissive and took a more educational approach to safety than did Mexican American parents, who tended to supervise their children more closely and who saw the world as a more dangerous place. Two hypotheses are suggested by these data. On the one hand, less acculturated Mexican American parents may lack information in regard to mediating childhood injury risks related to this environment; at the same time, their fear of danger may help them to compensate for material lack. Another hypothesis is that parents migrating from Mexico to the United States may have very different norms and expectations about child rearing than do native-born whites, a function of culture (Marín & Marín, 1991). If Mexican American parents cultivate dependency, then white parents encourage autonomy. Data suggest that parents need education about the developmental stages of their children to understand the capacity of children in the face of risks.

Culturally Informed Child Injury Prevention Programs

The studies described above are all oriented to understanding the cognitive and behavioral correlates of injury from a parental perspective, with special attention to issues of culture and norms of child rearing relevant to injury risk. Findings that parents misperceive threats to child safety and that ethnic group members rely more on supervision and less on safety devices are confirmed in the literature on this topic that takes account of cultural differences (Hsu & Williams, 1991; Mulligan-Smith, Puranik, & Coffman, 1998). It should also be added that this may be as much a function of acculturation as of ethnic group membership. To understand how this information might inform interventions to reduce childhood injury, it is important to first characterize the injury intervention field.

It is estimated that as many as 90% of unintentional injuries can be prevented. Strategies that reduce financial barriers to safety devices, increase education efforts, and improve the safety of the environment are effective at reducing death and injury among populations at risk (NCHS, 1995). Over the past 25 years, a combination of educational efforts, environmental improvements, engineering modifications, enactment and enforcement of legislation and regulations, economic incentives, community empowerment, and program evaluation has been effective at reducing the incidence and severity of unintentional injury-related death and disability (O'Donnell & Mickalide, 1998). Although policy, engineering, and regulatory activities are highly effective at reducing child injury (Robertson, 1986), they do not prevent all injuries and thus must be supplemented by health promotion interventions that take place in schools, clinics, and communities or through the mass media.

Given the multicultural nature of some regions in the United States today, the fundamental questions are these: To what extent are cultural differences related to injury risk being documented? How are they being incorporated into childhood injury prevention efforts? Although there is a large literature on childhood injury prevention, the published literature that actually addresses cultural differences and cultural competency in injury prevention efforts in U.S. contexts is small. At the same time, both anecdotally and experientially, we have heard of many efforts that do take place in multicultural contexts and communities. To a large degree, the work is defined by the type of injury or type of intervention conducted rather than by cultural variables or "cultural scripts."

A few published injury intervention studies that have taken account of cultural issues and have reported positive effects are summarized here. A school-based program among Head Start children in South Central Los Angeles targeted the high rate of pedestrian injuries in this population of Hispanic and African American families. A program that used behavioral skill training using safety rodeos to teach safe pedestrian behavior also used low-literacy reading materials in English and Spanish to help parents better understand the issues (Glik, Weiss, Reis, Hu, & Zhang, 1997). Another educational intervention, a K through 8 curriculum call *Risk Watch* sponsored by the National Fire Protection Association, uses an interactive or participatory learning approach that is developmentally appropriate and that can be adapted for particular cultural or regional risks and groups. A clinic-based intervention in a south Florida emergency services department that serves a Hispanic, African American, and Haitian population uses community input and planning to fashion a program that focuses on emergencies and teaching parents CPR and more basic injury prevention skills. A community-based program in Philadelphia in an African American community worked with community leaders to create a "safe block" approach to reduce residential hazards in homes (Schwarz, Grisso, Miles, Holmes, & Sutton, 1993). Another community-based program in Central Harlem, New York City, worked with community members to give children alternative activities and safe environments to reduce overall injury rates (Durkin et al., 1994). Finally, the National SAFE KIDS Campaign has worked for the past decade to help create more than 250 state and local SAFE KIDS Coalitions, many in multicultural communities (e.g., Navaho Country, Harlem, Alaska, and Hawaii).

Thus, there have been interventions in explicit multicultural contexts, but little research has attempted to account for cultural differences of populations targeted or differential responses to interventions proposed. Moreover, in some sense, all the interventions just cited, as well as the research described earlier in this chapter, took place in multicultural contexts. This is because whatever the cultural makeup of populations of interest, a basic paradigmatic truth in current injury prevention and research activities is that organized injury control generally represents biomedical or positivist assumptions and ideologies, which generally diverge from lay and popular cultural ideas about injury causation (Girasek, 1999, p. 19). Layered over this is the fact that at present we live in multicultural communities with many different ethnically specific beliefs and practices vis á vis injury prevention and causation. Hence, although not holding a young child's hand while crossing a street may be a fact of life in a rural village, in U.S. culture the practice may be important, given the heavy volume of cars on street surfaces as well as issues of confronting strangers in public places.

Not only must traditional versus modern conceptions of risk be considered but also the ethnic and cultural differences that may account for variations in injury rates. However, rarely are these issues considered, because most injury research is either epidemiological or behavioral in orientation. Moreover, not accounted for within the existing research is how beliefs and practices about childhood injury are changing within multiethnic communities, where intergenerational transmission of knowledge or practice may be altered by exposure to other cultural ideas or practice. For example, emblematic of this resistance is grandmothers' refusal to place children on their back to sleep, despite evidence of its salutory benefits.

If interventions in multicultural contexts are to succeed, care must be taken to account for the structural cognitive systems, or explanatory models, that direct thought and action in contexts for which the intervention is designed (Kleinman, 1980). All cultural systems have an underlying logic: It is the task of the worker in these contexts to define basic assumptions about reality and the practices these imply. For knowledge or new ideas to be communicated and processed, there must be some shared understanding between change agent and recipient. Hence, although within a modern Western medical view, injuries are seen to be preventable, within traditional cultures, risk and danger may be linked to many factors other than those defined epidemiologically. Rather than linking injury risk to environment, development, or behavior of a parent or child, risk may be viewed as caused by luck, fate or karma, jealous persons, restless spirits, or even God's will. Determining how these cultural predispositions influence injury prevention is a daunting task but certainly worth the effort if public health professionals are truly committed to reducing mortality and morbidity in our most vulnerable populations.

Thirty years after unintentional child injury was recognized as the leading killer of children in the United States, it is curious that most parents still do not recognize injury as the major risk to their children (Mickalide, 1993). Continued social and environmental change, geographic and social mobility, technological changes, shifting behavioral patterns, misinformation, and informational overload all serve to exacerbate uncertainty and the risk of injury to children in both urban and rural environments. On the basis of elevated injury statistics, children within distinct ethnic and cultural groups appear to be more vulnerable and less able to combat these risks. Growing recognition of cultural issues in injury control should serve to create more effective interventions for these children.

References

Agran, P. F. (1987). Injuries to children: The relationship of child development to prevention strategies. *Public Health Reports, 102*(6), 609-610.

Agran, P. F., Winn, D., & Castillo, D. (1991). Unsupervised children in vehicles: A risk for pediatrics. *Trauma Pediatrics, 87*(1), 70-73.

Anderson, R. N., Kochanek, K. D., & Murphy, S. L. (1997). Table 15: Number of deaths and death rates for the 10 leading causes of death for Hispanic and white non-Hispanic origins, for specified ages groups: Total of 49 reporting States and the District of Columbia. *Report of Final Mortality Statistics, 45* (11 Suppl. 2), 52-54.

Baker, S., & Waller, A. (1989). *Child injury: State by state mortality facts.* Washington, DC: U.S. Department of Health and Human Services, Office of Maternal and Child Health.

Baker, S. P., O'Neill, B., Ginsburg, M. J., & Li, G. (1991). *The injury fact book* (2nd ed.). New York: Oxford University Press.

Bass, J., Mehta K. A., & Ostrovsky, M. (1985). Educating parents about injury prevention. *Pediatric Clinics of North America, 32*(1), 233-242.

Bussing, R., Menvielle, E., & Zima, B. (1996, January). Relationship between behavioral problems and unintentional injuries in US children. *Archives of Pediatric and Adolescent Medicine, 150*, pp. 50-56.

Christoffel, K. K., Christoffel, T., & Tanz, R. (1988, November). *Biopsychosocial development: Critical to injury Analysis and Prevention.* Paper presented at the meeting of the American Public Health Association, Boston, MA.

DiGuiseppi, C. G., Rivara, F. P., Koepsell, T. D., & Polissar, L. (1989). Bicycle helmet use by children. *Journal of the American Medical Association, 262*, 2256-2261.

DiSorbo, A. (1995, Fall-Winter). Equity: Liberty and justice for all? *Harvard Journal of Minority Public Health, 1*(1), 16-19.

Division of Injury Control, Center for Environmental Health and Injury Control, Centers for Disease Control. (1990). Childhood injuries in the United States. *American Journal of Diseases of Children, 144*, 627-646.

Dunne, R. G., Asher, K. N., & Rivara, F. P. (1992). Behavior and parental expectations of child pedestrians. *Pediatrics, 89*, 486-490.

Durkin, M. S., Davidson, L. L., Kuhn, L., O'Connor, P., & Barlow, B. (1994). Low-income neighborhoods and the risk of severe pediatric injury: Small area analysis in Northern Manhattan. *American Journal of Public Health, 84*(4), 587-592.

Eichelberger, M. R., Gotschall, C. S., Feely, H. B., Harstad, P., & Bowman, L. M. (1990). Parental attitudes and knowledge of child safety. *American Journal of Diseases of the Child, 144*, 714-720.

Elders, M. J. E. (1995 Fall-Winter). Making prevention work for the poor and underserved. *Harvard Journal of Minority Public Health, 1*(1), 4-5.

Ellis, A. A., & Trent, R. B. (1997). Swimming pool drownings and near-drownings among California preschoolers. *Public Health Reports, 112*, 73-77.

Fingerhut, L. (1991-1992). *Unintentional injury death rates for children 0-14 years: United States, 1991-1992.* National Vital Statistics System, Compressed Mortality File. Unpublished raw data, National Center for Health Statistics.

Fingerhut, L. A., & Warner, M. (1997). *Injury chartbook health, United States, 1996-97.* Hyattsville, MD: National Center for Health Statistics.

Garling, A. & Garling, T. (1993). Mothers' supervision and perception of young children's risk unintentional injury in the home. *Journal of Pediatric Psychology, 18*, 105-114.

Garling, T., Garling, A., Mauritzon-Sandberg, E., & Bjornstig, U. (1989). Child safety in the home: Mother's perceptions of dangers to young children. *Architecture & Comportement/Architecture & Behavior, 5*, 293-304.

Geertz, C. (1973). *The interpretation of cultures.* New York: Basic Books.

Girasek, D.C. (1999). How members of the public interpret the word *accident*. *Injury Prevention, 5, 19-25.*

Glik, D., Greaves, P., Kronenfeld, J., & Jackson, K. (1993). Safety hazards in households with young children. *Journal of Pediatric Psychology, 18*(1), 115-131.

Glik, D., Kronenfeld, J., & Jackson, K. (1991). Predictors of risk perceptions of injury among parents of preschoolers. *Health Education Quarterly, 18*(3), 285-302.

Glik, D., Kronenfeld, J., & Jackson, J. (1993). Safety behaviors among parents of pre- schoolers. *Health Values, 17*(1), 18-27.

Glik, D., Weiss, B., Reis, L., Hu, F., & Zhang, W. (1997). *Evaluation of a preschool pedes- trian injury prevention program in an inner city community.* Manuscript submitted for publication.

Graves, E. J., & Gillum, B. S. (1996, October 3). *1994 Summary: National hospital dis- charge survey* (Advance data from vital and health statistics, No. 278). Hyattsville, MD: National Center for Health Statistics.

Greaves, P., Glik, D. C., Kronenfeld, J. J., & Jackson, K. (1994). Determinants of control- lable in-home child safety hazards. *Health Education Research, 9*(3), 307-315.

Guyer, B., Talbot, A., & Pless, I. B. (1985). Pedestrian injuries to children and youth. *Pediatric Clinics of North America, 32,* 163-174.

Hoffman, R. E. (1986). Tracking 1990 objectives for injury prevention with 1985 NHIS findings. *Public Health Reports, 101,* 581-586.

Hsu, J. S. J., & Williams, S. D. (1991, November). Injury prevention awareness in an urban Native American population. *American Journal of Public Health, 81*(11), 1466- 1468.

Jacquess, D. L., & Finney, J. W. (1994). Previous injuries and behavior problems predict children's injuries. *Journal of Pediatric Psychology, 19*(1), 79-89.

James, S. (1994-1995). *Unintentional injury death rates for children 0-14 years: United States, 1994-1995.* National Vital Statistics System, Compressed Mortality File. Un- published raw data, National Center for Health Statistics.

Kleinman, A. (1980). *Patients and healers in the context of culture.* Berkeley: University of California Press.

Kogan, M. D., Overpeck, M. D., & Fingerhut, L. A. (1995). Medically attended nonfatal injuries among preschool-age children: National estimates. *American Journal of Pre- ventive Medicine, 11*(2), 99-104.

Kraus, J., Hooten, E. G., Brown, K. A., Peek-Asa, C., Heye, C., & McArthur, D. L. (1996, September). Child pedestrian and bicyclist injuries: Results of a community surveil- lance and case control study. *Injury Prevention, 2,* 212-218.

Kronenfeld, J. J., & Glik, D. C. (1990). Perceptions of risk: Its applicability in medical so- ciological research. In D. Wertz (Ed.), *Advances in the sociology of health care systems* (Vol. 9; pp. 303-330). Greenwich, CT: JAI.

Kronenfeld, J. J., Reiser, M., Glik, D. C., Allatore, C., & Jackson, K. (1997). Safety behaviors of mothers of young children: Impact of cognitive, stress and background factors. *Health, 1*(2), 205-225.

Langley, J. D., & Silva, P. A. (1982). Childhood accidents: Parents' attitudes to prevention. *Australian Pediatric Journal, 18,* 247-249.

Levine, R. A. (1988). Human parental care: Universal goals, cultural strategies, individual behavior. In R. A. Levine, P. M. Miller, & M. M. West (Eds.), *Parental behavior in diverse societies* (New Directions for Child Development, No. 40). San Francisco: Jossey Bass.

Levine, R. A., Dixon, S., Levine, S., Richman, A., Leiderman, P. H., Keer, C. H., & Brazelton, T. B. (1994). *Child care and culture: Lessons from Africa.* New York: Cambridge University Press.

Lyman, D. O., Acee, K., Kelter, A., & Trent, R. B. (1992). *Pediatric injuries in California.* Sacramento: California Department of Health Services, Emergency Preparedness and Injury Control (EPIC) Program.

Marín, G., & Marín, B. V. (1991). *Research with Hispanic populations.* Newbury Park, CA: Sage.

Mazurek, A. J. (1994). Epidemiology of pediatric injury. *Journal of Accident and Emergency Medicine, 11*(1), 9-16.

McLouglin, L., & McGuire, A. (1990). The cause, cost, and prevention of childhood burn injuries. *American Journal of Childhood Disease, 144,* 677-683.

Mead, M. (1930). *Growing up in New Guinea.* New York: William Morrow.

Mickalide, A. D. (1993). Parents' perceptions and practices concerning childhood injury: 1987 vs. 1992. *Childhood Injury Prevention Quarterly, 4*(4), 29-32.

Miller, T. R. (1993). *Children's safety network, annual report.* Landover, MD: Economics and Insurance Resource Center.

Miller, T. R. (1996). *Children's safety network, annual report.* Landover, MD: Economics and Insurance Resource Center.

Mulligan-Smith, D., Puranik, S., & Coffman, S. (1998). Parental perception of injury prevention practices in a multicultural community. *Pediatric Emergency Care, 14*(1), 10-14.

National Center for Health Statistics. (1995). *National vital statistics system: Compressed mortality file.* Unpublished raw data.

National SAFE KIDS Campaign. (1997). *A national survey among parents of children age 14 or younger on child safety issues.* Washington, DC: Peter D. Hart Research Associates.

O'Donnell, G. O., & Mickalide, A. D. (1998, April). *SAFE KIDS at home, at play & on the way: A report to the nation on unintentional childhood injury.* Washington, DC: National SAFE KIDS Campaign.

Olson, L. M., Sklar, D. P., Cobb, L., Sapien, F., & Zumwat, R. (1993). Analysis of childhood pedestrian deaths in New Mexico, 1986-1990. *Emergency Medicine, 22,* 512-516.

Pless, I. B., Peckham, C. S., & Power, C. (1989). Predicting traffic injuries in childhood: A cohort analysis. *Journal of Pediatrics, 115,* 932-938.

Rivara, F. P. (1990). Child pedestrian injuries in the United States: Current status of the problem, potential interventions, and future research needs. *American Journal of Diseases of Children, 144,* 692-696.

Rivara, F. P. (1995, October). Developmental and behavioral issues in childhood injury prevention. *Developmental and Behavioral Pediatrics, 16*(5), 362-370.

Rivara, F. P., Bergman, A. B., & Drake, C. (1989). Parental attitudes and practices toward children as pedestrians. *Pediatrics, 84,* 1017-1021.

Robertson, L. S. (1986). Injury. In B. S. Edelstein & Michelson (Eds.), *Handbook of prevention* (pp. 343-360). New York: Plenum.

Santer, L. J., & Stocking, C. B. (1991). Safety practices and living conditions of low-income urban families. *Pediatrics, 88*(6), 1112-1118.

Scheidt, P. C., Harel, Y., Trumble, A. C., Jones, D. H., Overpeck, M. D., & Bijur, P. E. (1995, July). The epidemiology of nonfatal injuries among US children and youth. *American Journal of Public Health, 85*(7), 932-938.

Schwarz, D. F., Grisso, J. A., Miles, C., Holmes, J. H., & Sutton, R. L. (1993). Injury prevention in an African American community. *American Journal of Public Health, 83*(5), 675-680.

Singh, G. K., & Yu, S. M. (1996). US childhood mortality, 1950 through 1993: Trends and socioeconomic differentials. *American Journal of Public Health, 86*(4), 505-512.

Stussman, B. J. (1997, April 15). *National hospital ambulatory medical care survey: 1995 emergency department summary* (Advance data from vital and health statistics, No. 285). Hyattsville, MD: National Center for Health Statistics.

U.S. Department of Health and Human Services, Indian Health Service. (1995). *Trends in Indian health.* Rockville, MD. Program Statistics Team.

Valsiner, J. (1997). *Culture and the development of children's action: A theory of human development.* New York: John Wiley.

Warnecke, C. L., & Cooper, S. P. (1994). Child and adolescent drownings in Harris County, Texas, 1983-1990. *American Journal of Public Health, 84*(4), 593-598.

Woodwell, D. A., & Schappert, S. M. (1997, May 8). *National ambulatory medical care survey: 1995 summary* (Advance data from Vital and Health Statistics No. 286). Hyattsville, MD: National Center for Health Statistics.

7

The Usefulness of the *Health Diary*

Findings From a Case Study of Six Healthy Start Sites

Karen Thiel Raykovich
James A. Wells
Clifford Binder

The U.S. infant mortality rate, 7.2 per 1,000 live births in 1997, is a symptom of many underlying problems that extend beyond physical health (U.S. Department of Health and Human Services, 1999). Data indicate much higher infant mortality rates for some minority populations and confirm the association between disparities in socioeconomic factors and poor perinatal outcomes. African American infants continue to die at approximately twice the rate of the population of U.S. infants. The postneonatal death rate of 7.7 per 1,000 live births among American Indian infants in the Northern Plains is approximately 3 times the national average (Howell, 1998). Low-income mothers are more likely to enter prenatal care later and show a higher incidence of inadequate prenatal care. Providing health education to pregnant women at risk of poor birth outcomes is a challenge because of underlying issues of poverty, illiteracy, and access to culturally relevant materials.

In response to these challenges, the Onmibus Budget Reconciliation Act of 1989 (P.L. 101-239) included Section 6509, which provided for the Department of Health and Human Services (DHHS) secretary to develop a maternal and child health handbook. The section also provided for a field test and evaluation of the maternal and child health handbook. Furthermore, the authorizing legislation stipulated that the handbook was to be made available to pregnant women in maternal and child health programs that serve high-risk women.

Responsibility for the design of the *Health Diary* was assigned to the Health Resources and Services Administration's (HRSA) Maternal and Child Health Bureau (MCHB) in consultation with a number of public and private groups and the National Commission to Prevent Infant Mortality. The *Health Diary* was designed to contribute to efforts to reduce the U.S. infant mortality rate by increasing the involvement of women in their pregnancies and in caring for their infants. The *Health Diary* is an 82-page, interactive health education tool aimed at improving a woman's understanding of her pregnancy, encouraging communication with health care providers, and providing support for the care of her infant. The *Health Diary* also has space to help a woman chart both the progress of her pregnancy and her child's early health record. Sections of the *Health Diary* include following:

- My Pregnancy, My Baby and My Family
- How to Get the Prenatal Care I Need
- What Happens at Prenatal Care Visits
- What I Can Find Out From the Tests I Have
- How to Take Care of My Own and My Baby's Health
- Warning Signs
- Tracking My Weight Gain
- What to Eat for a Healthy Baby
- Fetal Growth and Development Chart
- Before My Baby Is Born

- Before I Become Pregnant Again
- After My Baby Is Born
- What to Feed My Baby
- When to Take My Baby to the Doctor or Clinic
- How to Take Care of Minor Problems
- When to Call the Doctor/How to Deal With Emergencies
- Tracking My Baby's Growth

In both its content and presentation, the focus of the *Health Diary* is pregnancy and infant care. The *Health Diary* was designed for a multicultural audience. There are no separate chapters for particular racial or ethnic groups, and the illustrations of infants and mothers reflected a variety of racial groups.

HRSA's Office of Planning, Evaluation, and Legislation (OPEL) contracted with the Center for Health Policy Studies (CHPS) to conduct an evaluation of the *Health Diary* to determine how useful it was as a health education tool for high-risk pregnant women and how it could best be used as a component of an overall perinatal care program. The agency was interested in learning whether the *Health Diary* would have broad appeal to a variety of racial/ethnic groups and whether its content and presentation would be perceived as sensitive to the health education needs of women served by HRSA programs. The *Health Diary* evaluation was undertaken during the winter of 1994-1995 as it was pilot-tested at six federally funded Healthy Start project sites, serving African American, Caucasian, Latina, and American Indian clients.

Healthy Start is major federal initiative, begun in 1991 and designed to reduce infant mortality in each of 15 original project sites with disproportionately high rates of infant mortality. These projects aim to provide access to comprehensive and continuous prenatal, postpartum, and infant care to increase the chances for healthy babies, but the focus extends beyond prenatal care and beyond the infant, to promote holistic health in families and communities. Healthy Start programs provide a variety of services to meet the specific needs of their target communities. In addition to access to prenatal and infant care, some of the key activities and services offered through Healthy Start include (a) smoking cessation and substance abuse treatment services, (b) nutrition counseling, (c) parenting and early childhood development classes, (d) family planning classes, (e) home visits and family support services, (f) literacy development and career training, (g) case management, (h) child care,

(i) transportation services, and (j) services to aid in eligibility determination for public assistance programs.

Each of the six participating Healthy Start sites identified a random sample of 50 women from clients who were given a copy of the *Health Diary* during their pregnancy or during their child's infancy (up to age 2). Women in the sample were invited to assist in the evaluation by participating in a 45-minute interview about their reactions, concerns, comments, and use of the *Health Diary.* Data from these client interviews, as well as from interviews with health care providers and Healthy Start staff members, were used in the evaluation of the *Health Diary.* Six Healthy Start sites volunteered to participated in this evaluation:

- Birmingham Healthy Start (Birmingham, Alabama)

- Great Expectations (New Orleans, Louisiana)

- Northern Plains Healthy Start (Aberdeen Area Tribal Chairmans' Health Board, Aberdeen, South Dakota)

- Northwest Indiana Healthy Start (Lake County, Indiana)

- Philadelphia Healthy Start (Philadelphia, Pennsylvania)

- Washington, D.C. Healthy Start (District of Columbia)

The population of the Healthy Start project areas (see Table 7.1) in four of these communities was predominately African American, ranging from 68.8% in Philadelphia to 94% in Washington, D.C. The Northwest Indiana Healthy Start project area was 45.5% African American and 13.9% Latino. The Northern Plains Healthy Start Project area was 100% Native American.

The overall purpose of the evaluation was to assess the usefulness of the *Health Diary* as a health education tool for Healthy Start clients and other pregnant women. In addition, attention was focused on the most effective methods to disseminate the *Health Diary,* train clients in it use, and involve health care providers in working with clients who use the *Health Diary.* Due to the multiracial compostion of the Healthy Start client population in these project sites and the focus of these interventions on high-risk pregnant women, these interviews provided valuable information on the health education needs of high-risk minority women.

Table 7.1   Project Area Characteristics

	Population, 1990				
Projects	*Total*	*Percentage African American*	*Percentage Latino*	*Percentage of Adults with < High School Education*	*Infant Mortality Rate 1989-91*
Birmingham	182,788	81.5	0.3	36.9	19.6
New Orleans	174,282	87.0	2.6	47.8	17.4
Northern Plains					
Northwest Indiana	248,673	45.5	13.9	34.6	12.0
Philadelphia	301,699	68.8	1.3	34.7	15.2
Washington, D.C.	141,062	94.0	1.1	37.1	23.5

SOURCE: Howell et al. (1997, p. 6).

Evaluation Methodology

The strategy selected for evaluating the *Health Diary* used elements of a case study and sample survey design. A field test conducted at the Washington, D.C. Healthy Start site was used to test the interview guides, logistics, interviewee recruitment procedures, and other aspects of the evaluation. Once Office of Management and Budget clearance was obtained, the remaining site visits, including completion of the Washington, D.C. site visit, were scheduled.

Figures 7.1 and 7.2 graphically present a model of the evaluation design. Interviews were conducted with three groups of *Health Diary* users: clients, Healthy Start staff members, and maternal and child health providers who worked with clients. As displayed in Figure 7.1, the client-level evaluation methodology assessed how the *Health Diary* was distributed to clients, how much training in using the *Health Diary* was given to Healthy Start staff members and providers, how much training clients were given in using the *Health Diary,* and the degree to which maternal and child health providers were encouraged to use the *Health Diary.* From the assessment of how the *Health Diary* was distributed to clients, the client-level evaluation approach moved to con-

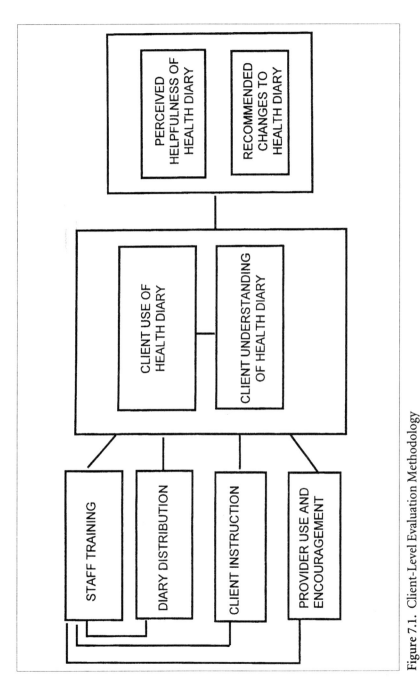

Figure 7.1. Client-Level Evaluation Methodology

SOURCE: Center for Health Policy Studies (1995, p. 3-2).

170

sideration of whether and how much clients used and understood the *Health Diary.* The final stage of the client-level evaluation methodology was to measure clients' impressions of the usefulness of the *Health Diary* and the need for changes.

As illustrated in Figure 7.2, the project-level evaluation methodology followed a similar approach. The process for distributing the *Health Diary* was assessed, including staff members and health care provider training and client instruction. These distribution factors were used to measure staff members' perceptions of whether clients were better informed, whether clients were more likely to follow staff member and provider recommendations, and whether there were problems in understanding the *Health Diary.* These staff perceptions were then compiled to determine if changes were needed or whether projects would continue to use the *Health Diary* or switch to other health education materials.

Questions Pertaining to Clients' Use of the Health Diary

The evaluation addressed the following questions about clients' use of the *Health Diary:*

- How is the *Health Diary* distributed to clients?
- What is the perceived impact of the *Health Diary* on clients?
- How has maternal and child health provider/client communication been affected by use of the *Health Diary?*
- Do clients use the *Health Diary?*
- Is the *Health Diary* understandable?
- How helpful is the *Health Diary?*
- How do clients believe use of the *Health Diary* is affected by maternal and child health provider interaction?
- What changes in the *Health Diary* do clients recommend?

Questions Pertaining to Staff and Provider Use of the Health Diary

The evaluation also addressed the following questions regarding Healthy Start staff members' and maternal and child health providers' use of the *Health Diary:*

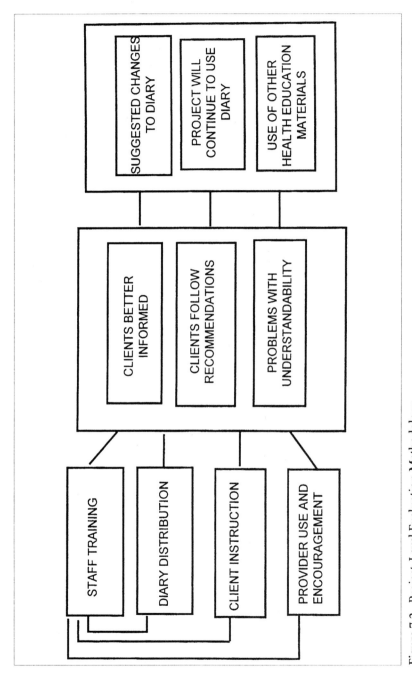

Figure 7.2. Project-Level Evaluation Methodology

SOURCE: Center for Health Policy Studies (1995, p. 3-3).

- Were project staff members trained in the use of the *Health Diary?*
- How do providers use the *Health Diary?*
- Do project staff believe that clients understand the material in the *Health Diary?*
- Do maternal and child health providers think that the *Health Diary* is useful?
- What changes would project staff make in the *Health Diary?*

The Sample

One of the goals of the site visit protocol was to help ensure that a random sample of 50 women from each site would be recruited from the total number of clients who received the *Health Diary.* The emphasis on a random sample was necessary to avoid selecting only clients who were favorably disposed to use the *Health Diary* and comply with the Healthy Start program's policies and practices. A randomly selected sample also would be representative of the Healthy Start client population at these sites and might permit some inferences to be drawn about how the *Health Diary* would be used by a larger, similar audience. Healthy Start sites were contacted 6 to 9 months prior to the scheduled site visits. These calls were used to outline the project, describe the schedule for site visits, and emphasize the importance of tracking clients so that sites could later identify which clients received the *Health Diary.* A proposed tracking form was sent to each site to help Healthy Start staff develop a process for tracking clients.

It also was recommended that the staff members who worked most closely with clients actually contact clients to be interviewed, because it was felt that staff members who had a relationship with clients would be better able to recruit participants. A $10 cash incentive to cover expenses such as transportation to the interview or child care was promised to each client. A similar process was recommended for recruiting maternal and child health care providers, although no cash incentive was offered. Schedules, draft telephone scripts, draft reminder letters, and other supporting documents, including random selection procedures, were provided in the site visit protocol.

Because only an English version of the *Health Diary* was available at the time of the field test and evaluation, non-English-speaking clients were not included in the sample.[1] It was acknowledged that this design feature would limit the applicability of the findings for non-English-speaking clients.

Table 7.2   *Health Diary* Interviews, By Site

Healthy Start Site	Client Interviews	Staff and Provider Interviews
Birmingham	35	11
New Orleans	51	5
Northern Plains	45	14
Northwest Indiana	57	12
Philadelphia	40	9
Washington, D.C.	39	9

SOURCE: Center for Health Policy Studies (1995, p. 31).

Client Interviews

Once arrangements were made to interview the sample of clients at each site, client interviews were conducted by a team of two interviewers. Each interview consisted of a structured 30- to 45-minute dialogue between the interviewer and a Healthy Start client. An interview guide was used to ensure that the interviews followed a consistent and comprehensive format. Each client was asked to sign a consent agreement prior to the interview and given a Certificate of Appreciation and $10 at the end of the interview.

Although the design was to interview at least 50 clients per site, fewer clients actually were interviewed in four of the six sites. In some cases, the $10 incentive was inadequate to induce women to participate. Other factors also contributed to the variation in the number of interviews that could be scheduled, including poor weather, the organization of the health care delivery system in different areas, the person who contacted women to participate (e.g., a staff member at a clinic or a case manager versus a Healthy Start staff person who was unknown to the client), and the determination of the staff who recruited study participants. In general, however, Healthy Start staff members were exceptionally supportive of the study, and their energetic recruitment of study participants was a key factor in the success of the conduct of the interviews on site.

Healthy Start Staff and Maternal
and Child Health Provider Interviews

At most sites, Healthy Start staff and provider interviews (see Table 7.2) were completed in 2 or 3 days. The length of the staff and provider interviews varied from 15 minutes to more than 2 hours, although the vast majority of the interviews required about an hour. A wide range of time was necessary to interview staff members and providers because of their varying involvement in using the *Health Diary*. For instance, some providers were very supportive of the *Health Diary* but had little firsthand experience working with clients who used it. The comments of these providers were more general than the comments of providers who had firsthand experience working with *Health Diary* users.

Which staff members and providers were selected to be interviewed was determined by how each site had elected to use the *Health Diary*. At some of the participating Healthy Start programs, the *Health Diary* was distributed to clients during an intake visit by home visitors or other layworkers but, subsequently, was not used as a systematic part of prenatal or child care visits. At other programs, the *Health Diary* was fully integrated into a prenatal and infant care health promotion program. A broader range of discussion about the usefulness, content, and any needed refinements was more possible at programs where the *Health Diary* was more completely integrated into the program.

Data Collection and Analysis

Table 7.3 summarizes key sociodemographic characteristics of clients who participated in this evaluation. A total of 267 women were interviewed for the evaluation, ranging from 57 at the Northwest Indiana site to 35 at the Birmingham Healthy Start site. Half (51%) of the clients had given birth by the time of the interview. The interview participants ranged in age from 13 to 44; however, over two thirds (69%) of the participants were aged 24 or younger. The racial and ethnic mix of the interview sample predominantly consisted of representatives from minority groups. Approximately 91% of the participants were African American (non-Latina), Latina, or American Indian. Almost half of the sample clients had household incomes of $10,000 or less, and an additional 10% had household incomes below $15,000. The educational status of the group was diverse, but the majority of women (59%) had completed high school, earned a GED, or attended some college. More than half of the women in the sample (62%) had not been married.

The sample of clients who participated in the evaluation of the *Health Diary* was representative of the overall Healthy Start population. The racial and ethnic mix of clients was consistent with the overall distribution of clients in the participating projects. The number of adolescents who participated was a little greater than what might be expected at one site and fewer at another, but when all clients are considered as a group, the distribution of adolescents was consistent with their representation in these Healthy Start sites.

How Is the Health Diary Distributed to Clients?

Healthy Start sites were free to develop their own process for using and distributing the *Health Diary,* so a number of approaches were used by the six participating sites. For all of the sites, clients reported that a health care provider usually gave them the *Health Diary.* Case managers and outreach workers, respectively, were the second and third most common staff members to distribute the *Health Diary.*

In Birmingham, the *Health Diary* was distributed to clients through the city health department's clinics. Prenatal, postpartum, and pediatric nurses distributed the *Health Diary* to clients during an intake visit. Although clients were encouraged to bring the *Health Diary* with them to subsequent prenatal and infant care visits, not all clinic providers used the *Health Diary.*

In New Orleans, the *Health Diary* was distributed at a neighborhood pregnancy care clinic located in a public housing complex and at a community health center. Although clients were encouraged to bring the *Health Diary* to subsequent appointments, most clients did not bring it with them.

The Northern Plains project consisted of 19 affiliated programs in four states. Four sites were included in the evaluation. At each site, nursing staff or outreach workers distributed the *Health Diary* to new clients during an intake or orientation visit. One of the four sites engaged in a formal effort to encourage maternal and infant health care providers to use the *Health Diary* with clients. In that site, clients earned points for bringing the *Health Diary* to prenatal appointments; the points could be used to purchase merchandise from a "store" run by the Healthy Start project.

The Northwest Indiana Healthy Start site included the cities of East Chicago, Gary, Hammond, and Lake Station. Nurses affiliated with the Healthy Start project in each city distributed the Health Diary to clients and coordinated its use with providers. Clients were encouraged to bring the *Health Diary* to prenatal and infant care visits, and providers spent considerable time during orientation and follow-up appointments explaining the *Health Diary* and responding to clients' questions.

The Philadelphia Healthy Start project encompassed a wide range of locations and providers. Seven providers participated in the *Health Diary* evaluation. The *Health Diary* was distributed during intake at the client's home or in a provider's office. Staff members at all of the participating agencies encouraged clients to bring the *Health Diary* to health care visits, but follow-up tended to be more consistent with health care providers.

The Washington, D.C., Healthy Start project consisted of Wards 7 and 8 in the District of Columbia. Case managers, resource parents, and nurse midwives distributed the *Health Diary* to clients. Resource parents were trained in the use of the *Health Diary,* and they encouraged clients to bring it to prenatal and infant care appointments as part of their effort to facilitate clients' compliance with Healthy Start project goals, such as keeping appointments, abstaining from alcohol and drugs, and adhering to a healthy diet.

What Is the Perceived Impact of the Health Diary on Clients?

The *Health Diary* seemed to have an important impact on the Healthy Start women who participated in the evaluation. Clients' initial reactions to the *Health Diary* were overwhelmingly positive. More than 90% of clients said they liked the *Health Diary.* Women who used the *Health Diary* were impressed with a number of specific features as well as with the overall concept. A number of women said that they especially liked the idea of having space to write down their comments or to note questions. There were many other positive comments about the colors, layout, and graphics. Many women liked the fetal growth and development chart.

Another measure of the impact of the *Health Diary* is the number of women who thought that they would have healthier babies because they used the *Health Diary.* Two thirds of clients said that they thought that by using the *Health Diary* their babies would be more likely to be healthy.

How Has Maternal and Child Health Provider/Client Communication Been Affected by Use of the Health Diary?

The evidence that the *Health Diary* helped to facilitate communication between clients and maternal and child health care providers was mixed. Improved communication between clients and providers may increase client

Table 7.3 Key Sociodemographic Characteristics of *Health Diary* Evaluation Clients

Client Characteristics	Birmingham		New Orleans		Northern Plains		Northwest Indiana		Philadelphia		Washington, D.C.		Total[a]	
	Number	%	Number	%	Number	%	Number	%	Number	%	Number	%	Number	%
Clients interviewed	35	100	51	100	45	100	57	100	40	100	39	100	267	100
Age groups														
13–15	3	9	1	2	2	4	3	5	3	8	1	3	13	5
16–19	12	34	17	33	9	20	19	33	9	23	15	38	81	31
20–24	13	37	20	39	17	38	20	35	11	28	7	18	88	33
25–29	4	11	7	14	7	16	9	16	7	18	5	13	39	15
30–34	1	3	1	2	9	20	5	9	6	15	10	26	32	12
35+	1	3	2	4	1	2	1	2	4	10	1	3	10	4
Racial/ethnic groups														
Black, non-Hispanic	33	94	51	100			19	33	38	95	39	100	180	67
American Indian	1	3			41	91	1	2					43	16
Hispanic							21	37					21	8
White, non-Hispanic	1	3			3	7	15	26	2	5			21	8
Other					1	2	1	2					2	1
Household income														
Less than $5,000	12	34	31	61	4	9	17	30	9	23	8	21	81	30
$5,000–10,000	8	23	5	10	8	18	9	16	10	25	10	26	50	19

	C1	C2	C3	C4	C5	C6	C7	C8	C9	C10	C11	C12	C13	C14
$10,001–15,000	6	17	2	4	6	13	6	11	3	8	5	13	28	10
$15,001–20,000	2	6	4	8	7	16	4	7	3	8	3	8	19	7
$20,001–25,000	1	3	3	6	2	4	4	7	2	5	1	3	12	4
Greater than $25,000	4	11			5	11	4	7	3	8		3	17	6
Don't know	2	6	6	12	13	29	17	30	10	25	12	31	60	22
Education														
6–7th grade	1	3	1	2	1	2	1	2					4	1
8–9th grade	3	9	6	12	7	16	8	14	5	13	6	15	35	13
10–11th grade	7	20	21	41	6	13	14	25	9	23	13	33	70	26
12th grade or GED	14	40	17	33	15	33	16	28	15	38	16	41	93	35
Some college	10	29	6	12	16	36	18	32	11	28	4	10	65	24
Marital status														
Married	3	9	6	12	17	38	14	25	4	10	1	3	45	17
Never married	30	86	30	59	22	49	28	49	32	80	24	62	166	62
Separated	2	6	1	2	2	4	3	5			1	3	9	3
Divorced			2	4	2	4	3	5					7	3
Live with someone			12	24	2	4	9	16	4	10	13	33	40	15
Delivery status														
Prenatal	22	63	23	45	18	40	37	65	15	38	16	41	131	49
Postpartum	13	37	28	55	27	60	20	35	24	60	22	56	134	50

a. Due to rounding and elimination of missing values, totals may not sum.

179

involvement in their prenatal care. In addition, better communication can help providers to identify and reduce unhealthy behaviors, such as poor diet, smoking, drug abuse, and other social and environmental risks. It was difficult, however, to determine the direct effect of using the *Health Diary* on communication between clients and their health care providers. It was assumed that communication between providers and clients was improved if providers were involved in the use of the *Health Diary*. Furthermore, if clients brought their *Health Diary* or asked questions and their physician or nurse talked about the *Health Diary* or made notes in it, then there was thought to be improved communication.

With the exception of a few sites, there was a general lack of formal procedure for clients and providers to interact regarding the *Health Diary*, although clients seemed to be more eager to communicate with their health care providers. Nearly 67% of clients said they brought their *Health Diary* to at least some of their prenatal or infant care visits. About 56% of clients also indicated they asked questions at least sometimes at their health care visits.

Providers, on the other hand, did not seem to be as involved in using the *Health Diary*. Less than a third of clients reported that their health care providers asked, at least sometimes, that they bring their *Health Diary* to prenatal or infant care checkups; only about a third said that their health care provider talked, at least sometimes, to them about sections of the *Health Diary;* and fewer than a third of clients said that their health care providers wrote in their *Health Diary*. One third of clients said that they never brought their *Health Diary* to health care provider visits.

Do Clients Use the Health Diary?

Healthy Start clients who participated in the evaluation of the *Health Diary* made considerable use of it. A significant portion of clients regularly read and wrote in their *Health Diary*. Nearly 64% of clients read their *Health Diary* at least once a week. Clients were much more likely to have written in the sections containing biographical or more general information, such as "My Health Diary," "My Health History," "Prenatal and Postpartum Appointments," and "My Weight Gain," than in sections that had space for recording more medically oriented information.

Is the Health Diary Understandable?

Most clients in this sample said that they were able to understand the material in most *Health Diary* sections. This may be because almost 60% of the sample had graduated from high school, earned a GED, or had taken some college courses and another 26% of the sample indicated they had completed 10th or 11th grade. However, a substantial portion of the women interviewed (from 21 to 29%) said they had difficulty understanding some material in sections of the *Health Diary.*

How Helpful Is the Health Diary?

Clients' responses suggested that they believed the *Health Diary* gave them factual, more detailed information about their pregnancy and infant care. Half of the clients said that the *Health Diary* provided information that was new to them, and 89% said the *Health Diary* provided more detailed information than they had previously read on some topics related to pregnancy and infant care.

More clients rated the prenatal sections of the *Health Diary* as helpful than they did infant care sections. For example, 67% of clients said that the fetal growth and development chart was helpful, 60% said the section on what happens at prenatal care visits was helpful, and 58% said the section on "warning signs" was helpful. In contrast approximately 40% of clients rated each of the infant care sections of the *Health Diary* as helpful. This difference in rating, however, may be more an artifact of the pregnancy status of clients at the time of the interview. Approximately half of the clients were still pregnant at the time of the interview, so it may be that sections on infant care were not yet salient for these clients.

How Do Clients Believe Use of the Health Diary Is Affected by Maternal and Child Health Provider Interaction?

Health Diary clients were split in their assessment of whether more interaction with their health providers would increase their use of the *Health Diary.* Only a little more than half of clients (52%) said that more interaction with providers in the form of instruction would increase their use of the *Health Diary.*

Similar results were obtained from another question about whether additional provider encouragement would increase clients' use of the *Health Diary.* The hypothesis underlying this question was that if a physician or nurse actively used the *Health Diary* or asked if the client bought it, clients would be more likely to bring the *Health Diary* to their appointments, read it, and use it. In the opinion of clients, encouragement, interactions, and involvement in the use of the *Health Diary* would help about half of them to use their diaries.

Table 7.4   Clients' Opinions About the Need for More Information on Selected Topics

Topic	Percentage of clients indicates the need for more information
Sex (during and after pregnancy)	34
What to eat (alternative for meals and snacks)	31
Amniocentesis	31
Family planning (deciding whether and when to have another baby)	29
Exercise	29
Medical tests and why they are necessary	25
Not using drugs	24
Warning signs	20
Signs of labor	18
A plan for getting to the hospital	15

What Changes in the Health Diary Do Clients Recommend?

In general, clients were very pleased with the *Health Diary*; 89% believed it was about the right length, and 96% thought it was written "about right." In addition, as noted in the responses to questions about whether they used, understood, or found the *Health Diary* helpful, clients seemed to be satisfied with the content of the *Health Diary*.

However, clients also recommended that more material be added on a number of topics (see Table 7.4), including sex during and after pregnancy (34%), what to eat/alternatives for meals and snacks (31%), amniocentesis (31%), family planning (29%), exercise (29%), and medical tests and why they were necessary (25%).

Were Project Staff Members Trained in the Use of the Health Diary?

The *Health Diary* was distributed to Healthy Start clients by a number of different staff members and providers. The distribution process ranged from including the *Health Diary* along with a number of public relations and health promotion materials to issuing the *Health Diary* as part of a formal, comprehensive health education program focused around the *Health Diary* as an educational vehicle. In the former distribution process, there was little training or direction for clients, Healthy Start staff members, or providers. In the latter, there was training and follow-up discussion, as well as encouragement for all *Health Diary* users. At one site, the project even went so far as to provide clients with incentive rewards for completing the *Health Diary* as evidence that they attended prenatal health care appointments and other activities. Several different distribution and training approaches worked well or at least better than an unsystematic approach. The three most common distribution approaches were distribution by health providers, distribution by layworkers, and distribution by professional case managers.

Health Provider Model

When health care providers, such as nurse midwives and clinical nurse specialists, were responsible for distributing the *Health Diary,* there seemed to be little need to train them in health education. In the health provider distribution process, there was also reduced need for coordination between Healthy Start staff members and providers, although that could have been a liability in that there was less opportunity to reinforce similar messages or discuss problem cases and other information.

When nurses distributed the *Health Diary,* however, there was a need to explain or create a model so that the busy clinic and health provider staff could understand how using the *Health Diary* helped to reinforce common Healthy Start themes that clients would be hearing elsewhere. The failure to coordinate with nurses or to develop a model for distribution and training was the most common failing of the programs where health providers distributed the *Health Diary.* The nurses and other staff members essentially created their own individualized training programs, which may or may not have encouraged clients to use the *Health Diary* or reinforced common themes, goals, and expectations. Health providers would have been better able to use the *Health Diary* had they had at least some outline of the distribution process and the intent in using the *Health Diary.* In practice, many Healthy Start programs had only marginal control or input into the staffing, materials, and other activities conducted at health provider sites, which may have impeded the creation of a more formal, comprehensive, and consistent *Health Diary* distribution process. In addition, some health providers who had developed their own medical model for patient education might have had difficulty integrating the *Health Diary* into their programs.

Lay Healthy Start Staff Model

In the *Health Diary* distribution and training process in which a lay home visitor, outreach worker, or other nonprofessional staff (e.g., resource parent, health advocate) distributed the *Health Diary,* integration of the *Health Diary* into prenatal and infant care visits was less certain. In this model, lay-workers were trained to distribute the *Health Diary* to clients and to review the *Health Diary* with their clients at subsequent visits. Clients were encouraged to bring the *Health Diary* to their health care appointments. This model also required that maternal and child health providers were made aware of the *Health Diary* and its use as part of an effort to inform, motivate, and track clients. However, health care providers sometimes were not aware of the need to include the *Health Diary* in their interactions with clients. In addition, some layworkers, despite considerable training, were not capable of explaining the medical issues outlined in the *Health Diary.*

Professional Case Manager Model

The model in which professional case managers, such as social workers and public health nurses distributed the *Health Diary* and trained clients in its use worked well. Unlike the distribution and training model that relied on lay staff, professional staff could easily master the medical content of the *Health Diary,* with limited training. If the *Health Diary* was to be used throughout a Healthy Start client's pregnancy and the infancy period, and health education and other goals of Healthy Start were to be reinforced and sustained, there was still a need to include health providers in the *Health Diary* process. To include providers so that the *Health Diary* would be used during prenatal and infant care visits, some training, orientation, or other coordination was necessary so providers could understand the process and their role.

For all approaches to the use of the *Health Diary,* there was a need to ensure continuity between the prenatal, postpartum, and infancy periods. Healthy Start clients often switched providers after their babies were born, and there was a tendency for clients to fall away from the program. Health education during the infancy period can also be very important, yet there are fewer opportunities to maintain contacts with clients and their infants. This transition problem was reflected somewhat in the distribution and training for the

Health Diary. Infant care providers seldom seemed to be involved in the process. A process for training and distribution of the *Health Diary* that included infant care providers would have helped to maintain clients' use of the *Health Diary.*

How Do Providers Use the Health Diary?

Most maternal and child health providers used the *Health Diary* to help reinforce information and training they were giving to their clients. Many maternal and child health providers explained that the *Health Diary* was a very useful summary, and its appealing presentation, language, and concept made it ideal for getting and holding the young mother's attention, which helped providers to teach women about proper nutrition and the importance of maintaining their own health and well-being. In most cases, providers connected with the Healthy Start program said the *Health Diary* did not present any information they were not already giving to their clients, but it did help to organize, focus, reinforce, and maintain continuity of their maternal and infant care educational efforts. In a few instances, health providers, either independently or in concert with their Healthy Start program, integrated or built a maternal and child health program around the *Health Diary.* However, even these programs used a number of resources to supplement specific components of the information in the *Health Diary.* Some of the topics on which supplementary information was used included obtaining social services and financial support, nutrition, specific medical tests and procedures, exercise, infant care, parenting, medical care, high-risk conditions, drug and alcohol abuse, sexually transmitted diseases, and family planning.

Do Project Staff Believe That Clients Understand the Material in the Health Diary?

Healthy Start staff members and maternal and child health providers generally said that clients could understand most of the material in the *Health Diary.* They reported that the concept of the *Health Diary* and the information available seemed to be accessible and understandable to most Healthy Start clients. However, staff members and providers offered a number of qualifications to this overall assessment. One of the principal qualifications was that clients could understand the *Health Diary* but probably would not use or comprehend most of the material without some assistance, coaching, or other support from providers, case managers, home visitors, or other staff members. Staff members and providers often remarked that the sections that contained full pages of text were too complicated or that the key points needed to be highlighted or otherwise emphasized by bulleted text.

Most staff members and providers said that it was difficult to estimate the percentage of their clients who could not read well. Some said it was a high as 40%, but most estimated that the number of clients who could not read well was no more than 20%, and probably closer to 10% to 15%. As several interviewees noted, however, it was difficult to judge the reading level of clients without specific tests, because poor readers often develop skills to camouflage their reading deficiencies.

Do Maternal and Child Health Providers Think the Health Diary Is Useful?

Like the Healthy Start clients, virtually all staff members and providers were positive in their assessment of the usefulness of the *Health Diary*. Many interviewees praised specific features or sections, such as the fetal growth and development chart, the pocket in the back, the section on warning signs, the immunization record, and dos and don'ts, to name a few. Many providers said that they did not have or know of any other comparable source for the same information and they were pleased to have the *Health Diary*. There were a number of comments such as these: "We love it." "I use it with patients all the time." "It's worth it for the fetal growth and development chart alone." "The infant care information is very good; we have lots of first-time mothers who need this information."

A question related to clients' use of the *Health Diary* was whether the *Health Diary* reflected cultural diversity. The *Health Diary* was created for a diverse cultural and racial audience and was successful in appealing to the range of racial and ethnic groups that participated in the Healthy Start program. Healthy Start staff members and providers of maternal and infant care said that the *Health Diary* was culturally neutral in that it did not overly emphasize any cultural or racial group. Some of these *Health Diary* users thought the pictures of minority women and their families should be moved closer to the beginning of the book. However, most interviewees thought the information, presentation, tone, concept, and other characteristics were culturally neutral. It seemed that there was a consensus that maternal and infant care was an experience with which most women could relate, so it was unnecessary to emphasize the symbols or concerns of any particular group to encourage use of the *Health Diary*.

What Changes Would Project Staff Make in the Health Diary?

Healthy Start staff suggested a number of changes that could be made to the *Health Diary*. These suggestions could be classified into three different groups of suggested changes: (a) philosophy/design changes, (b) content changes, and (c) enhancements and refinements. The most common complaint with the underlying philosophy of the *Health Diary* was the reading level.

In the analysis of client interview data it was clear that, overall, clients believed the *Health Diary* was "understandable." In looking at specific sections, however, it was also clear that clients did not fully understand some sections, at least without assistance from Healthy Start staff members or providers.

A number of staff members considered the language, content, and design of the *Health Diary* beyond the reading comprehension level of the most needy Healthy Start clients and thought the *Health Diary* should be rewritten at a lower reading level.

Another less common comment with the philosophy and design of the *Health Diary* related to the division of the book into prenatal and infant care sections. Some staff members and providers said that it would be preferable to have two books with more information about what they perceived to be two different phases of child health. Some interviewees also said that the woman's health and well-being are hardly mentioned in the infant care section so that the *Health Diary* failed to integrate infant care and the mother's health. These interviewees thought the concept of a diary of the woman's pregnancy developed in the prenatal care section seemed to diverge more into a baby keepsake in the infant care section.

Some of the changes suggested by Healthy Start staff members and providers concerned the content of the *Health Diary*. A number of staff members and providers said that the *Health Diary* did not go far enough. The *Health Diary* contained considerable information on many important topics, but few topics were covered in sufficient detail that additional prenatal and infant care education material could be omitted. In addition, many staff members and providers said that the message in the *Health Diary* was not strong enough. Topics such as breast-feeding, exercise, birth control and family planning, and safety needed more emphasis. Other recommendations included adding information about common myths, common discomforts of different stages of pregnancy and the postpartum period, and more detailed nutritional information.

Most of the suggested *Health Diary* changes were refinements rather than substantive changes, such as suggestions to add features to enhance the *Health Diary's* utility and flexibility. There were a number of suggestions to add features to make it easier for clients to use the *Health Diary*, including adding more pockets to hold supplementary health information, birth certificates, immunization records, and other materials that would help clients to maintain all their documents in one place and to bring them to checkups and other health care appointments.

Healthy Start staff members and providers also suggested including more information on the role of the baby's father or the client's male partner to help include him in the experiences of pregnancy, child birth, and child rearing. Staff members at the one project that served Latina clients also recommended that the *Health Diary* be translated into Spanish.

Several staff members noted that part of the *Health Diary*'s usefulness was that it made prenatal and infant care information available. In areas where bookstores, libraries, and health providers were common, prenatal and infant care information was plentiful. However, in many neighborhoods served by Healthy Start programs, there were limited prenatal and infant care resources. The *Health Diary* met a need for information and was provided at no cost to clients. It was also praised for being nonauthoritarian, reassuring in tone, culturally neutral, more comprehensive than many sets of alternative materials, and appealing in design. The diary format could be kept as a keepsake of the mother's pregnancy and the child's early years.

Discussion

This evaluation demonstrates that there was a clear perception of the usefulness of the *Health Diary* as a component of a perinatal health education program. Clients were enthusiastic about using the *Health Diary*. Most health care providers thought the *Health Diary* was a useful health education tool, and most were supportive of Healthy Start efforts to use it. Most providers thought it could be a useful component of a general maternal and child health promotion program, but they noted that there would be a need to supplement the material provided in some sections of the *Health Diary*. The *Health Diary* tended to be regarded as a tool with which to organize and focus a maternal and infant care education program. Regardless of the site, clients, staff members, and providers agreed that they would like to see more information on family planning, exercise, and nutrition. In addition, the *Health Diary* could be used to structure a program, sustain client contact, and maintain continuity of health education.

The usefulness of the *Health Diary* was closely connected to the ability of clients to understand and use the *Health Diary*. Clients said they understood most sections of the *Health Diary* without assistance from providers or Healthy Start staff. However, when asked about individual sections, many clients indicated they had trouble understanding some sections. There was considerable variation in the opinions of Healthy Start staff members and maternal and infant care providers about whether the *Health Diary* is written at too high a reading level for many Healthy Start clients to use. A number of staff members and providers thought the *Health Diary* required too high a reading comprehension level for the most needy clients. These staff members thought the *Health Diary* should be rewritten at a lower reading comprehension level so that it could be accessible to all Healthy Start clients.

Probably, a number of Healthy Start clients were unwilling to take the time or were unable to comprehend some of the *Health Diary* material. However, it also seemed likely that the material was accessible to most clients, which suggests that the issue was whether a handbook like the *Health Diary* should be targeted at the lowest, highest, or some midpoint of reading levels of the target audience. The most prevalent opinion among Healthy Start and providers was that the reading level of the *Health Diary* was appropriate.

The incentive program used in the Northern Plains site seemed to add considerable interest and enthusiasm for using the *Health Diary*. In this site, clients were awarded "credits" for attending prenatal care appointments, health classes, and other activities, such as smoking cessation and abstaining from alcohol and drugs. The credits could be refunded for gifts and infant care supplies. The *Health Diary* was used as a method of verifying that clients had attended appointments. The strength of the incentive program was that it created a vehicle for sustaining client contact and interaction with the Healthy Start program and its goals and objectives. Many Healthy Start staff members and providers indicated that maintaining contact with clients and reinforcing maternal and child health promotion messages were the strongest techniques they had with clients.

Summary

The *Health Diary* is a popular and useful health education tool that is well suited to the needs of Healthy Start programs but could also be appropriate in other public health settings where pregnant women receive services. The overwhelmingly positive reaction to the *Health Diary* by the multicultural sample of women who participated in this case study is also encouraging for the development of health education materials with broad application to diverse groups of women. Several "lessons" from this case study could be significant for the field of multicultural health education. First, evaluating health education materials in public health settings provides an opportunity for health communications researchers to test materials as they are being used by diverse populations in actual health care settings. This case study illustrates the variety of ways in which one health education manual was used in prenatal patient care settings. The women who were interviewed in the evaluation of the *Health Diary* were clients of six Healthy Start grantees located in urban as well as rural settings. They were African American, Caucasian, Latina, and American Indian women interacting with health care professionals, case managers, and layworkers in clinics and social service agencies. Understanding the experience of these women and their providers with a federally funded maternal and infant health manual should aid in the development of other health education materials for low-income multicultural populations.

Second, the success of the *Health Diary* in its appeal to a culturally diverse audience supports the idea that health education materials, when carefully developed, can have universal appeal. Despite the ethnic diversity in the sample of women interviewed, 90% of the clients said they liked the *Health Diary*, 89% said it provided more detailed information on some topics related to pregnancy and infant care than they had previously received, and 64% read the *Health Diary* at least once a week. Many of the providers explained this widespread appeal of the *Health Diary* to their clients by noting that it was "culturally neutral." These findings suggest that health communication programs should be careful not to assume that special cultural approaches are necessary without formative research to suggest a need for these approaches.

A third implication of this evaluation relates to the underlying intent of health education materials. Is the goal of a publication like the *Health Diary* intended to extend beyond education to support behavior change? If so, the information from this case study of the various modes providers used to integrate the *Health Diary* into their health education efforts is important. Although almost all the women interviewed used the *Health Diary*, not all providers used it during their appointments with these women. This was particularly the case with infant care providers. There were also variations in the way that health providers, layworkers, and professional case managers interacted with clients around the *Health Diary.* If health education materials are to become an integral part of patient care and are to affect behavioral change, training materials and suggested models for patient/provider use of health education materials that emphasize systematic and comprehensive approaches should accompany the distribution of these materials.

A fourth lesson learned from the evaluation of the *Health Diary* was what additional information the pregnant women interviewed would like to learn about their pregnancy. One quarter to a third of all women interviewed wanted information on medical tests and the reasons these tests were necessary, sex during and after pregnancy, family planning, nutrition, and exercise. This information is important to any pregnant woman in terms of being a well-informed patient and having better reproductive health and a healthier lifestyle.

Finally, even health education materials as useful as the *Health Diary* may not be appropriate for a substantial subset of low-income pregnant women. There were concerns among Healthy Start staff members and providers about the ability of all of their clients to read and understand the health education materials presented in the *Health Diary.* Most providers estimated that between 10% and 20% of clients would have problems reading the material. These estimates correspond with those of the women themselves. Depending on the Healthy Start site, between 21% and 29% of the women interviewed said that they had difficulty understanding some of the material in the *Health Diary.* Clearly, other forms of health education materials written at a lower reading level or other modes of communicating health education material intended for broad distribution are needed. Group presentations or recordings and video presentations of material as well as follow-up reviews and explanations by trained providers and health educators may help to bring the information on pregnancy and infant care contained in the *Health Diary* to this group of women.

Note

1. The *Health Diary* subsequently has been translated into Spanish and a second printing of a revised version of the *Health Diary* has been distributed to Healthy Start grantees and other maternal and child health programs funded through the Title V MCH Block Grant.

References

Center for Health Policy Studies. (1995). *Final Report: Health Diary Case Study Evalua-tion.* Columbia, MD: Author.

Howell, E., Devaney, B., Foot, B., Harrington, M., Schettini, M., McCormick, M. C., Hill, I., Schwalberg, R., & Zimmerman, B. (1997). *The implementation of Healthy Start: Lessons for the future.* Princeton, NJ: Mathematica Policy Research. (Available from Jan Watterworth, Librarian, Mathematica Policy Research, P.O. Box 2393, Princeton, NJ 08543-2393; 609/275-2350 or 609/275-2334 or from the World Wide Web: http://www.mathematica-mpr.com)

Howell, E. M. (1998, May). *The Northern Plains Healthy Start Project.* Draft report. (Can be ordered on the World Wide Web at http://www.mathematica-mpr.com/northplains.pdf)

U.S. Department of Health and Human Services. (1999). *Child Health U.S.A. 1999.* Washington, DC: Author.

8

Parent–Child Communication in Drug Abuse Prevention Among Adolescents

Gauri Bhattacharya

In a 1996 survey (*National Survey*, 1996), American adolescents and their parents identified drugs as the biggest problem they face. However, they differed significantly in their perceptions of the discussions they had on the

AUTHOR'S NOTE: This study was supported by a grant from the National Institute on Drug Abuse (DA09982: Gauri Bhattacharya, principal investigator). The views expressed herein do not necessarily reflect the positions of the granting agency or of the institution by which the author was employed. At the time of this study, the author was a principal investigator at the National Development and Research Institutes, New York. Address correspondence to the author at the University of Illinois at Urbana-Champaign, School of Social Work, 1207 West Oregon Street, Urbana, IL 61801. Phone: 217 244-5222; E-mail: gbhattac@uiuc.edu dangers of drug use; 94% of the parents reported that they had discussions with their children about the risks of drug use, but only 64% of the adolescents confirmed that these discussions took place. This finding raises a critical question: What could explain the differences in the perceptions of the communication of messages between parents and adolescents regarding the harmful consequences of drug use?

Parent-child communication is an interactive process that influences behavior directly through the social reinforcement of positive behavior (the clear communication of pro-social behavior and positive consequences) and the development of values and attitudes against drug use. Previous researchers have indicated that youths' perceptions of their family's attitude toward drug use and abuse influence youths' own perceptions of norms and attitudes regarding the use of drugs. The process of distilling and integrating any messages, including those on drug abuse prevention, however, varies among individuals. These differences are determined by individuals' perceptions and beliefs, based on sociocultural, familial, and environmental factors. This situation, in turn, may lead to variations in the impact of messages among individuals. To gain a better understanding of the efficacy of the parent-child communication process in the context of drug use prevention among adolescents, researchers need to examine the following questions:

1. What factors could promote the efficacy of parents' communication with their adolescent children?

2. Is this parent-child communication process similar in all cultural groups?

3. What are the issues from practice, research, and policy perspectives that can improve this communication process?

To address these questions, I first identify the risk factors that may influence the use and abuse of drugs among adolescents. Knowledge of the risk factors informs parents of the areas in which their children are vulnerable to drug use and abuse from a developmental perspective. Once these areas are known, parents can target them in their messages about drug abuse prevention to their children. Second, I examine the communication process among Asian Indian adolescents and their parents—by presenting a study on Asian Indian adolescents that examined the extent to which similar and unique family variables rooted in cultural contexts may differently affect the messages conveyed. Third, I consider the ways in which the efficacy of the communication process can be improved and present a range of issues from research, practice, and policy perspectives to guide future studies.

Risk Factors Contributing to Adolescent Drug Use

Previous theoretical and empirical findings have shown that the onset, severity, and pattern of drug use and abuse are positively associated with multiple risk factors (biological, social, familial, personality, behavioral, and environmental) present in the individual and the environment (Ellickson & Hays, 1992; Hawkins, Catalano, & Miller, 1992; Newcomb, 1995). Because adolescence is the period of socialization or transition from childhood to adulthood, when emotional, psychological, and sociocultural skills are learned, it is a critical time for implementing interventions against drug use. In particular, studies have shown that adolescents' behavior (pro-social or antisocial, including drug use and abuse) is positively associated with the predominant behaviors, cultural orientations, norms, and values of the families to whom the adolescents are bonded (Brook & Brook, 1992; Jessor & Jessor, 1977; Kandel, 1982). To develop strategies to prevent drug use and abuse, these underlying mechanisms (individual as well as contextual) of family relationships and drug use/abuse must first be understood.

Previous researchers found a positive correlation between the characteristics of peer networks (peers' drug use and school achievement) and adolescents' drug use (Adler & Lotecka, 1973; Brook, Balka, Gursen, Brook, & Shapiro, 1997; Oetting & Beauvais, 1990). Adolescents who associate with deviant peers follow a similar pattern of behavior and thus reinforce one another's deviant behavior. Recent research on drug abuse established a link between academic success/school achievement and low drug use by adolescents (Swaim, Beauvais, Chavez, & Oetting, 1997) and emphasized that adolescents who stay in school are less likely than those who drop out to use illicit drugs.

Although peer influence is a final pathway to drug abuse among adolescents, studies indicate that pro-social family interactions and strong, positive parent-child relationships can reduce risks and protect adolescents' association with drug-abusing and otherwise deviant peers (Brook, Brook, Gordon, Whiteman, & Cohen, 1990; Newcomb & Felix-Ortiz, 1992; Resnick et al., 1997; Swaim, Oetting, Edwards, & Beauvais, 1989). A pro-social family interaction process entails parents' supervision and monitoring of children's activities. Parents who supervise and monitor their children's behavior at home, grades in school, and network of peers are often the first persons to notice any behavioral changes in their adolescents (such as cutting classes and bonding with deviant peers). Often, they are also the first persons to be able to find out if those changes are related to drug use and abuse and can then act immediately to intervene in the process (Kumpfer & Alvarado, 1995). Parents can decide on the optimal timing, contents, and mechanisms for influencing adolescents' behavior. In the case study presented in this chapter, effective monitoring entailed the parents' knowledge of their children's activities at home, at school, and with peers. Following this model, drug use prevention messages and early intervention programs recommend focusing on developing parent-child communication strategies.

Racial/Ethnic Differences in Communicating Messages

Previous researchers indicated that adolescents' perceptions of their family's attitude toward drug use and abuse influence youths' own perceptions of norms and attitudes regarding the use of drugs and may influence their decisions to use (or not to use) drugs (Brook, 1993; Dishion, Reid, & Patterson, 1988; Kumpfer & Turner, 1990-1991). Particularly, adolescents' perceptions of their family's beliefs about the use of alcohol and its effects for socializing purposes have been cited as a critical factor in group differences in alcohol use among Caucasians, African Americans, and Hispanic adolescents (Johnson & Johnson, 1999).

In addition, studies have emphasized that parents' style of monitoring and supervision of their children may be associated with the efficacy of parent-child communication on drug use prevention (Barnes & Farrell, 1992; Dishion & Loeber, 1985). However, they did not associate any particular type of parenting style (such as authoritarian) with less drug abuse across the ethnic groups. For example, Baumarind (1991) found that the authoritarian parenting style was associated with the increased use of alcohol among Caucasian adolescents, but not among African American or Hispanic adolescents (Canino & Zayas, 1997). Thus, the communication of a clear, consistent message about the rules and norms of pro-social behavior, *not* a particular style of discipline and monitoring, can buffer the risks of drug use. Messages that emphasize the negative consequences of drinking alcohol and the disciplinary consequences of violating the behavioral rules have been found to be effective in preventing alcohol abuse among African American adolescents (Peterson, Hawkins, Abbott, & Catalano, 1995).

A Case Study of Asian Indian Adolescents

This study aimed (a) to identify the factors that are age appropriate and critical for conveying drug abuse prevention messages effectively by parents to their children and (b) to examine the relationships of those factors to the use and abuse of drugs among Asian Indian adolescents. Adolescents who were born in the United States and their parents who emigrated from India are referred to as Asian Indians. Grounded in family relationship theory and previous research on drug use and abuse among adolescents, this study assessed the influence of three elements in parent-child communication—harmful consequences of drug use, expectations of high grades in school, and approval of the peer network. Because the effectiveness of any communication mechanism depends on how the target audience validates the importance of the message, this community-based survey examined (a) Asian Indian adolescents' perceptions of their parents' concerns about children's drug abuse and (b) the extent to which the adolescents cared about their parents' concerns (details of this study have been published in Bhattacharya, Cleland, & Holland, 1999).

Method

Sampling Procedure

The sample for this community-based study consisted of 200 Asian Indian adolescents, 116 males and 84 females, aged 13 to 18, who were born in the United States and resided in the greater New York metropolitan area. The data were part of a larger research project funded by the National Institute on Drug Abuse (NIDA) to examine the relationships between generational conflicts and drug abuse among the same subjects.

A two-stage stratified sampling procedure was used to collect data based on place of birth (the United States or another country) and age. The subjects were interviewed using a semistructured instrument adapted from relevant validated scales and items used by previous researchers (Center for Therapeutic Community Research, 1993). The Institutional Review Board of the National Development and Research Institutes approved the measurement protocols. Both the parents and subjects provided informed consent. The questionnaire was field-tested for cultural relevance, reliability, and validity for Asian Indian adolescents. A single interviewer administered the instrument in a group setting. Data were collected from May 1997 to February 1998, the interview protocol took 40 to 60 minutes to complete, and each subject was paid $15 as compensation for his or her time.

Semistructured Survey Questionnaire

Adolescent-reported data included sociodemographic characteristics for themselves (such as age, gender, and grades in school) and their parents (marital status, education, and occupation). Additional data were collected in three domains: (a) adolescents' characteristics—drug use/abuse and concerns for their parents' expectations of their grades and drug use/abuse; (b) parents' communication of their awareness/concerns for the adolescents' school grades, consequences of drug use, and peer networks; and (c) characteristics of peer networks—education and drug abuse. Response patterns followed the Likert-scale format. Examples of items included parents' awareness about drug abuse ("How much does *your family* care if *you* smoke cigarettes?"), what parents talked about ("To what extent has *your family* talked to *you* about the dangers of smoking cigarettes?"), parents' approval of the adolescents' peer network ("Does *your family* approve of *your* friends?"), and the adolescents' caring about their parents' concerns ("How much do *you care* about *your family's* concerns about *you using drugs?*"). Adolescent-reported data were analyzed using descriptive and multiple-regression techniques.

Drug Use and Abuse

A section on drug use/abuse documented the extent of the adolescents' involvement (frequency and quantity) with cigarettes, alcohol, marijuana, and other "hard" drugs (cocaine, opiates, hallucinogens, and amphetamines/speed and the nonmedical use of prescription drugs). In addition, data were collected on the context (variety of times and places) of drug use, drug use partners, reasons for use, and history of use (age at first use) for a variety of drugs, including alcohol and cigarettes. Drug use was measured for the following periods: ever (lifetime), in the past 12 months, and 30 days before the interview. The frequency and quantity of use were measured separately for each of the three drugs commonly used by adolescents (cigarettes, alcohol, and marijuana) and all other drugs. Frequency was measured on a 7-point scale, ranging from 1 (*never used*) to 7 (*used more than once every day*), and quantity was measured from 1 (*no ingestion*) to 7 (*heavy use*—two or more packs of cigarettes, five or more alcoholic beverages at one sitting, or six or more marijuana cigarettes a day).

Results

Description of the Sample

The sample consisted of 58% males and 42% females with a mean age of 16, 93% of whom were living with both parents. More than 70% of both parents were high school graduates and 83% of both parents were currently employed. With regard to employment categories, 62% of the fathers and 50% of the mothers were employed as professionals, and 25% of the mothers and 22% of the fathers were managers or salespersons

Extent, Frequency, and Quantity of Drug Use

The data in Table 8.1 show the prevalence of drug use in this sample. Of the 200 adolescents, 33 (16.5%) had smoked *cigarettes* at least once (ever). Of these, 5 smoked less than one cigarette per day, and 4 smoked less than half a pack per day. Of the 200 adolescents, 56 (28%) had ever tried (at least once) some kind of *alcoholic beverage,* primarily wine (20.5%) and beer (18%). Of these, 78% had used wine and wine coolers at least once in the past 12 months, 75% had used liquor, and 69% had used beer. Of the 5 adolescents who reported ever having tried *marijuana,* 3 had smoked it in the past 12 months before the interview. Two of the 5 adolescents reported smoking marijuana several times during that period, and the remaining 3 reported smoking about once per week. Finally, of the 7 adolescents who reported having ever tried a *hard drug* in the past 12 months, one had used cocaine several times, 1 had used both crack and heroin about once a month, and 1 had used an "upper" (amphetamines, speed, or prescription diet pills) one time.

Relationships Between Adolescents' Drug Use and Parents' Concerns

Users Versus Nonusers of Drugs. To explore which variables may be related to drug use, 65 (32.5%) adolescents who had tried some form of tobacco, alcohol, or other drug were compared with the remaining 135 (67.5%) adolescents who did not report drug use of any kind (see Table 8.2). The results indicated that the adolescents who reported having tried tobacco, alcohol, marijuana, or other drug seemed to have peers with lower academic performance, peers who had used drugs, and peers of whom their parents were less likely to approve. In

Table 8.1 Drug Use Among Asian-Indian Adolescents—Prevalence Rate, by Type of Drug ($N = 200$)

Type of Drug	Ever Used[a]		Used in the Past 12 Months[b]	
	Percentage	n1	Percentage	n2
Cigarettes	16.5	33	27.3[c]	9[c]
Beer	18.0	36	69.4	25
Wine	20.5	41	78.0	32
Wine cooler	11.5	23	78.3	18
Liquor	10.0	20	75.0	15
Marijuana	2.5	5	60.0	3
Other drugs	3.5	7	85.7	6

SOURCE: Bhattacharya, Cleland, and Holland (1999). Reprinted with permission from Kluwer Academic/Plenum Publishers.
NOTE: Percentage ever used: n1 as a percentage of N; percentage used in the past 12 months: n2 as a percentage of n1.
a. Ever used—used at least once
b. Used in the past 12 months—used at least once in the 12 months prior to the survey.
c. Used in the past 30 days.

addition, the parents of these adolescents were less concerned about drug use than were the parents of adolescents who had never used any kind of drug.

Parental Concerns and Drug Abuse. The parents' concerns for education and the adolescents' academic performance were positively and significantly related ($r = .26$; $p < .05$). The parents' communication of the harmful consequences of drug use was correlated ($p < .05$) with less drug use by the adolescents, and the parents' concern about the adolescents' drug use was positively related to the parents' approval of the adolescents' friends ($r = .28$; $p < .05$). A greater level of parental concern about drug use was associated with less drug use by the adolescents ($r = .27$; $p < .05$). Adolescents' caring about their parents' concerns predicted users versus nonusers of drugs ($p < .005$).

Table 8.2 Characteristics of Peers, Parents, and Adolescents: Differences Between Drug Users and Nonusers

Characteristics	Nonusers (n = 135)		Users (n = 65)				
	Mean	SD	Mean	SD	t	df	p
Peers' academic performance	.16	.86	−.34	1.18	3.29	185	.001
Parents' educational concern	3.83	.29	3.76	.44	1.32	197	.188
Parents' drug use concern	3.46	.56	3.13	.58	3.88	194	.000
Parents' approval of friends	.11	.96	−.22	1.06	2.17	195	.032
Peers' substance use	.44	.66	.7461	.62	−3.12	194	.002
Adolescents' caring for parents' concerns	3.74	.57	3.48	.67	2.81	194	.005
Adolescents' academic performance	4.03	.79	4.16	.71	−1.11	193	.270

SOURCE: Bhattacharya, Cleland, and Holland (1999). Reprinted with permission from Kluwer Academic/Plenum Publishers.

Discussion

This study identified three critical factors in parental communication and monitoring associated with Asian Indian adolescents not using drugs. First, the parents' awareness of their children's educational performance and success in school was associated with the adolescents' bonding with nondrug users. Second, parents' communication of the harmful consequences of drug use was linked with adolescents' nonuse of drugs. Third, parents' approval of their children's peer networks significantly influenced the adolescents' nonassociation with drug-using peers. The findings of this study thus corroborated those of previous studies that a parent-child communication strategy must address the importance of academic success, the harmful consequences of drug abuse, and association with nondeviant peers.

The findings reaffirm that adolescents' perception of their parents' concern and the extent to which adolescents' care about their parents' concern are determinants of the effectiveness of the communication strategy. The development of a drug prevention communication strategy must address two components: (a) content—communicators delivering specific messages to the target audience—and (b) perceived importance—the audience recognizing the importance of the contents of the message. These two components contribute to the need to understand that communication is a process and that these two components work together. For example, to be effective, parent-child communication must counter false perceptions among adolescents that drug use is normative and is a part of growing up (Flay, 1987). At the same time, adolescents must accept the negative consequences of drug use and the positive benefits of not doing drugs (e.g., in regard to health, school achievements, sports).

Implications for Research, Practice, and Policy

The findings of this and other studies substantiate the importance of parent-child communication as a mechanism for influencing drug use behavior among adolescents. Although there is a general agreement among program developers and researchers that parent-child communication is a critical mechanism, many questions regarding the ways in which this process can be made effective remain unanswered. This observation takes us back to the survey findings that mentioned the wide gap between the perceptions of parents and adolescents on parents' communication of messages against the use of drugs. For optimal and effective use of the parent-child communication process, the following issues are presented from research, practice, and policy perspectives.

Research

Research in the areas of family beliefs and the pathways explaining ethnic group differences in drug abuse is currently in its initial stage. Parent-child communication has been linked to group differences in buffering alcohol drinking, but this link has not been found in tobacco and marijuana smoking.

Studies are warranted to examine the different components of the communication process and how they affect, in isolation and in combination, the use of different substances—alcohol, tobacco, marijuana, and other drugs.

Studies are also needed to understand the unique and universal risk factors and their impact on drug use in different ethnic groups. Empirically based longitudinal studies indicate that the effects of risk factors are not likely to be the same or equally powerful across all ethnic groups, although there may be similarities (Brook, 1993; Etz, Robertson, & Ashery, 1998; Gfroerer & De La Rosa, 1993). Currently, research does not recommend developing separate parent/child-based communication strategies for each ethnic group but emphasizes that communication strategies must be tailored to specific cultural contexts.

The parent-child communication issue seems to be critical in the context of understanding the acculturation process and immigrant families. A pertinent question is this: To what extent are cultural variables entangled with the various dimensions of the parent-child communication process? For example, the beliefs of Asian Indian adolescents who were born in the United States about socialization and alcohol drinking may differ from those of their parents, because adolescents' beliefs may be shaped by the norms prevailing in the United States. Thus, the question arises: Would immigrant parents' disciplining and monitoring style be equally effective for first- and second-generation immigrant children? As mentioned earlier, the bonding and attachment between parents and children buffer children from drug abuse. Indeed, more information is needed to elucidate the parent-child relationships among immigrant children. Another related question in understanding the effectiveness of the parent-child communication process is this: Do sociocultural factors influence adolescents' compliance with parents' disciplining system? Often, sociocultural variables prescribe behavioral norms and expectations for family members. For example, the concept of self is integrated more with familial and community components for individuals in Asian, Hispanic, and African American families than for those in Caucasian families. In Asian families, parents explicitly express their children's duties and responsibilities in the family structure. Moreover, adolescents' socializing with peers from the same ethnic group may further reinforce the rules and norms expressed by their parents. Parents' delineation of their children's behavior with the expectations of enhancing family pride may indicate the family's attitude toward pro-social behavior and can mediate drug use among adolescents.

Previous research focused broadly on family relationships variables and drug abuse prevention interventions (Brook, 1993). For guiding prevention/intervention programs on communication, data are needed to examine the elements and dimensions of the communication process. Data are needed on the content (what is said) of the messages, context (where communication takes place), and style (how the messages are presented). Research on risk and protective factors can assist parents to convey age-appropriate messages to their children. Contexts for discussing the harmful consequences of drug use may contribute to the effectiveness of the messages. For example, discussion at the dinner table in the presence of parents, other siblings, and extended family members can energize and heighten the value and the importance of the messages. Style indicates the mechanisms that parents adopt to convey the harmful consequences of drug use, the criteria parents use to approve peer networks, and how children react when peers are not approved. Data are also needed to determine why some adolescents value their parents' concerns and others do not.

Another critical area that requires further research is whether the parent-child communication process is gender specific. Gender-specific role expectancies regarding no or less drug use among females prevail cross-culturally. However, recent data on drug abuse among American adolescents indicate that the rate of drug use among females is increasing (Johnston, Bachman, & O'Malley, 1998). Research findings must delineate if the effectiveness of the parent-child communication process is different for males and females and if the differences are related to sociocultural and familial factors.

One promising trend in research is studies on the family practices of various ethnic groups. Researchers recognize the importance of examining the family communication processes in ethnic groups (such as African Americans, Hispanics, and Asian Indians) in which drug use among adolescents is lower than among "mainstream" Caucasians. A comparison of the lifetime use of cigarettes, alcohol, and marijuana by racial/ethnic groups was the lowest among African Americans (cigarettes, 47.3%; alcohol, 71.9%; marijuana, 42.7%), followed by Hispanics (cigarettes, 63.0%; alcohol, 82.5%; marijuana, 50.2%), and Caucasian Americans (cigarettes, 69.8%; alcohol, 84.2%; marijuana, 60.9%) (Johnston et al., 1998). Most of the research on family practices has been done on alcohol-related problems, but research needs to be extended to the use of other drugs.

Practice

There is a broad societal consensus on issues such as preventing drug abuse among adolescents. However, parents often lack the skills to discuss sensitive issues with their children, such as drug use and related deviant behavior, including sexual promiscuity. Communication strategies must be developed not merely as a medium of prevention and intervention but to ensure that parents are able to execute the messages effectively (Leshner, 1996). In particular, communication among adolescents born in the United States and their immigrant parents regarding norms of drug use may be difficult because of their differential cultural orientations. Differential acculturation levels that may enhance the gap in the parent-child communication process include (a) cultural identity conflict, (b) value conflict because of changes in roles and responsibilities, and (c) the lack of functional skills, including linguistic constraints, leading to socialization problems. This conflict in views between adolescents and parents may affect family relationships and create parent-child communication problems. The lack of communication, conflicts in communication, or both may lead to the adolescents' alienation from their parents, which may subsequently lead adolescents to use drugs as a way of ameliorating these conflicts. Therefore, understanding the parent-child communication process in the context of specific sociocultural characteristics is a special need that should be addressed for developing drug abuse prevention communication strategies (Bhattacharya, 1998b).

Enhancing Parents' Communication Skills. Techniques, such as enhancing interactive communication skills and involving parents in children' activities, have been found to be effective in conveying messages to adolescents and are recommended (Bhattacharya, 1998a). Although the content of the messages is crucial, equally powerful are parents' efforts to facilitate and reinforce their children's capability to follow the directions they give. Three areas identified in the content of messages are dispelling the myths of (a) socializing and alcohol use, (b) the use of cigarettes and marijuana as a part of growing up, and (c) that everyone is doing drugs. However, for the messages to be effective, it is imperative that adolescents perceive the negative consequences of drug use. The mechanisms that convert external meanings into internal beliefs determine whether adolescents will adhere consistently to the positive beliefs of pro-social behavior. Studies indicate that (a) youths' perceptions of the norms of drug use are shaped by observing and imitating (social learning) the drug use and attitudes of closely bonded persons (such as their parents and peers) and (b) the motivation to comply with the perceived norms is influenced by youths' cultural and social bonding with their families, school, and peers. Parents' modeling of drug use behavior may encourage children to contextualize pro-social behavior within the family unit.

Studies have found that perceived norms and attitudes regarding the use of drugs influence the decision to use (or not to use) drugs. Thus, parent-child communication mechanisms need to guide adolescents in this decision-making process and to develop self-efficacy so that children learn effective ways to avoid these harmful situations.

Enhancing Parents' Management Skills. Parental supervision and monitoring require parents' direct involvement with adolescents' activities at home, in school, and with peers. To learn to do so, parents may need to be educated to provide consistent discipline and nurturance at home. Previous research (Rogoff, 1990) noted that guided family participation (like going on outings and doing yard work together) and assigned responsibilities communicate feelings of connectedness to children that they are important contributing members in the family. Researchers identified the following predictors of less substance abuse: (a) praise and clear rule setting, (b) practices regarding monitoring and punishment, (c) attachment to parents, and (d) parents' disapproval of drug abuse (Catalano et al., 1992). This study also emphasized that ethnic differences are important in understanding the influence of parenting and other family factors on drug abuse.

Policy

Parent-child communication is recognized as a critical protective factor in the prevention of substance use/abuse. Parents' transmission of values and attitudes toward drugs (influencing demand) and their imposition of physical impediments to the availability of drugs (controlling supply) directly affect the demand for drugs as well as their supply. Within this broad policy, two recommendations are suggested for future policy directions: (a) Adapt a universal prevention policy from a multicultural perspective, and (b) target intervention policies to both adolescents and their parents. The family is the first socializing unit in a child's life. Because the early use of drugs is found to be a predictor of future drug abuse, family-based early intervention is recommended for drug abuse prevention. A universal prevention policy requires structuring communication strategies that will map the specific and appropriate mechanisms for all cultural groups. To achieve this objective, research must delineate the similar and unique sociocultural factors that can influence the decision to use (or not to use) drugs. A comprehensive approach based on a theoretical conceptualization with a practical perspective is recommended for this purpose.

Educating parents on how to develop communication patterns, in general with their adolescent children—particularly about drug use prevention—is a component that has not yet received full consideration at the policy level.

Researchers indicate that parent-based intervention programs allow parents to make value judgments and decisions about the content, context, and style of presentation (Jaccard & Turrisi, 1999). The influences of parents as change agents during adolescence has now been established in studies. The variables that can impede parents' influence on their children include low levels of control and empowerment, the lack of awareness of what is happening in children's lives, and poor communication skills. Maintaining a balance between assertive discipline and bonding is essential in communicating sensitive issues, such as the harmful consequences of drug use. The availability of information from the media and community-based organizations can have an impact in this context.

Conclusion

Three critical factors that promote parents' effective communication with and monitoring of their adolescent children are (a) parents' awareness of children's educational performance and success in school, (b) parents' clear communication of the harmful consequences of drug use, and (c) parents' approval of their children's peer networks. Future studies are needed to understand the contents, context, and style of presentation of parent-child communication in family settings. Because cultural orientations, values, and norms influence communication patterns, the effectiveness of the same messages in different cultural groups may differ. A multicultural perspective in research, practice, and policy areas is recommended to filter the pro-social drug use/abuse prevention messages in parent-child communication strategies.

References

Adler, P. T., & Lotecka, L. (1973). Drug use among high school students: Patterns and correlates. *International Journal of the Addictions, 8,* 537-548.

Barnes, G. M., & Farrell, M. P. (1992). Parental support and control as predictors of adolescent drinking, delinquency, and related problem behaviors. *Journal of Marriage and Family, 54,* 773-776.

Baumarind, D. (1991). The influence of parenting style on adolescence competence and substance abuse. *Journal of Early Adolescence, 11,* 56-95.

Bhattacharya, G. (1998a). Communicating to prevent drug use among adolescents: Linking social work practice with public health strategies. *Health promotion and education database.* Atlanta, GA: Centers for Disease Control and Prevention.

Bhattacharya, G. (1998b). Drug use among Asian-Indian adolescents: Identifying protective/risk factors, *Adolescence, 33,* 169-179.

Bhattacharya, G., Cleland, C., & Holland, S. (1999). Peer networks, parental attributes, and drug use among Asian-Indian adolescents born in the United States, *Journal of Immigrant Health,* 1 (3), 14

Brook, D. W., & Brook, J. S. (1992). Family processes associated with alcohol and drug use and abuse. In E. Kaufman & P. Kaufman (Eds.), *Family therapy of drug and alcohol abuse* (pp. 15-33). Boston: Allyn & Bacon.

Brook, J. S. (1993). Interactional theory: Its utility in explaining drug use behavior among African-American and Puerto Rican youth. In M. R. De La Rosa & J-L Recio Adrados (Eds.), *Drug abuse among minority youth: advances in research and methodology* (NIH Publication No., 93-3479; pp. 79-97). Washington, DC: Government Printing Office.

Brook, J. S., Balka, E. B., Gursen, M. D., Brook, D. W., & Shapiro, J. (1997). Young adults' drug use: A 17-year longitudinal inquiry of antecedents. *Psychological Reports, 80,* 1235-1251.

Brook, J. S., Brook, D. W., Gordon, A. S., Whiteman, M., & Cohen, P. (1990). The psychosocial etiology of adolescent drug use: A family interactional approach. *Genetic, Social, and General Psychology Monograph, 116* (Whole No. 2).

Canino, I., & Zayas, L. H. (1997). Puerto Rican children. In G. Johnson-Powell & J. Yamamoto (Eds.), *Transcultural child development: Psychological assessment and treatment* (pp. 61-79). New York: John Wiley.

Catalano, R. F., Morrison, D. M., Wells, E. A., Gillmore, M. R., Iritani, B., & Hawkins, J. D. (1992). Ethnic differences in family factors related to early drug initiation. *Journal on the Study of Alcohol, 53,* 208-217.

Center for Therapeutic Community Research. (1993). *Drug abuse among adolescents: Survey protocol.* New York: National Development and Research Institutes.

Dishion, T. J., & Loeber, R. (1985). Adolescent marijuana and alcohol use: The role of parents and peers revisited. *American Journal of Drug and Alcohol Abuse, 11,* 11-25.

Dishion, T. J., Reid, J. B., & Patterson, G. R. (1988). Empirical guidelines for a family intervention for adolescent drug use. *Journal of Chemical Dependency Treatment, 1,* 189-214.

Ellickson, P. L., & Hays, R. D. (1992). On becoming involved with drugs: Modeling adolescent drug use over time. *Health Psychology, 11*(6), 377-385.

Etz, K. E., Robertson, E. B., & Ashery, R. S. (1998). Drug abuse prevention through family-based interventions: Future research. In R. S. Ashery, E. B. Robertson, & K. L. Kumpfer (Eds.), *Drug abuse prevention through family interventions* (NIH Publication No., 99-4135; pp. 1-11). Washington, DC: Government Printing Office.

Flay, B. R. (1987). Mass media and smoking cessation: A critical review. *American Journal of Public Health, 77,* 153-160.

Gfroerer, J. & De La Rosa, M. (1993). Protective and risk factors associated with drug use among Hispanic youth. *Journal of Addictive Diseases, 12*(2), 87-107.

Hawkins, J. D., Catalano, R. F., & Miller, J. Y. (1992). Risk and protective factors for alcohol and other drug problems in adolescence and early adulthood: Implications for substance abuse problems. *Psychological Bulletin, 112,* 64-105.

Jaccard, J., & Turrisi, R. (1999). Parent-based intervention strategies to reduce adolescent alcohol-impaired driving. *Journal of Studies on Alcohol, 13,* 84-93.

Jessor, R., & Jessor, G. L. (1977). *Problem behavior and psychosocial development: A longitudinal study of youth.* New York: Academic Press.

Johnson, P., & Johnson, H. (1999). Cultural and familial influences that maintain the negative meaning of alcohol. *Journal of Studies on Alcohol, 13*(13), 79-83.

Johnston, L. D., Bachman, J. G., & O'Malley, P. M. (1998). *Monitoring the future study.* Ann Arbor: University of Michigan, Institute for Social Research, Survey Research Center.

Kandel, D. B. (1982). Epidemiological and psychosocial perspectives on adolescent drug use. *Journal of the American Academy on Clinical Psychiatry, 21,* 328-347.

Kumpfer, K. L., & Alvarado, R. (1995). Strengthening families to prevent drug use in multiethnic youth. In G. J. Botvin, S. Schinke, & M. A. Orlandi (Eds.), *Drug abuse prevention with multiethnic youth* (pp. 255-283). Thousand Oaks, CA: Sage.

Kumpfer, K. L., & Turner, C. (1990-1991). The social ecology model of adolescent substance abuse: Implications for prevention. *International Journal of the Addictions, 25,* 435-463.

Leshner, A. (1996). NIDA seeks new keys to preventing drug abuse among adolescents. *NIDA NOTES, 11*(3), 3-4.

National Survey of American Attitudes on Substance Abuse and Addiction II: Teens and their Parents [Press release]. (1996, September 9). New York: Columbia University, National Center on Addiction and Substance Abuse.

Newcomb, M. D. (1995). Drug use etiology among ethnic minority adolescents: Risk and protective factors. In G. J. Botvin., S. Schinke., & M. A. Orlandi (Eds.), *Drug abuse prevention with multiethnic youth* (pp. 105-126). Thousand Oaks, CA: Sage.

Newcomb, M. D., & Felix-Ortiz, M. (1992). Multiple protective and risk factors for drug use and abuse: Cross-sectional and prospective findings. *Journal of Personality and Social Psychology, 63,* 280-296.

Oetting, E. R., & Beauvais, F. (1990). Adolescent drug use: Findings of national and local surveys. *Journal of Consulting and Clinical Psychology, 58,* 385-394.

Peterson, P. L., Hawkins, J. D., Abbott, R. D., & Catalano, R. F. (1995). Disentangling the effects of parental drinking, family management, and parental alcohol norms on current drinking by black and white adolescents. In G. M. Boyd, J. Howard, & R. A. Zucker (Eds.), *Alcohol problems among adolescents: Current directions in prevention research* (pp. 33-57). Hillsdale, NJ: Lawrence Erlbaum.

Resnick, M. E., Bearman, P. S., Blum, R. W., Bauman, K. E., Harris, K. M., Jones, J., Tabor, J., Beuhring, T., Sieving, R. E., Shew, M., Ireland, M., Bearinger, L. H., & Urdry, R. (1997). Protecting adolescents from harm: Findings from the National Longitudinal Study on adolescent health. *JAMA, 278*(10), 823-832.

Rogoff, B. (1990). *Apprenticeship in thinking: Cognitive development in social context.* New York: Oxford University Press.

Swaim, R. C., Beauvais, F., Chavez, E. L., & Oetting, E. R. (1997). The effect of dropout rates on estimates of adolescent substance use among three racial/ethnic groups, *American Journal of Public Health, 87,* 51-55.

Swaim, R. C., Oetting, E. R., Edwards, R. W., & Beauvais, F. (1989). The links from emotional distress to adolescent drug use: A path model. *Journal of Consulting and Clinical Psychology, 57*(2), 227-231.

9

The Effectiveness
of Peer Education in
STD/HIV Prevention

Donald E. Morisky
Vicki J. Ebin

Accumulating evidence suggests that the HIV epidemic in the United States has shifted from high-risk subgroups of homosexual men to adolescents and young adults, particularly those who are gay and in racial/ethnic minorities (National Institutes of Health, 1997; Warren, Harris, & Kann, 1995). Using multiple data sources, including seroprevalence, clinical, and behavioral data, Hein (1993) estimates that the number of HIV infections among 13- to 21-year-olds doubles every 14 months. Conservative estimates for adolescent risk behavior—that is, those based on nationally representative studies of in-school youths, Grades 9 through 12 from 1990 to 1995 (Kann et al., 1996)—show a high prevalence of sexual risk-taking behaviors among youths. Even though some trends revealed by these studies are promising in that they demonstrate that previously increasing rates of sexual experience have stabilized and that condom use at last intercourse has increased (Kann et al., 1996), the stabilization does not affect the increasingly early age of sexual onset over the past 20 years (Ehrhardt, 1993). Furthermore, it does not reduce the number of in-school youths who have experienced sexual intercourse before their 18th birthday—approximately 56% of females and 73% of males (Warren et al., 1995). In addition, the positive trend across years 1990 to 1995 toward increased condom use is countered by the disturbing trend whereby condom use at last intercourse peaks at Grade 10 then decreases each year according to age and grade level (Doll, 1997), a pattern also found among Canadian (Nguyet, Maheux, Beland, & Pica, 1994) and Australian (Dunne et al., 1994) youths. Compared with national samples, urban and low-income African American and Hispanic youths have even earlier ages of sexual onset and are even less likely to have used condoms at first and last intercourse (Ford, Rubinstein, & Norris, 1994).

Significance

Additional evidence for high levels of unprotected intercourse can be found in the extremely high rates of pregnancy and sexually transmitted diseases (STDs) in the adolescent population. Of U.S. female adolescents, 40% become pregnant before reaching the age of 20, and 1 million become pregnant each year (Hayes, 1987). In 1996, over a half million females less than 20 years of age gave birth ("State-Specific Birth Rates," 1997). The Centers for Disease Control, Health Promotion and Disease Prevention (CDC) reports that the birth rates for teenage women in the United States have been steadily on the rise, increasing 40% from 1982 to 1992, with African American and Hispanic birth rates being on average twice that of the nation's overall rates (Warren et al., 1995). For at least the past decade, there have been higher rates of STD infection among adolescents than among adults (Haffner, 1996). Each year since then, 2.5 to 3 million U.S. teenagers have become infected with STDs and 1 in 4 sexually active youths has been infected with an STD by the time he or she reaches the age of 21 (Donovan & Stratton, 1994; CDC, 1993; U.S. Department of Health and Human Services [DHHS], 1991). For the past several years, the largest increase of sexually transmitted diseases has been among adolescents between the ages of 10 to 19 years. Furthermore, gonorrhea case rates for adolescents have been steadily on the increase this past decade (Krowchuk, 1997).

Adolescents who are sexually active constitute a population at considerable potential risk. Despite the fact that not all adolescents are sexually active, those who are often have multiple partners (especially in the context of short-term serial relationships), and most do not regularly use condoms (DiClemente, Boyer, & Morales, 1988; DiClemente, Forrest, & Miekler, 1990). Given the long latency between initial infection and onset of an AIDS diagnosis, it is apparent that a large number of these persons first contracted HIV while still teenagers. As is true for adults, risk is not uniform for all adolescents. The adolescent populations most imminently vulnerable for contracting HIV infection are probably those most vulnerable to teenage pregnancy, STDs, and involvement in drug use networks. Several adolescent populations have been identified as being at particular high risk. These include teenage males who engage in sex with male partners; adolescents who use drugs, especially cocaine or crack, and engage in sex with multiple or high-risk partners in exchange for drugs or through association with risk-taking peers; and runaway or homeless youths who, in addition to sexual contact with peers, may engage in "survival sex" with exploitative adults in exchange for money, drugs, or a place to live (Fullilove, Fullilove, Bowser, & Gross, 1990).

Adolescence is a time of rapid physical, emotional, and cognitive growth and development; unfortunately very few studies have focused on the progression of HIV virus through the American adolescent population. As a result, very little is known about how effectively or ineffectively adolescents can resist the disease and how the infection will affect their life spans. In the absence of a vaccine against HIV or a cure for AIDS, behavior modification through health education strategies is currently the only means available by which to halt or slow down the spread of this deadly and devastating infection.

Theoretical Framework and Applications for Educational Approaches

During the early part of the AIDS epidemic, very few adolescent HIV/AIDS risk reduction interventions had been rigorously evaluated and documented to demonstrate changes in risk-taking behaviors (Brown, DiClemente, & Reynolds, 1991; Kirby & DiClemente, 1994). At this same time, an emerging body of well-controlled studies has provided evidence for intervention effectiveness among adolescent populations (Choi & Coates, 1994; Jemmott & Jemmott, 1997). The interventions that have demonstrated program effectiveness are grounded in psychosocial theories—that is, social cognitive theory (Bandura, 1986, 1992), theory of reasoned action (Ajzen, 1988; Fishbein & Ajzen, 1975), social influence theory (Deutsch & Gerard, 1955; Fisher, 1988; Kandel, 1986, 1996)—or combinations of these approaches—for example, the AIDS risk reduction model (Catania, Kegeles, & Coates, 1990; Rotheram-Borus, Koopman, & Rosario, 1995). Although the most effective interventions have been based on solid theoretical frameworks and generally on formative research with target populations, they have also used different design characteristics and different delivery techniques—for example, educational videos (O'Donnell, Doval, Duran, & O'Donnell (1995) and skill training (Gillmore et al., 1997). Condom purchase rates were almost doubled when individuals participated in the combination of a culturally appropriate video-based presentation followed by group discussion compared with video presentation alone. However, many of these intervention studies are limited to adolescents at relatively low HIV/AIDS risk, whereas others are compromised by significant methodological limitations. For example, one study identified minimal effectiveness of specific condom motivation classes for teens; however, significant contamination effects may have compromised the randomization of the two study groups (Smith, Weinman, & Parrilli, 1997).

Social Influence Modeling

Social influence from peers has been examined as a determinant of numerous health-related behaviors among adolescents, including tobacco and alcohol prevention (Hansen, Malotte, & Fielding, 1988), sexual activity and pregnancy prevention (Davis, 1994; Steiner, Shields, Noble, & Bayer, 1994), HIV/AIDS risk reduction (Kipke, Boyer, & Hein, 1993; Podschun, 1993; Quirk, Godkin, & Schwenzfeier, 1993; Remafedi, 1994; Shafer & Boyer, 1991; Slap, Plotkin, Khalid, Michelman, & Forke, 1991), smokeless tobacco use (Gottlieb, Pope, Rickert, & Hardin, 1993), anabolic steroid use (Komoroski & Riskert, 1992), drinking and driving prevention (Klepp, Perry, & Jacobs, 1991), and substance abuse (Hansen & Graham, 1991; Kafka & London, 1991). Peer influence as a behavioral determinant can promote healthy practices or encourage risky behaviors. The suggested mechanism is the ability of social influence, through social norms, to affect perceptions on a variety of beliefs. Ransom (1992) has suggested that educational efforts should include consideration of the perceptions that adolescents hold of their peers' health behaviors.

A common feature of adolescence is the tendency to downplay one's susceptibility to the consequences of engaging in risky behaviors (Hansen & Malotte, 1986), commonly referred to as denial. Benthin, Slovic, and Severson (1993) report that adolescents who participated in a risk activity perceived the risk to be smaller, better known, and more controllable than did nonparticipants. The investigators also noted that participants perceived greater peer pressure to engage in the activity, greater benefits relative to risk, and a higher rate of participation by others. Denial of personal risk is illustrated in a survey of 11th-grade students at seven high schools in central Arkansas (Komoroski & Riskert, 1992). The findings revealed a denial of adverse effects in white adolescent males, who tended to be strongly motivated by social influences.

Social influences and social norms directly influence high-risk sexual behavior among adolescents. Kirby and DiClemente (1994) report that adolescents who perceive that their peers support condom use were more that 4 times as likely to be consistent condom users as those who thought their peers did not support condom use. Walter and Vaughn (1993) showed that norms and values interact to generate normative behavioral standards, which influence adoption and maintenance of HIV/AIDS prevention behaviors. Interventions that use peers as agents of change have social influence process as their underlying theoretical mechanism, and they capitalize on the process whereby people influence one another, directly and indirectly. The particular mechanism of social influence includes social norms, network membership, conformity pressures, media influences, social comparison, and modeling. Although differing in specifics, social influence approaches emphasize behavioral expectations and standards (social norms) present in the environment and prepare the learner to resist pressure to engage in risk-taking behaviors (such as using information to correct misperceptions about peer norms, using small groups of peers to guide decision-making processes, using role plays to model and practice prevention scripts, and using peer leaders to support prevention norms.

Peer-Based Approaches

STD/HIV prevention programs for adolescents have used different educational approaches to increase knowledge and awareness as well as to provide important communication skills required for safe sexual behaviors. Despite the relative success of some approaches, such as interactive school-based programs and role-playing activities, the most successful interventions have included components of peer-based interventions. In a peer-based approach, members of a social group or network communicate with, educate, or counsel members of their own group. The theory of social comparison states that behavior is determined through a comparison of others within one's social network (Festinger, 1954). This appears to be especially true within the adolescent age group in which individual behavior may be dictated by the normative beliefs of the social group.

One of the strongest theoretical factors leading to a focus on peer approaches includes peer credibility, in which young people often identify their peers as frequent, reliable, and preferred sources of information on sexuality-related topics, including STDs and AIDS (Perry & Sieving, 1991; Wren, Janz, Carovano, Zimmerman, & Washienko, 1997). The peer, demonstrating the behavioral action, can successfully direct individuals toward healthy lifestyles (Bandura, 1977). The practical issue relates to youths' high level of commitment, energy, and enthusiasm. When motivated for HIV/STD prevention and when provided with appropriate support, young people usually wish to share this information with other youths. When peer approaches are well conceived and implemented, young people can reach large numbers of their peers in a cost-effective, efficient, and effective manner.

STD/HIV prevention programs have used peer approaches to reach youths in a wide range of settings, including schools, venues in the community, and with high-risk groups (e.g., street youths) (Connolly & Franchet, 1993). Generally, such programs have various interrelated approaches, based on the function, intensity, cultural appropriateness, and objective of the peer activity. One approach, the peer information approach, undertakes specific information and education activities for large audiences. In New York City, for example, a youth theater group has developed a drama and a video on young people's sexual health, AIDS, and STDs. The troupe has performed numerous dramas to impart information and foster the development of social norms that support healthy lifestyles and preventive behaviors.

Peer education has been used as a strategy to reach hard-to-reach, vulnerable populations. Podschun (1993) reports on a teen peer outreach street project dealing with HIV prevention education for runaway and homeless youths. The teens used were "true" peers in that many of the youths had been former clients. Thus, it was felt that they would best be familiar with the issues and needs of the target population.

Rickert, Jay, and Gottleib (1991) examined possible advantages of using peers rather than adults. This investigation compared the effect of a peer-led versus an adult-led AIDS education program on the knowledge, attitudes, and satisfaction of the adolescents with their education. The findings revealed that although both adult and peer counselors were equally effective in promoting knowledge gains and appropriate attitude changes, more questions were asked of the peer counselors. The investigators suggest that when education is presented by peer counselors, adolescents may be more likely to see AIDS as a personal danger and that peer counselors should be considered when designing comprehensive AIDS education programs.

Perhaps, the most structured, most focused, and most intensive approach, the peer counseling approach, focuses on training adolescents as sexual health, STD, and HIV counselors to discuss personal problems and problem-solving strategies with other youths on an individual basis. This approach helps smaller groups of young people build their knowledge, attitudes, and safer sex skills through educational activities carried out by members of their peer group who are trained as peer educators. A detailed presentation of the implementation of a peer education program for high school youths in Los Angeles (PEP-LA) is presented later in this chapter. The PEP-LA program consists of a combination of peer education and peer counselor approaches.

Given the relatively successful results of peer leadership training (Booker, Robinson, Kay, Najera, & Stewart, 1997), several investigators have suggested that peer leaders might be necessary when changes in adolescent social behavior are sought (Botvin, Baker, Renichk, & Filazzola, 1984). Compared with school-based programs in which the teacher alone manages the classroom activities, peer leaders enhance the program's capacity by modeling health-enhancing behaviors outside the school setting (Perry, Kelder, & Komro, 1993). In addition, peer leaders are perceived as credible sources of social information, especially on sensitive topics such as sexuality and drug use (O'Hara, Messick, Fichter, & Parris, 1996). Even though prevention programs that use peers as agents of change have been shown to be effective in the prevention of adolescent drug use, such as cigarettes, alcohol, and marijuana, HIV/AIDS prevention programs that use adolescent peer leaders have been widely promoted but underevaluated (Kirby & DiClemente, 1994). Published evaluation programs of peer educators have been restricted to adult and young adult populations in general, not adolescents (Kegeles, Hays & Coates, 1993; Kelly et al., 1992) or late-adolescence populations such as college students (Fischer, Fisher, Williams, & Malloy, 1994). There are few evaluations of peer education programs for HIV prevention among early to mid-adolescence.

Strengths and Limitations
of Peer Education Programs

In reviewing research articles that employed peer educators as a major component of an educational program, several salient features were noted. These consist of methodology, generalizability, and program evaluation criteria. The following programs exemplify these issues.

An innovative HIV prevention project, Teen Peer Outreach-Street Work Project, was designed to address the specific needs of runaway and homeless youths in San Diego, California (Podschun, 1993). The adolescent peer educators closely reflect the multicultural nature of the target population. Many of the trained peers are former clients of the participating youth centers of this project. The project identifies leaders within the homeless youth community who are then trained to provide HIV education and skill development. The author did not elaborate on the training component, curriculum, or time needed to train the peer educators. This outreach project and its peer educators are integrated into established youth service provider programs; thus, HIV prevention messages are delivered on the street and reinforced within these service centers. The integration of an HIV prevention program into an existing youth service provider organization is an excellent method of linking a specific health issue into the entirety of issues faced by homeless youths.

The quantification of the number of outreach hours and clients reached was one process evaluation technique used in this project. Impact and outcome evaluation of this outreach project was problematic because of the transient nature of the target population. Focus group discussions were conducted with homeless youths to note changes in population norms.

SNAPP (Skills and kNowledge for AIDS and Pregnancy Prevention), a school-based program, was designed to delay the onset of intercourse and increase the use of condoms (Kirby, Korpi, Adivi, & Weissman, 1997). The curriculum used interactive tasks, emphasizing communication and negotiation skills. One hundred and two seventh-grade classrooms within six middle schools were randomly assigned to SNAPP or the control group. Ten peer educators, reflecting the ethnic diversity of the target population, were given extensive training and continual supervision throughout the program. However, these peer educators were between 15 and 22 years of age; five were teen mothers, and two were HIV positive. These were not "true peers" because they were older and had experiences not yet encountered by the target population. At the 17-month follow-up survey, increases in knowledge were maintained. However, SNAPP did not have a "significant impact upon any sexual or contraceptive behavior, including the initiation of intercourse, frequency of sex, number of sexual partners, use of condoms or use of birth control pills" (Kirby et al., 1997, p. 56). This well-designed program strictly adhered to treatment implementation yet did not affect HIV risk behavior.

Another example of a theory-based intervention examined the use of varied methods to decrease the risk of contracting HIV/AIDS and other sexually transmitted disease among heterosexually active adolescents (Gillmore et al., 1997). The peer group skills-building component was given to adolescents, 14 through 19 years of age, in an urban juvenile detention facility. The teens trained as peer tutors "were recruited from a local community group of teen peer educators who had already been trained to deliver HIV/AIDS prevention education in area high schools" (Gillmore et al., 1997, p. 28). The teens trained as peers were of similar ages and ethnicity but probably had never experienced juvenile detention and, therefore, were not true peers.

Several imitations of peer education programs have been identified. A generic problem is the lack of explicit terminology in defining the "peer educator." Often, a program will use any individual with similar experiences. Age, culture, gender, education, social class, and similar experiences must all be included. The inconsistency of the term *peer* prevents a comparison of programs in that one intervention will use true peers and another will use older teens as peers. It is difficult to determine whether or not the efficacious component of an intervention is due to the peer or due to the interpersonal communication aspect of the intervention.

A benefit of peer education is thought to be its cost-effectiveness. Teens do not demand the same payment as older people and are often willing to participate without payment. However, the peer training cost-effectiveness of a program is rarely analyzed. Questions that need to be addressed are these: What is the actual cost of training and using peers? What is the cost-benefit of peer-led programs? How long will the program effect be maintained following the conclusion of the program? How often are booster sessions needed to maintain the effect? Do the same peer educators need to administer these follow-up sessions? A recent economic evaluation of an HIV prevention intervention that included a peer component reports $6,180 additional savings of health care costs and improvement of quality of life (Tao & Remafedi, 1998).

Another limitation of many peer education programs is the lack of a conceptual rationale for the use of such a program. As seen in the previously described interventions, the assumption that a peer component is appropriate under all conditions has yet to be proved. As yet, research has not measured the effectiveness of peer programs in different settings, with different ethnic/cultural communities, or within varied age groups. Few studies have shown sustained behavior change attributable to a peer-led intervention (Milburn, 1995). Also lacking is a detailed peer educator training procedure and training content. The inability to specify training procedures across various peer-led programs prevents a complete comparison and evaluation of these programs. The ambiguity of program effectiveness may be a result of variable training techniques. A thorough description of the issues addressed in the training sessions, training time, and evaluation criteria of trainee completion success is of value to other program planners.

Finally, the provision of information and increase in knowledge do not automatically equate to a change in behavior (National Commission on AIDS, 1994). Too often, HIV/STD peer-led prevention programs evaluate pre-/posttest changes in knowledge, or intention to change behavior, as a measure of program success. Impact and outcome evaluation measures must be developed to demonstrate program effectiveness.

Haignere suggests that an assessment of a peer education HIV program may want to evaluate changes in knowledge and various psychosocial parameters of the peer educator (Haignere, Freudenberg, Silver, Maslanka, & Kelley, 1997). As the peer increases his or her self-esteem, it is hypothesized that more people will be contacted, thereby disseminating the prevention message to a wider audience.

Explicit information regarding the recruitment and retention of peer educators is an important addition to the process evaluation. Conclusions regarding the merit of using peer education as a component of an HIV/STD prevention program for adolescents should include peer training issues and ease of replicating the program.

Recruitment and Retention
of Peer Educators: Selection Criteria

The program tasks required of the peer counselor determine the selection criteria. As previously mentioned, the interpretation of a "peer" can vary, although most researchers describe peer counseling as being "provided by someone of equal standing with or similar age to the recipient" (Turner, 1995, p. 330). Other relevant selection factors include gender, language, communication skills, and the ability to work with peers as well as adults. A recurrent problem when serving immigrant populations is the need to find adolescent peers legally able to work in the United States. Finally, the adolescent chosen as a peer counselor must be responsible to job demands, possess excellent interpersonal and communication skills, be capable of learning the necessary skills to counsel, enjoy interacting with people, and desire to help others. Also, any program using adolescent peer counselors must address possible transportation and curfew issues.

Training Needs of Peer Educator

The training needs of the peer educator depend on the scope of the program and the functions required of the peer. Most training sessions will need to include dissemination of general health information, as well as information specifically related to the program topic. Often, the peer educator will have erroneous information regarding the health topic, and this must be assessed in the training session and addressed in the training curriculum.

Skills addressing interpersonal interactions are essential to a successful program. These should include telephone skills, public speaking skills, appropriate self-introductions to variable audiences and ages, and listening skills. Awareness and the ability to "read" nonverbal communication must be addressed in the training session from the standpoint of personal actions as well as learning to understand the recipient's actions. Inclusion of personal self-esteem and self-efficacy is an essential component of any skills training for adolescent peer educators.

Regardless of the worksite, every peer educator should be apprised of the general functioning and structural design of the site. This is invaluable when working with adolescents, who are often incapable of approaching adults and asking questions. Similarly, general adolescent resource guides should be created and made available to the peer educator. These resources must be updated continuously.

An ideal peer counselor-training curriculum would contain an overview of the adolescent program, goals of the project, importance of the peer counselor to the project, types of expected questions and appropriate answers to the problem, tangential issues relevant to the program, and related adolescent behaviors. Sessions should address all adolescent issues and problem indicators that might arise in the interaction. This includes addressing signs of suicidal ideology. Suicidal ideology is of growing concern within the adolescent population and needs to be addressed in any program serving this age group. The peer counselor should be familiar with specific danger signs and how to respond and should be given emergency resource telephone numbers.

Retention of Peer Counselors

As in any program, retention of well-trained counselors is essential to its continued viability and integrity. Ongoing maintenance sessions should be incorporated into the program. This allows for process evaluation of peer training. More seasoned peer counselors act as role models for the novices. These sessions provide group discussions on difficult cases and allow for problem solving. Finally, maintenance sessions can reignite peer counselor excitement for their tasks, renewing enthusiasm for counseling responsibilities.

Peer Education Program of Los Angeles

Wendy Arnold, President of the Peer Education Program of Los Angeles (PEP-LA), established this program in 1985 to target health education programs to the very vulnerable, high-risk population of adolescents in the Los Angeles area. Over the years, she has expanded her program to include peer education groups all over the world, including countries in Africa, Asia, and Europe. The purpose of the program is to educate and train multicultural adolescents to present and discuss STD/HIV transmission and prevention openly and accurately with their peers and to stress the reasons that teenagers are at risk. During presentations, an emphasis is placed on establishing good communication skills and behavioral risk reduction guidelines through a lecture/discussion format. Unfortunately, this type of format can limit the audience's possibility of exploring the key components for interactive decision making in high-risk situations. As a result, a research study was conducted to determine the effectiveness of two different educational approaches directed at improving knowledge, risk awareness, and communication/negotiation skills regarding STD/HIV among adolescents. A total of 30 students—25% Hispanic, 25% Asian, 20% African American, and 30% white—enrolled in the peer education training program. All students attended 6 hours of HIV/AIDS prevention lectures, conducted over a 3-week period and facilitated by the program director. Following the lecture series, students gave a 20-minute presentation to the class, addressing a particular aspect of STD/HIV prevention among adolescents (e.g., discussing condom use). All student presentations were videotaped, and the group of students randomized to the control group received comments from the director and participants following their presentation. Students randomized to the treatment group viewed their presentation and received specific feedback on their presentation using special freeze-framing techniques.

The specific objectives of this training program included the following:

- To develop and implement a peer-led training program among Los Angeles teenagers using audiovisual technology
- To evaluate the relative effectiveness of this approach versus the current lecture approach
- To export the successful components of this model to participating Los Angeles area high schools

Figure 9.1 presents the experimental design employed in this research study. A total of 30 high school adolescents were randomly assigned to either an oral feedback session following their presentation or to a video-based feedback session using freeze-framing techniques in which the video was stopped several times during the discussion to identify and reinforce important communication skills and teaching principles. Table 9.1 identifies the demographic characteristics of the study group, which was composed of mostly females (75%) with a mean age of 14.8 years. Of the participants, 40% were in the 9th grade, 40% in 10th grade, and 20% in the 11th grade. Ethnicity was mixed, with 25% Hispanic, 25% Asian, 20% black, and 30% white. All participants completed a basic knowledge assessment questionnaire prior to and following their training program. Examples of knowledge included the identification of the routes of HIV transmission and various prevention measures. Students were also assessed with respect to their attitudes toward AIDS. Following successful completion of the training program, students were sent to various high schools in the district to give a 1-hour presentation to students. Students from these participating schools also completed a basic knowledge and attitude assessment 3 days prior to the peer educator's presentation as well as a posttest assessment following the presentation. However, only data pertaining to the knowledge, attitudes, and performance skills of the peer educator are presented here.

Table 9.2 presents the results of the pretest/posttest according to randomized assignment—experimental or control group. There were no statistically significant differences between study groups at baseline or posttest assessment

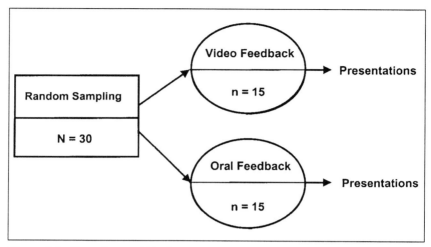

Figure 9.1. Experimental Design

Table 9.1	Demographic Characteristics of Peer Educators
Male	25%
Female	75%
Mean Age	14.8 years
Grade Level	
9th	40%
10th	40%
11th	20%
Ethnicity	
Hispanic	25%
Asian	25%
Black	20%
White	30%

Table 9.2 Results of Student Rating of Peer Educators According to
Study Group (in percentages)

Content Area	Pretest		Posttest		
	Experimental (n = 76)	Control (n = 80)	Experimental (n = 70)	Control (n = 74)	p
General Knowledge	72	75	87	82	ns[a]
Attitudes (% positive)	75	76	94	83	ns

a. ns = nonsignificant.

with respect to mean scores on knowledge or attitudes toward AIDS. However, individuals assigned to the video feedback were found to exhibit higher change scores from pretest to posttest compared with the control group. For example, the intervention group recorded a 15% increase in knowledge (72% to 87%) at posttest, whereas the control group recorded a 7% increase (75% to 82%). Similar differences were noted with respect to attitudes toward AIDS, with intervention participants recording a 19% increase in attitudes (75% to 94% posttest), and the control group recording only a 7% increase (76% to 83%) posttest. However, the *p* value for both these differences was statistically nonsignificant.

The form used by high school students to rate the presentation skills of the peer educator is presented in Table 9.3. Results of these ratings are presented in Table 9.4. Again, it is noted that study groups did not differ significantly according to general and medical knowledge of HIV/AIDS as measured by a subjective measure rated by the students. However, highly significant differences were found in each of the skill areas, including a 16% differential in command of questions, a 12% differential in ease of comprehension, a 12% differential overall in organization and body language, and a 16% differential in their overall rating of the presentation.

Table 9.3   Students Rating of Peer Educators' Knowledge and Skills
             During Presentation

Content Area	Excellent (100%)	Good (90%)	Fair (80%)	Needs Work (70%)
General overview of HIV/AIDS	_____	_____	_____	_____
Medical knowledge	_____	_____	_____	_____
Command of questions	_____	_____	_____	_____
Overall organization	_____	_____	_____	_____
Ease of comprehension	_____	_____	_____	_____
Sensitivity to subject (nonjudgmental)	_____	_____	_____	_____
Body language (eye contact, gestures)	_____	_____	_____	_____
Overall rating of presentation	_____	_____	_____	_____

What do you feel were the speaker's greatest attributes?

_____

What do you feel the speaker needs to work on?

_____

_____

_____

Consequently, we can conclude that the training program was a success as indicated by significantly improved communication skills as rated by the student attending the presentations of peer educators. In addition, a second objective of integrating the successful components of this training program has been realized in two participating schools. A health education counselor from each of these schools has become formally linked to the PEP/LA program and has identified students from these respective schools to become trained as peer

Table 9.4   Results of Student Rating of Peer Educators According to Study Group

Content Area	Experimental (n = 70)	Control (n = 74)	p
Peer Educator Communication Skills			
General knowledge of HIV/AIDS	90	85	ns[a]
Medical knowledge	90	88	ns
Command of questions	96	80	< .05
Ease of comprehension	94	82	< .05
Overall organization	96	84	< 05
Body language	98	86	< .05
Overall rating of presentation	98	82	< .01

a. ns = nonsignificant.

educators. Now, each of these schools has the continuity of a resident peer educator who can provide the initial presentation as well as follow up with student concerns over time. This mechanism has worked very well and is being expanded to other participating high schools in the district. An additional effort has recently been initiated to include targeted outreach to minority communities in the district, including schools with predominately Hispanic and Asian populations.

Peer Education: The Panacea for Adolescent STD/HIV Risk Reduction?

The use of adolescent peers as a conduit to reduce STD/HIV health risks has been implemented in diverse communities and age groups. Often, the decision to use peer educators is driven more by practice rather than by theory. Program findings are often inconclusive as to the specific benefits derived from peer education. Definitions of *peers* vary among the programs—some using true peers, others using older peers. Peer counseling programs may also suffer from lack of sustainability within a community. PEP/LA is one example of a peer education program that has created strong community links, sustained and expanded its implementation to international settings, and maintained institutional affiliations.

Finally, program effectiveness measures need to include immediate changes in knowledge, attitudes, beliefs, and practices as well as change over longer periods of time. Evaluation designs must be implemented to assess the level of maintenance of STD/HIV risk reduction behaviors over time. Furthermore, how should programs institute booster sessions across the dynamic period of adolescent development? These and other issues must be addressed before peer education is shown to be the most appropriate method of reducing adolescent STD/HIV risk.

Implications for Multicultural Communication Research, Policy, and Action

The specific interventions employed in the several studies cited above indicate a variety of diagnostic, educational, and communication approaches. The theoretical underpinnings of peer-based techniques identify social network analyses, group dynamics, interpersonal communication skills, and social comparisons as a basis for the content and application of intervention programs. For example, programs that employ adolescent peer educators targeting Hispanic populations often employ a multicultural communication technique using several approaches, including group dynamics, interpersonal communications, theater, and the *fotonovella,* or picture story book. This combination of multicultural approaches has been shown to benefit the larger community of individuals identifying with the same health concern.

In addition, these research actions often lead to policy implementation based on the relative success of the intervention. For example, the Los Angeles County Health Department is considering the integration of peer counseling as one of the innovative approaches for achieving completion of care for chemoprophylactic tuberculosis among Hispanic and Asian adolescents. Also, PEP-LA has produced numerous theater presentations targeting communication and social skills found to be effective in reducing risk-taking behaviors among Asian, Hispanic, and African American youths. These programs all employ commonly shared cultural beliefs and attitudes found among high-risk youths. The concept of the interventions is shared among all population groups; however, the specificity of the content areas provides the uniqueness of the tailored messages that addresses the knowledge, cultural beliefs, and the background of the study population. This fine-tuning of the communication approach has often proven to be the essential ingredient that separates a good intervention program from an outstanding program. Programs employing a combination of educational learning opportunities based on scientifically validated needs analysis and a strong, theoretical/conceptual framework generally rank among the noteworthy programs. We strongly recommend the inclusion of these planning components into the conceptualization, implementation, and evaluation of programs involving multicultural communication approaches.

References

Ajzen, I. (1988). *Attitudes, personality and behavior.* Milton Keynes, UK: Open University Press.

Bandura A. (1977). Self-efficacy: Toward a unifying theory of behavioral change. *Psychological Review, 84,* 191-215.

Bandura, A. (1986). *Social foundations of thought and action.* Englewood Cliffs, NJ: Prentice Hall.

Bandura, A. (1992). A social cognitive approach to the exercise of control over AIDS infection. In R. DiClemente (Ed.), *Adolescents and AIDS: A generation in jeopardy* (pp. 890-116). Newbury Park, CA: Sage.

Benthin, A., Slovic, P., & Severson, H. (1993). A psychometric study of adolescent risk perception. *Journal of Adolescence, 16*(2), 153-168.

Booker, V. K., Robinson, J. G., Kay, B. J., Najera, L. G., & Stewart, G. (1997). Changes in empowerment: Effects of participation in a lay health promotion program. *Health Education and Behavior, 24*(4), 452-464.

Botvin, G., Baker, E., Renichk, N., & Filazzola, A. (1984). A cognitive-behavioral approach to substance abuse prevention. *Addictive Behaviors, 9,* 137-147.

Brown, L., DiClemente, R., & Reynolds, L. (1991). HIV prevention for adolescents: Utility of the Health Belief Model. *AIDS Education and Prevention, 3*(1), 50-59.

Catania, J., Kegeles, S., & Coates, T. (1990). Towards an understanding of risk behavior: An AIDS risk reduction model. *Health Education Quarterly, 17*(1), 53-74.

Centers for Disease Control. (1993). "Sexually transmitted diseases guidelines." *MMWR: Morbidity and Mortality Weekly Report, 42* (no. RR-14).

Centers for Disease Control. (1997, September 12). State-specific birth rates for teen-agers—United States 1990-1996. *MMWR: Morbidity and Mortality Weekly Report, 46,* 837-842.

Choi, K., & Coates, T. (1994). Prevention of HIV Infection. *AIDS, 8,* 1371-1389.

Connolly, M., & Franchet, C. N. (1993). Manila street children face many sexual risks. *Network: Family Health International, 14,* 24-25.

Davis, A. J. (1994). The role of hormonal contraception in adolescents. *American Journal of Obstetrics and Gynecology, 170*(5), 1581-1585.

Deutsch, M., & Gerard, H. (1955). A study of normative and informational social influ-ences on individual judgment. *Journal of Abnormal and Social Psychology, 51,* 629-636.

DiClemente, R. J., Boyer, C., & Morales, E. (1988). Minorities and AIDS: Knowledge, at-titudes and misconceptions among black and Latino adolescents. *American Journal of Public Health, 78,* 55-57.

DiClemente, R. J., Forrest, K. A., & Miekler, S. (1990). College students' knowledge and attitudes about AIDS and changes in HIV preventive behavior. *AIDS Education and Prevention, 2,* 201-212.

Doll, L. (1997). Epidemiology of HIV-related behaviors in risk populations. In National Institutes of Health, *Interventions to prevent HIV risk behaviors: Programs and ab-stracts* (pp. 27-31). Washington, DC: National Institutes of Health.

Donovan, C. A., & Stratton, E. (1994). Changing epidemiology of AIDS. *Canadian Fam-ily Physician, 40,* 1414-1420.

Dunne, M., Donald M., Lucke, J., Nilsson R., Ballard, R., & Raphael, B. (1994). Age re-lated increase in sexual behaviors and decrease in regular condom use among adoles-cents in Australia. *International Journal of STD & AIDS, 5*(1), 41-47.

Ehrhardt, A. (1993). Sex education for young people. *National AIDS Bulletin, 6,* 32-35.

Festinger, L. (1954). A theory of social comparison processes. *Human Relations, 7,* 117-140.

Fischer, J., Fisher, W., Williams, S., & Malloy, T. (1994). Empirical tests of an informa-tion-motivation-behavioral skills model of AIDS prevention behavior. *Health Psy-chology, 13,* 238-250.

Fishbein, M., & Ajzen, I. (1975). *Belief, attitude, intention and behavior: An introduction to theory and research.* Reading, MA: Addison-Wesley.

Fisher, J. (1988). Possible effects of reference group-based social influence on AIDS-risk behavior and AIDS prevention. *American Psychologist, 43,* 914-920.

Ford, K., Rubinstein, S., & Norris, A. (1994). Sexual behavior and condom use among urban, lower-income African American and Hispanic youth. *AIDS Education and Prevention, 6*(3), 219-229.

Fullilove, R. E., Fullilove, M. T., Bowser, B., & Gross, S. (1990). Risk of sexually transmitted disease among black adolescent crack users in Oakland and San Francisco, California. *JAMA, 262,* 851-855.

Gillmore, M. R., Morrison, D. M., Richey, C. A., Balassone, M. L., Gutierrez, L., & Farris, M. (1997). Effects of a skill-based intervention to encourage condom use among high-risk heterosexually active adolescents. *Aids Education and Prevention, 9*(1 Suppl), 22-43.

Gottleib, A., Pope, S. K., Rickert, V. I., & Hardin, B. H. (1993). Patterns of smokeless tobacco use by young adolescents. *Pediatrics, 91*(1), 75-78.

Haffner, D. (1996). Sexual health for America's adolescents. *Journal of School Health, 66*(4), 151-152.

Haignere, C. S., Freudenberg, N., Silver, D. R., Maslanka, H., & Kelley, J. T. (1997). One method for assessing HIV/AIDS peer-education programs. *Journal of Adolescent Health, 21,* 6-79.

Hansen, W. B., & Graham, J. W. (1991). Preventing alcohol, marijuana, and cigarette use among adolescents: Peer pressure resistance training versus establishing conservative norms. *Preventive Medicine, 20,* 414-430.

Hansen, W. B., & Malotte, C. K. (1986). Perceived personal immunity: The development of beliefs about susceptibility to the consequences of smoking. *Preventive Medicine, 15,* 363-372.

Hansen, W. B., Malotte, C. K., & Fielding, J. (1988). Evaluation of a tobacco and alcohol abuse prevention curriculum for adolescents. *Health Education Quarterly, 15,* 135-154.

Hayes, C. (1987). *Risking the Future: Adolescent Sexuality, Pregnancy, and Childbearing.* Washington, DC: National Academy Press.

Hein, K. (1993). Risky business: Adolescents and human immunodeficiency virus. *Pediatrics, 88,* 1052-1054.

Jemmott, J., & Jemmott, L. (1997). Behavioral interventions with heterosexual adolescents. In National Institutes of Health, *Interventions to Prevent HIV Risk Behaviors: Program and Abstracts* (pp. 75-80). Washington, DC: National Institutes of Health.

Kafka, R. R., & London, P. (1991). Communication in relationships and adolescent substance use: The influence of parents and friends. *Adolescences, 26*(103), 587-598.

Kandel, D. (1986). Processes of peer influences in adolescence. In R. Silbereisen, K. Eyferth, & G. Rudinger (Eds.), *Development as action in context* (pp. 203-227). New York: Springer-Verlag.

Kandel, D. (1996). The parental and peer contexts of adolescent deviance: An algebra of interpersonal influences. *Journal of Drug Issues, 26*(2), 289-315.

Kann, L., Warren, C. W., Harris, W. A., Collins, J. L., Williams, B. I., Ross, J. G., & Kolbe, L. J. (1996). Youth risk behavior surveillance—United States, 1995. *Journal of School Health, 66*(10), 365-377.

Kegeles, S., Hays, R., & Coates, T. (1993, June). *A community-level risk reduction intervention for young gay and bisexual men.* Paper presented at the Eighth International Conference on AIDS, Amsterdam.

Kelly, J., St. Lawrence, J., Stevenson, Y., Hauth, A. C., Kalichman, S. C., Diaz, Y. E., Brasfield, T. L., Koob, J. J., & Morgan, M. G. (1992). Community AIDS/HIV risks reduction: The effects of endorsements by popular people in three cities. *American Journal of Public Health, 82,* 1483-1489.

Kipke, M. D., Boyer, C., & Hein, A. (1993). An evaluation of an AIDS risks reduction education and skills training (ARREST) program. *Journal of Adolescent Health, 14*(7), 533-539.

Kirby, D., Korpi, M, Adivi, C. & Weissman, J. (1997). An impact evaluation of Project SNAPP: An AIDS and pregnancy prevention middle school program. *AIDS Education and Prevention, 9*(Supplement A), 44-61.

Kirby, D., & DiClemente, R. (1994). School-based interventions to prevent unprotected sex and HIV among adolescents. In R. DiClemente & J. Peterson (Eds.), *Preventing AIDS: Theories and methods of behavior interventions* (pp. 117-139). New York: Plenum.

Klepp, K. I., Perry, C. L., & Jacobs, D. R. (1991). Etiology of drinking and driving among adolescents: Implications for primary prevention. *Health Education Quarterly, 18*(4), 415-427.

Komoroski, E. M., & Riskert, V. I. (1992). Adolescent body image and attitudes to anabolic steroid use. *American Journal of Diseases of Children, 146*(7), 823-828.

Krowchuk, D. P. (1997). Sexually transmitted diseases in adolescents: What's new? *Southern Medical Journal, 91,* 124-131.

Milburn, K. (1995). A critical review of peer education with your people with special reference to sexual health. *Health Education Research, 10*(4), 407-420.

National Commission on AIDS. (1994). Preventing HIV/AIDS in adolescents. *Journal of School Health, 64*(1), 39-51.

National Institutes of Health. (1997). *NIH consensus development conference on interventions to prevent HIV risk behaviors: Conference statement.* Washington, DC: Author.

Nguyet, N. T., Maheux, B., Beland, F., & Pica, L. A. (1994). Sexual behaviors and condom use: A study of suburban male adolescents. *Adolescence, 29*(113), 37-48.

O'Donnell, L. N., Doval, A. S., Duran, R., & O'Donnell, C. (1995). Video-based sexually transmitted disease patient education: Its impact on condom acquisition. *American Journal of Public Health, 85*(6), 817-822.

O'Hara, P., Messick, B., Fichter, R., & Parris, D. (1996). A peer-led AIDS prevention program for students in an alternative school. *Journal of School Health, 66*(5), 176-182.

Perry, C., Kelder, S., & Komro, K. (1993). The social world of adolescents: Family, peers, schools, and the community. In S. Millstein, A. Petersen, & E. Nightingale (Eds.), *Pro-*

moting the health of adolescents: New directions for the twenty-first century (pp. 73-96). New York: Oxford University Press.

Perry, C. L., & Sieving, R. (1991). *Peer involvement in global AIDS prevention among adolescents.* Geneva: World Health Organization, Global Programme on AIDS.

Podschun, G. D. (1993). Teen peer outreach-street work project: HIV prevention education for runaway and homeless youth. *Public Health Reports, 108*(2), 150-155.

Quirk, M. E., Godkin, M. A., & Schwenzfeier, E. (1993). Evaluation of two AIDS prevention interventions for inner-city adolescent and young adult women. *American Journal of Preventive Medicine, 9*(1), 21-26.

Ransom, M. V. (1992). Peer perceptions of adolescent health behaviors. *Journal of School Health, 62*(6), 238-242.

Remafedi, G. (1994). Cognitive and behavioral adaptations to HIV/AIDS among gay and bisexual adolescents. *Journal of Adolescent Health, 15*(2),142-148.

Rickert, V. I., Jay, M. S., & Gottleib, A. (1991). Effects of a peer-counseled AIDS education program on knowledge, attitudes, and satisfaction of adolescents. *Journal of Adolescent Health, 12*(1), 38-43.

Rotheram-Borus, M. J., Koopman, C., & Rosario, M. (1995). Predicting patterns of sexual acts among homosexual and bisexual youths. *American Journal of Psychiatry, 152*, 588-595.

Shafer, M. A., & Boyer, C. B. (1991). Psychosocial and behavioral factors associated with risk of sexually transmitted diseases, including human immunodeficiency virus infection, among urban high school students. *Journal of Pediatrics, 119*(5), 826-833.

Slap, G. B., Plotkin, S. L., Khalid, N., Michelman, D. F., & Forke, C. M. (1991). A human immunodeficiency virus education program for adolescent females. *Journal of Adolescent Health, 12*(6), 434-442.

Smith, P. B., Weinman, M. L., & Parrilli, J. (1997). The role of condom motivation education in the reduction of new and reinfection rates of sexually transmitted diseases among inner-city female adolescents. *Patient Education and Counseling, 31*(1), 77-81.

Steiner, B. D., Shields, C. G., Noble, G. L., & Bayer, W. H. (1994). Associations with high-risk sexual behavior: A survey of young men of color attending urban youth centers. *Journal of the American Board of Family Practices, 7*(3), 189-195.

Tao, G., & Remafedi, G. (1998). Economic evaluation of an HIV prevention intervention for gay and bisexual male adolescents. *Journal of Acquired Immune Deficiency and Human Retrovirology, 17*(1), 83-90.

Turner, G. M. (1995). Peer counseling. *Pediatric Annals, 24*(6), 330-333.

U.S. Department of Health and Human Services. (1991). *Healthy people 2000: National health promotion and disease prevention objectives* (DHHS Publication No. 91-50212). Washington DC: Government Printing Office.

Walter, H., & Vaughn, R. (1993). AIDS risk reduction among a multiethnic sample of urban high school students. *JAMA, 270*, 725-730.

Warren, C. W., Harris, W. A., & Kann, L. (1995). *Pregnancy, sexually transmitted diseases, and related risk behaviors among U.S. adolescents* (Adolescent Health: State of the Nation monograph series, No. 2; CDC Publication No. 099-4630). Atlanta, GA: Centers for Disease Control and Prevention.

Wren, P. A., Janz, N. K., Carovano, K., Zimmerman, M. A., & Washienko, K. M. (1997). Preventing the spread of AIDS in youth: principles of practice from 11 diverse projects. *Journal of Adolescent Health, 21*(5), 309-317.

10

Health Communication for HIV Risk Reduction Among Homeless Youth

Lisa A. Russell

To gain a clearer understanding of the cultural heterogeneity of homeless youth populations and their reference groups, one can begin by considering definitions of culture and ethnicity. Culture can be defined broadly as "a

AUTHOR'S NOTE: Project ABLE was conceptualized by Lisa Russell, Gary Bess, Linda Fleischman, Pamela Smith, and Henry Rodriguez and was supported initially by the California Department of Health Services Offices of AIDS, Contract No. 89-97339; the California Community Foundation; and the Los Angeles Free Clinic. The views expressed herein are those of the author and do not necessarily represent those of the sponsoring agencies. The author thanks the following individuals and groups for their participation and support of Project ABLE and its evaluation during the program's first years of operation: the homeless youth of Los Angeles County, Don Morisky, Nina Mancina, Kergan Edwards, Jack Carrel, Alex Acuna, the original peer actors/educators: Valerie Allerme, Heidi Van Lier, Ricardo Alfaro, Rowdy Metzger, Brian Bowen, Debbie Meyerson, Charles Joo, and Seidy Lopez; staff members at the Los Angeles Free Clinic and at the many agencies who serve homeless youth in Los Angeles County and who invited Project ABLE to perform at their organizations. Dr. Russell wrote her chapter while she was an Assistant Professor at Indiana University in Bloomington.

tool which defines reality for its members" (Kagawa-Singer & Chung, 1994). Furthermore, culture provides a sense of identity as well as a set of beliefs, values, behaviors, rules, and communication patterns and is learned by socialization. Ethnicity refers to a sense of identity based on common ancestry and national, religious, tribal, linguistic, or cultural origins (Huff & Kline, 1999). Although there is conceptual overlap between culture and ethnicity, they are not synonymous (Slonim, 1991). For homeless youths, one could argue that there may exist a street culture to which youths can become acculturated through socialization as well as an ethnic (or other primary) culture to which youths have been acculturated during childhood. Understanding the relative influences of multiple reference groups (cultural and other) on beliefs, values, norms, and behavior for the purpose of health communication requires collaboration between the population and practitioners. One aspect of collaboration includes use of peer educators.

Although much has been published regarding peer health education among adolescents, particularly in school settings, little has been published documenting the effects of peer education among homeless youths (Podschun, 1993). To my knowledge, nothing has been published describing peer education using theater among homeless youths. This chapter describes an evaluation of the HIV risk reduction efforts of Project ABLE: a peer health education project that uses theater as the primary component of its intervention.

HIV Risk Among Homeless Youths

Estimates of HIV seroprevalence among homeless youths have ranged from 4% to 11.5% (Pfeifer & Oliver, 1997; Shalwitz, Goulart, Dunnigan, & Flannery, 1990; Stricof, Novick, & Kennedy, 1990). Nearly half the homeless youths surveyed in Los Angeles reported prior behavior that places them at risk for HIV infection (Robertson, 1990). Among runaway and homeless youths, the prevalence of involvement in prostitution or survival sex has ranged from 19% to 29% (Russell, 1998; Sugerman, Hergenroeder, Chacko, & Parcel, 1991; Yates, MacKenzie, Pennbridge, & Cohen, 1988). Rotheram-Borus and her colleagues (1992) found that 47% of the male runaways and 16% of the female runaways sampled in New York City disclosed histories of 10 or more opposite-sex sexual partners. Only 14% to 20% of homeless youths report consistent use of condoms (Rotheram-Borus et al., 1992; Sugerman et al., 1991), and only 34%

report use of a condom at their last sexual encounter (Greenblatt & Robertson, 1993). Sugerman and colleagues (1991) reported that homeless youths claimed to engage in HIV risk behavior because of low perceived risk of infection. Of homeless young women interviewed in Los Angeles, 44% reported histories of pregnancy (Robertson, 1991), and between 19% and 71% of homeless youths in California disclosed ever having a sexually transmitted disease (Robertson, 1991; Shalwitz et al., 1990). History of intravenous drug use has been reported by 25% to 30% of some samples (Robertson, 1991; Sugerman et al., 1991). The high prevalence of HIV risk behaviors coupled with above-average rates of drug and alcohol use and mental disorders, multiple placements in institutional care, and exposure to physical and sexual violence and other severe stressors and survival needs may place homeless youths in uniquely vulnerable positions with regard to HIV infection compared with other adolescents.

Project ABLE:
AIDS Beliefs Learned Through Education[1]

In 1988, the script *The Street Where I Live* was developed by Oliver Goldstick, a professional playwright, and was based on focus group interviews with homeless youths in Los Angeles as well as on an understanding of the life experiences of homeless youths as documented in the scholarly literature. *The Street Where I Live* emphasizes personal vulnerability, decision making, communication, and role modeling of risk prevention in portrayals of multiethnic peer characters living on the streets. The intervention included a 30-minute performance of *The Street Where I Live* followed by a 20-minute didactic and question-and-answer period. The language level of the play was tailored for the local homeless youth audience with an average English reading and comprehension level of Grade 8. Actors used language common to the street and the ethnic culture of their characters. Performances were scheduled in shelters and drop-in centers serving homeless and runaway youths between the ages of 9 and 25 years. Most of the performance sites had ongoing HIV risk reduction discussion groups, which would presumably reinforce the play's message. Limited funding did not permit follow-up visits to conduct small-group activities as originally planned.

The Project ABLE teen theater AIDS education project was planned using the PRECEDE (predisposing, reinforcing, and enabling constructs in educational and environmental diagnosis and evaluation) framework (Green, Kreuter, Deeds, & Partridge, 1980) and was based on constructs from social cognitive theory (Bandura, 1986), the persuasion literature (McGuire, 1985), the health belief model (Rosenstock, 1974), and the theory of planned behavior (Ajzen & Fishbein, 1985). It was thought that by using the dramatic format of a play and by having the content and story characters accurately reflect the lives and cultures of homeless youths, the project could attract the active attention of the homeless youth audience. Selection of young adult (i.e., persons in their late teens or early 20s) actor/educators whose own experiences and ethnic and cultural backgrounds overlapped with those of homeless youths was intended to increase the audience's ability to identify with the actor/educators, with their characters and their situations, and with the attitudes, behaviors, and consequences being modeled. Using *peer* actor/educators was thought to have a potential impact on normative beliefs about HIV risk and prevention behaviors. The scenes and relationships are set in the context of heterosexual and homosexual relationships, sex work, the lure of the entertainment industry, sexual and physical assault, pregnancy, and intravenous drug use.

Counterarguments to the HIV risk and prevention message were presented and refuted in the play, sometimes with humor to provide anxiety relief and maintain attention. Various factors that may be considered during decision making regarding strategies to avoid potential HIV exposure during sexual activity, the negotiation of using condoms, and the potential outcomes of HIV antibody testing were presented during the course of the play. Communication skills relevant to HIV risk reduction were modeled in scenes depicting peer relationships of homeless youths as well as survival relationships (e.g., prostitution) of homeless youths. The behavioral skills required for using condoms and for disinfecting intravenous drug equipment were modeled during the didactic/question-and-answer period following the play. The immediate and longer-term consequences of the decisions made by the characters portrayed were depicted in the play. Other enabling factors addressed during the didactic session following the play included referrals for local HIV antibody testing and treatment sources, numbers for local and national AIDS information hotlines, distribution of free condom and bleach kits, and frank discussion of the efficacy of proper condom use as well as creative and pleasurable methods of incorporating condom use into sexual activities.

The Effects of Project ABLE

After completion of their training and demonstration of proficiency in HIV-related knowledge and skills, the original eight peer actor/educators were confidentially surveyed about their perceptions of any personal effects resulting from their involvement in the program. Most peer actor/educators reported increased feelings of confidence and comfort discussing HIV prevention with friends, peers, parents, siblings, and sexual partners and had already initiated HIV prevention conversations with friends. Several peer actor/educators who were sexually active had discussed condom use with their partners and had begun using condoms. A few peer educators reported initiating discussions of HIV prevention with their parents. At least two of the original peer actors/educators completed college degrees and worked in community health programs after leaving the project; one of these actor/educators spontaneously disclosed that his involvement with Project ABLE had significantly affected his career choice.

The impact of Project ABLE on homeless youth audience members was evaluated using a separate sample pre-/posttest, quasi-experimental design. Pretests and posttests were conducted throughout each funding year. Audience members anonymously completed questionnaires that contained items to measure HIV-related knowledge, beliefs, attitudes, behavioral intentions, and risk activities. The questionnaires were written at an eighth-grade reading level and were accompanied by a recitation of each item by a peer actor/educator to accommodate youths with low literacy skills. The specific constructs measured included[2] (a) HIV-related knowledge (10 items); (b) attitudinal barriers to condom use (a 3-item scale, Cronbach's α = .66); (c) attitudinal reinforcers or benefits for condom use (a 3-item scale; Cronbach's α = .66); (d) condom efficacy (2 items); (e) condom access; (f) past safer sex efforts; (g) condom use (2 items); (h) general willingness to try condoms; (i) intention to use condoms; (j) self-efficacy regarding consistency of condom use; (k) comfort asking partner to use a condom or "negotiation efficacy" (2 items); (l) beliefs about people who use condoms (a 3-item scale, Cronbach's α = .61); (m) belief about friends' attempts to avoid HIV infection; and (n) perceived vulnerability (2 items).

Evaluation results from 211 homeless youths exposed to the play *The Street Where I Live* during Project ABLE's fiscal years 1989-90 and 1991-92 follow.[3]

The data from the two periods were aggregated to permit greater statistical power. One hundred fifty-one youths were surveyed before exposure to the play, and 60 youths were surveyed after exposure. Although all audience members were given the evaluation survey, approximately 10 youths returned surveys that were mostly incomplete and therefore were eliminated from the analyses.

Evaluation participants ranged in age between 10 and 25 years with a mean age of 17.2 years. Of the respondents, 52% were women. Respondents were distributed among six racial/ethnic categories in the following way: Hispanic/Latino (25%), black/African American (25%), white/Caucasian (31%), Asian American (4%), Native American (1%), and multi/other (14%). Of the participants, 91% reported ever having sex, and 67% had used a condom during sex; 14% disclosed histories of intravenous drug use, and 47% had become intoxicated by drugs and/or alcohol to the point of "losing control" over behavior. Thirty-six percent of the participants reported having been tested for HIV antibodies. The treatment group (i.e., posttest group) was comparable to the comparison group (i.e., pretest group) on all of the above characteristics except age. The treatment group was significantly older than the comparison group (18.9 years of age vs. 16.5 years of age, respectively). Consequently, age was controlled as a covariate when analyzing treatment effects when age was significantly associated with the dependent variable. Inclusion of age as a covariate significantly influenced only one analysis; the remaining analyses of treatment effects are reported as one- or two-way analyses of variance (ANOVA).

To assess the impact of exposure to Project ABLE, a series of one-way analyses of variance using the general linear model (GLM) were run using exposure status (i.e., treatment or comparison group) as the fixed factor and the other constructs as separate dependent variables.[4] Exposure to Project ABLE significantly predicted a decrease in attitudinal barriers to condom use ($F_{1,187} = 9.285$; $p < .005$; $\eta^2 = .05$), a general willingness to try condoms ($F_{1,198} = 6.547$; $p < .05$; $\eta^2 = .03$), and an increase in intention to use condoms ($F_{1,198} = 6.547$; $p < .05$; $\eta^2 = .03$). Factorial two-way GLM ANOVAs were run using exposure status and ethnicity as fixed factors and the other constructs as dependent variables. The two-way ANOVAs revealed a significant interaction between ethnicity and intervention exposure when predicting variation in perceived HIV risk ($F_{2,142} = 5.633$; $p < .005$; $\eta^2 = .07$). Whereas Caucasians and African Americans reported higher levels of perceived HIV risk following exposure to the intervention, Latinos/Hispanics reported lower levels of perceived HIV risk. ANOVAS testing main and interaction effects of respondent sex by exposure status yielded no significant relationships with the dependent variables.

Intervention exposure status was not significantly associated with aggregate changes in HIV knowledge or other measures of attitudes and beliefs.

Although the modest sample size did not allow for simultaneous testing of main and interaction effects of respondent sex, ethnicity, age, and exposure status, some trends were suggested by the data.[5] Project ABLE appeared to have the most influence on HIV-related knowledge and perceived norms among male respondents. There were trends for respondents who were male, younger, and/or African American or Latino/Hispanic to improve the most on HIV-related knowledge. Audience members who were male, older, and/or Caucasian or African American demonstrated increases in perceived risk. Scores on the perceived barriers scale were lowest at baseline among African American youths, with the most change observed among Caucasians and males. Scores on the perceived reinforcers scale were most improved among Caucasian and African American males. There was a trend for Latino/Hispanic men to indicate stronger beliefs in condom efficacy following program exposure. Condom negotiation efficacy was most increased among older respondents with a positive trend among Latino/Hispanics and men. Self-efficacy regarding consistent future condom use was most increased among female youths and was equally increased across the three predominant ethnic groups in the sample: Latino/Hispanic, African American, and Caucasian. Audience members who were younger, Latino/Hispanic, and/or female seemed to have the most aggregate increase in willingness to try condoms. Stronger positive trends were observed between program exposure and intention to use condoms among younger and Latino/Hispanic participants compared with others.

Several hierarchical regressions were run on the baseline data to determine which independent variables were significant predictors of the dependent variable, behavioral intention to use condoms, and whether their effects were direct or mediated by other independent variables. Behavioral intention (the distal dependent variable) was regressed onto (Block 1) age, prior condom use, past safer sex efforts, and HIV-related knowledge and (Block 2) condom efficacy, negotiation efficacy, self-efficacy, perceived risk, attitudinal reinforcers and barriers, beliefs about others' use of condoms, condom access, and willingness to try condoms. Negotiation efficacy, condom efficacy, and willingness to try condoms were significant predictors of intention to use condoms ($F_{3,142} = 32.999$; $p < .001$; adjusted $R^2 = .40$). When behavioral intention was regressed on the four predictors for each ethnic group, willingness to try condoms remained a significant predictor of intention to use condoms for Latinos/Hispanics, Caucasians, and African Americans. General willingness to try condoms was conceptualized to be a potential mediator of the effects of the other independent variables and was regressed on the blocks of independent variables used in the regression for behavioral intention. The regression was done on the entire baseline sample and revealed the following significant predictors of willingness to try condoms: condom efficacy, attitudinal reinforcers and barriers, and negotiation efficacy ($F_{4,141} = 21.803; p < .001$; adjusted $R^2 = .36$).

Implications for Communication Interventions and Research

The evaluation data suggested that Project ABLE had a differential impact on respondents' aggregate HIV-related knowledge and may have favorably influenced selected beliefs, attitudes, and intentions. Specifically, Project ABLE appeared to have a weak impact on perceived attitudinal barriers to condom use as well as on a general willingness to try condoms and behavioral intention to use condoms. Exposure-related influence on perceived risk was moderated by ethnic group. Project ABLE had no statistically significant impact on the tested indicators of HIV knowledge, attitudinal reinforcers for condom use, perceived condom efficacy, perceived condom access, self-efficacy for future condom use, negotiation efficacy, beliefs about friends' attempts to avoid HIV infection, or beliefs about people who use condoms.

Methodological Considerations

Three threats to causal validity must be considered with this quasi-experimental design:

1. Although intervention sites were randomly assigned to pretest and posttest conditions throughout the fiscal years, it is possible that the aggregate pretest group was not comparable to the posttest group in ways other than exposure to the intervention (such as the observed mean age differences).

2. Contamination of the pretest group may have occurred by interpersonal diffusion of the Project ABLE innovation among the homeless youth community.

3. Other HIV risk communication interventions in the community and mass media may have been partially or wholly responsible for any observed changes.

The design did not allow for testing of delayed or sleeper effects or for deterioration of change. Notwithstanding the above-mentioned caveats to drawing any causal conclusions about Project ABLE, it may be remarkable that a one-shot intervention is able to demonstrate any significant immediate effect, given the complexity of determinants of change in attitudes and behavioral intention. At the very least, Project ABLE may have served to favorably predispose the audience to subsequent exposures to HIV prevention messages and efforts.

The intervention and its evaluation were not designed to test the theoretical models on which they were based or the adequacy of those models for the cultures represented in the audience. Although the measures used demonstrated acceptable levels of internal reliability, they may not have been adequate representations of the targeted theoretical constructs, particularly for a culturally diverse audience, and measures were not taken of all constructs of the models used. Consequently, one cannot conclude that the intervention's apparent modest effects were necessarily due to weaknesses of a specific theory or construct. Although there is much scholarly literature that documents the association between behavioral intention and behavior and some evidence of strong relationships between intentions and actual use of condoms among ethnically diverse adolescents (Kennedy, O'Hara, Fichtner, & Fishbein, 1996), program-related impact on actual condom use was not assessed in this study.

All of the evaluations were conducted at service sites; therefore, the findings may not be generalizable to youths who do not use such services. The evaluation sample was relatively small and may not have permitted adequate statistical power to detect some program effects. Although there appeared to be few nonrespondents, no information was obtained that would allow a comparison of characteristics of nonrespondents with respondents.

Despite attempts at data transformation, the statistical assumption of homoscedasticity could not be met for two of the ANOVAs (i.e., general willingness to try a condom and intention to use condoms), and the use of imbalanced ANOVA designs may have exaggerated the effects of any departures from normality in the data. However, associations between program exposure and transformations of the two dependent variables listed above were significant among younger participants (i.e., 10-17 years old) when examined by cross-tabulation using Fisher's Exact Test.

Furthermore, the evaluation process could have benefited from greater col-laboration with representatives from the cultural, ethnic, and other reference groups represented in the audience. For instance, the pilot testing of the play and the focus group testing of the evaluation instrument could have had a more thorough assessment of ethnic relevance and validity. Measures of accul-turation to the major referent and ethnic groups of the homeless youth audi-ence and measures of stages of change (Prochaska & DiClemente, 1983) were not taken but may have been useful in guiding and understanding the cultural and change stage dimensions of the intervention's development, implementa-tion, and evaluation.

Conceptual Considerations

Because the participants had fairly high levels of HIV knowledge at base-line (mean score of 87% for comparison/pretest group vs. 91% for treatment/posttest group), it is not surprising that the project had no measurable effect on aggregate knowledge. With regard to the apparent differential program impact by age, several explanations are possible:

1. The data suggest that the mediators of the program's effects on attitudes and behavioral intentions may differ for younger adolescents compared with older adolescents.

2. Age may be a proxy for moderators of program effects such as develop-mental stage, stage of change, length of lifetime homelessness, depen-dency on the street economy, degree of acculturation to street life, and level of psychological distress.

3. A youth's developmental stage or change stage may influence responsive-ness to specific types or aspects of interventions (e.g., characteristics of the source, message, channel, etc.), exposure requirements, and the eco-logical comprehensiveness required for the intervention.

Project ABLE appeared to have more impact on most of the independent variables and intention to use condoms among male respondents and more influence on self-efficacy regarding consistent condom use and general will-ingness to try condoms among female respondents. Because male and female respondents were equally likely to report prior use of condoms, one possi-ble explanation is that, as female participants' perceived access to condoms increased with exposure to the intervention, so did their willingness to try condoms. Female audience members may have been at more advanced stages of change than the male participants before program exposure and, thus, responded to the more action-oriented aspects of the intervention and evaluation.

With regard to the project's differential effects by ethnic group, program exposure seemed to be associated with more change in beliefs about individuals who use condoms, condom efficacy, HIV-related knowledge, negotiation efficacy, willingness to try condoms, and behavioral intention to use condoms among Latinos/Hispanics compared with Caucasians and African Americans. Several explanations are possible. The highly attractive and engaging nature of one of the Latina educators may have contributed to the observed effect through her social influence as a reference group member. Data collected during pilot testing of the script suggest that audience members may have found the ethnic, sexual orientation, social class, experience, physical, and interpersonal characteristics of the peer educators/actors to be the most salient aspects of the intervention. It is possible that the observed impact was due to the story characters' reflections of core health values, perspectives, and attitudes held by Latino/Hispanic and other audience members. On the other hand, ethnicity may be related to stage of change; Latino/Hispanic participants may have been at stages of change that were more responsive to Project ABLE. It is not known what impact, if any, other specific intervention variables—such as setting, group exposure, or changes in peer educators/actors—may have had on the processing of the messages or on resistance or receptiveness to the content.

Intervention exposure was significantly associated with increases in perceived HIV risk among African American and Caucasian youths and decreases in perceived risk among Latino/Hispanic youths. Because the largest improvements in behavioral intention and willingness to try condoms were observed among Latino/Hispanic youths, the observed decrease in perceived risk appears to be a paradox. However, the indicator for perceived risk was not a significant direct predictor of either willingness to try condoms or intention to use condoms in the study sample. In addition, for some populations, high levels of perceived risk may immobilize rather than facilitate risk reduction intentions and efforts.

Implications for Interventions

Several general lessons were learned during the planning, implementation, and evaluation processes for Project ABLE.

Cultural Competence and Cultural Context

- Program planning and evaluation works best when it reflects the value and practice of collaborative decision making between participants, agency staff, planners, funding agencies, and other stakeholders.

- There must be a safe and culturally acceptable way to express disagreement or constructive criticism by each participant in the program planning and evaluation decision-making process.

- A thorough strengths/needs assessment of the target audience and its segments and collaboration with current representatives of each major segment (including cultural groups) of the target audience are essential to effective program planning and evaluation.

- The strengths/needs assessment must include a thorough understanding of the histories, various beliefs, attitudes, behaviors, and values related to health, prevention and protective behaviors, disease causality, non-Western and Western health services, sexuality, sexual behavior, and HIV transmission that are represented in a multicultural audience as well as the various levels of acculturation within the audience.

- Program staff members need to increase their cultural competencies and abilities to respond to different interpersonal and communication styles and needs when working in cross-cultural settings.

- Program staff should recognize and respect the heterogeneity within any classification of individuals.

- Members of some cultural groups may be reluctant to offer constructive criticism when asked to preview a developing intervention. Soliciting feedback from audience members should be done in culturally acceptable and meaningful ways.

- Certain subpopulations may have negative perceptions about the agency(ies) providing the intervention.

- Conflict may arise among program staff and audience members as diverging cultural perspectives are expressed.

- Selection of the best-fitting health behavior theory(ies) and intervention planning model should take into account the variety of perspectives, expectations, strengths, and needs of the cultural groups represented in the audience as well as the health issue and intervention setting.

- Homeless youth populations are heterogeneous on dimensions of homelessness; ethnicity; social class; education and literacy; income and poverty; employment skills; sex; gender and sexual orientation; psychological, intellectual, social, moral, and physical development; family histories; institutionalization histories; physical and mental health; and affiliation and acculturation to macrolevel and microlevel reference groups.

Peer Health Education, in General

- The characteristics of the health problem as well as the characteristics, strengths, and needs of the audience change over time and require monitoring to adjust the message content and delivery as necessary.

- Assessment of program fidelity and quality and potential mediating and moderating factors are essential to understanding impact data.

- Adequate resources and organizational support for all phases of program evaluation must be available.

- Peer actors/educators may be more comfortable and effective in collaborative rather than leadership roles in the development of a health communication script.

- The turnover of peer actors/educators is slowed and motivation is higher when the positions are paid rather than voluntary.

- In-service training for the peer actors/educators needs to be ongoing to update knowledge and maintain efficacy, especially when turnover is rapid.

Finally, health communications for homeless youths might be most effective if considered in the context of the competing and more immediate needs and motivations inherent in the experience of homelessness as well as the levels of intervention required to affect the social ecology of homelessness.

Notes

1. Project ABLE still serves the adolescents of Los Angeles County from its home at the Los Angeles Free Clinic and continues to expand its repertoire of interventions and health topics as well as its target audiences.

2. To minimize the length of the questionnaire, the constructs listed were measured using single questions unless otherwise noted.

3. Results from the fiscal year 1990-91 are not presented due to data collection errors. In addition, respondents who recalled prior completion of the evaluation survey were eliminated from the sample.

4. Significant interaction was found between age and intervention exposure status in predicting differences in perceived reinforcers for condom use; this finding suggests that age, rather than the intervention, may have caused the observed differences. Age did not produce significant covariate or interaction effects in any of the other ANOVAs.

5. No significant relationships were found between respondent gender and ethnicity or age.

References

Ajzen, I., & Fishbein, M. (1985). From intentions to actions: A theory of planned behavior. In J. Kuhl & J. Beckman (Eds.), *Action control from cognition to behavior* (p. 11-38). Heidelberg, Germany: Springer.

Bandura, A. (1986). *Social foundations of thought and action: A cognitive social theory.* Englewood Cliffs, NJ: Prentice Hall.

Goldstick, O. (1988). *The street where I live.* Unpublished script.

Green, L. W., Kreuter, M. W., Deeds, S. G., & Partridge, K. B. (1980). *Health education planning: A diagnostic approach.* Palo Alto, CA: Mayfield.

Greenblatt, M., & Robertson, M. J. (1993). Lifestyles, adaptive strategies, and sexual behaviors of homeless adolescents. *Hospital and Community Psychiatry, 44*(12), 1177-1180.

Huff, R. M., & Kline, M. V. (1999). Health promotion in the context of culture. In R. M. Huff & M. V. Kline (Eds.), *Promoting health in multicultural populations* (pp. 3-22). Thousand Oaks, CA: Sage.

Kagawa-Singer, M., & Chung, R. (1994). A paradigm for culturally based care in ethnic minority populations. *Journal of Community Psychology, 22,* 192-208.

Kennedy, M. G., O'Hara, P., Fichtner, R. R., & Fishbein, M. (1996). Can intentions to use condoms predict condom use among high-risk, multicultural youth in a Miami alternative school? In I. I. Schenker, G. Sabar-Friedman, & S. S. Francisco (Eds.), *AIDS education* (pp. 195-201). New York: Plenum.

McGuire, W. J. (1985). Attitudes and attitude change. In G. Lindzey & E. Aronson (Eds.), *Handbook of social psychology* (Vol. 2). New York: Random House.

Pfeifer, R. W., & Oliver, J. (1997). A study of HIV seroprevalence in a group of homeless youth in Hollywood, California. *Journal of Adolescent Health, 20*(5), 339-342.

Podschun, G. (1993). Teen peer outreach-street work project: HIV prevention education for runaway and homeless youth. *Public Health Reports, 108*(2), 150-155.

Prochaska, J. O., & DiClemente, C. C. (1983). Stages and process of self-change of smoking: Toward an integrated model of change. *Journal of Consulting and Clinical Psychology, 51,* 390-395.

Robertson, M. J. (1990, August). *Homeless youth in Hollywood: Patterns of alcohol use.* Paper presented at the annual meeting of the American Psychological Association, Boston.

Robertson, M. J. (1991). Homeless youth: An overview of the recent literature. In J. H. KryderCoe, L. M. Salamon, & J. M. Molnar (Eds.), *Homeless children and youth* (pp. 33-68). New Brunswick, NJ: Transaction Publishers.

Rosenstock, I. M. (1974). Historical origins of the health belief model. In M. H. Becker (Ed.), *The health belief model and personal health behavior.* Thorofare, NJ: Charles B. Slack.

Rotheram-Borus, M. J., Meyer-Bahlburg, H. F., L., Koopman, C., Rosario, M., Exner, T. M., Henderson, R., Matthieu, M., & Gruen, R. (1992). Lifetime sexual behaviors among runaway males and females. *Journal of Sex Research, 29*(1), 15-29.

Russell, L. A. (1998). *Child maltreatment and psychological distress among urban homeless youth.* New York: Garland.

Shalwitz, J., Goulart, M., Dunnigan, K., & Flannery, D. (1990, June). *Prevalence of sexually transmitted diseases and HIV in a homeless youth medical clinic in San Francisco.* Paper presented at the International Conference on AIDS, San Francisco, CA.

Slonim, M. (1991). *Children, culture, and ethnicity: Evaluating and understanding the impact.* New York: Garland.

Stricof, R. L., Novick, L. F., & Kennedy, J. T. (1990, June). *HIV1 seroprevalence in facilities for runaway and homeless youth adolescents in four states (FL, TX, LA and NY).* Paper presented at the International Conference on AIDS, San Francisco, CA.

Sugerman, S. T., Hergenroeder, A. C., Chacko, M. R., & Parcel, G. S. (1991). Acquired immunodeficiency syndrome and adolescents: Knowledge, attitudes, and behaviors of runaway and homeless youth. *American Journal of Diseases in Childhood, 145,* 431-436.

Yates, G., MacKenzie, R., Pennbridge, J., & Cohen, E. (1988). A risk profile comparison of runaway and nonrunaway youth. *American Journal of Public Health, 78,* 820-821.

11

The Community as Classroom

A Health Communication Program Among Older Samoan and American Indian Women

Lené Levy-Storms
Steven P. Wallace
Fran Goldfarb
Linda Burhansstipanov

The Problem

This case study focuses on communication and health issues within two "minority-minority" groups who have often been lost within classifications of other larger minority groups: Samoans and American Indians. Because of their

AUTHORS' NOTE: This study was made possible by support from the California Wellness Foundation. The authors wish to thank the Center for Healthy Aging, the (formerly) Bellflower American Indian Clinic, the Office of Samoan Affairs, and the Samoan Federation of America for their assistance in this program. In particular, the authors appreciate the leadership and efforts of Chief Pelé Faletogo.

relatively small numbers, these two groups have traditionally been included under "Asian/Pacific Islanders" and "other." Both groups have a history of migration from their native lands to more urbanized settings. One setting, Los Angeles County, provides access to otherwise "invisible" populations. In migrating, each group encountered personal, social, and economic stressors that have left them at risk for the development of chronic diseases. Paradoxically, neither group inherently faced such risks in their native lands, but they do so in their more urbanized environments largely because of alterations in their traditional cultural lifestyles (Pawson & Janes, 1982; Wykle & Kaskel, 1991).

A brief review of Samoan and American Indians' migration histories places their health risks in context. As a result of their participation in the military and defense industry during World War II, Samoans experienced a surge of migration in the 1950s to Los Angeles (among other places). The "Great Migration of 1950" marked the first significant movement of Samoans to the U.S. mainland from both the U.S. territory of American Samoa and the larger, independent Western Samoa (Pouesi, 1994). In migrating, they sought to take advantage of educational and employment opportunities in the United States (Pouesi, 1994). Samoan migration patterns generally flowed from Western Samoa to the semi-urban environments of American Samoa and Hawaii and then to the U.S. mainland. Many older Samoans have lived in the U.S. mainland for the latter third of their lives.

American Indians share with Samoans a history of migration; however, American Indians' migration patterns flowed back and forth directly from their rural reservation settings to more urbanized settings beginning in the early 1930s. Their migration incentives largely arose from federal policies throughout the mid-20th century designed to assimilate native peoples into Western culture and partly from a better job market in urban settings (Kramer, 1991). A study on American Indian women in Los Angeles County found that most of them had lived in an urban setting for less than 10 years and often returned to reservations for ceremonies (Farmer, Barnett, & Bouchard, 1993).

Neither Samoans nor American Indians expected the health disadvantages that they faced as a consequence of their migration. In adapting to Western culture and practices, both groups developed chronic health problems, including obesity, hypertension, and diabetes—health problems traditionally unheard of among them (Hodge, 1994). These problems contributed to each group's major causes of mortality. Among American Indian women, heart disease, cancer, and diabetes are the first, second, and fourth leading causes of death (Indian Health Service, 1992). Major causes of mortality specifically among Samoans are not available. However, data on Samoans' health status documents common chronic health conditions such as stress, cardiovascular disease, diabetes, and cancer (Crews, 1989; Crews & MacKeen, 1982; Janes, 1990a; Paksoy, Bouchardy, & Parkin, 1991) with a disproportionate number of articles on obesity and hypertension (McGarvey, 1979, 1991; McGarvey & Baker, 1979).

Often in research studies, Samoans and American Indians have been combined with larger minority groups, resulting in less attention to their diversity and individual health needs. For example, American Indians have been termed "the invisible minority" and have often been categorized as Hispanic (Kramer, 1992), and Samoans have usually been "lost" under the Asian Pacific Islander (API) rubric where there is an assumption of a "typical API" (Tanjasiri, Wallace, & Shibata, 1995). Unlike Samoans, the American Indian community is very diverse, both in location and tribal affiliation.

The 1990 U.S. census provides some insight into the numbers and socioeconomic status of Samoan and Native American populations. There were a total of 63,000 Samoans in the United States; 55,000 of them live in the western region (primarily California), although they make up only 0.9% of the large group of Asian/Pacific Islanders Americans. However, from 1980 to 1990, the number of Samoans in the United States grew by 50% compared with the total population percentage growth of 9.8% (U.S. Bureau of the Census, 1993). The census is probably a low estimate because migrants frequently return to their native Samoa and because of language and educational barriers to the census. Janes and Pawson (1986) estimate that the census undercounts Samoans by about 20%. However, their concentration in California provides ample access to their communities. For example, Samoans made up 41% of Pacific Islanders in Los Angeles County or 12,000 in 1990 (Hornor, 1995; U.S. Bureau of the Census, 1993). The largest concentration of Samoans in California resides in the Los Angeles Basin, especially near the community of Carson (Pouesi, 1994).

Likewise, in the Southern California area, the largest concentration of Native Americans resides in Los Angeles County. There were an estimated 45,508 American Indians, Eskimo, and Aleutians in Los Angeles County in 1990; American Indians made up 96% of the Native population and .5% of the total population in Los Angeles County (U.S. Bureau of the Census, 1992). Unlike Samoans, American Indians live all over the county with no concentrations in any particular geographic area. For example, there is no "Little Indian Country" in Los Angeles, although Los Angeles has the largest urban Indian population of any nonreservation county in the country and includes people from over 200 tribes (Kramer, 1992). Like Samoans, the American Indian population has substantially increased in the last decade. From 1980 to 1990, the number of American Indians in the United States grew by 38% compared with the total population growth of 9.8% (U.S. Bureau of the Census, 1993). These estimates are debatable for reasons including high mobility of the Native American populations, language barriers, and resistance to government questionnaires. For example, the Indian Alcoholism Commission of California proposes that over 100,000 American Indians reside within Los Angeles County (Department of Health Services, 1992).

Prior research on these populations has typically favored problem-oriented rather than intervention-oriented approaches (John, 1991). The Community Action for Women's Health (CAWH), a health promotion program, addressed these two populations' chronic health problems by creating "community classrooms." In these classrooms, women learned about preventive health concepts and practices relevant to general health and specific chronic diseases such as hypertension, diabetes, and cancer. A review of the specific links between Samoan and American Indian's chronic disease risk factors and their lifestyles will set the stage for the program communication processes and effects later in this case study.

Chronic Disease Risk Factors

Samoans and American Indians alike exhibited changes in specific health-related behaviors as they adapted after migrating to more urbanized environments. Subsequent changes in their lifestyles increased their risk for the development of chronic, noninfectious health problems and diseases, such as obesity, hypertension, diabetes, coronary heart disease, and some cancers (Hodge, 1994; Janes & Pawson, 1986; John, 1991; Kramer, 1991). Following migration, Samoans experienced increased stress levels, changes in diet, decreased physical activity, and a lack of access to medical care (Pearson, James, & Brown, 1993), which was similar to the American Indian experience. American Indians faced an especially acute risk for hypertension and diabetes mellitus regardless of their residing on reservations or urbanized areas.

There are links between stress and chronic disease (Kramer, 1992). Migrant Samoans' stress levels increase because of both cultural and environmental factors. Samoans extensively depend on their kin networks following migration for monetary support, employment opportunities, finding housing, and negotiating with the administrative bureaucracies (Hanna, Fitzgerald, Pearson, Howard, & Hanna, 1991). In turn, migrant Samoans are expected to send money back to Samoa as part of *Fa'aa Samoa* or the Samoan way of life (Fitzgerald & Howard, 1990). The conflict between the Samoan culture, which values collectivism and groups, and the migrant Samoans' adaptation to a Westernized culture, which values individualism, operates as a source of stress (Janes & Pawson, 1986). Their lifestyle changes, in turn, are exacerbated by their need to adapt to an urban and Western environment despite their lack of labor force skills, limited education, and language barriers (Pouesi, 1994). One study that compared stress levels among Korean, Filipino, and Samoan immigrants to Hawaii found that Samoans experienced the greatest amount of stress (Kincaid & Yum, 1987).

American Indians shared some of the same challenges as Samoans in adapting to Western society in that they also lacked labor force skills and had low levels of educational attainment. Many American Indian elders live with their children, and these multigenerational households have an increased risk for poverty compared with whites (Kramer, 1991). These socioeconomic factors contribute to their high risk for poor health and contribute to high stress levels (Chovan & Chovan, 1985; Hodge, 1994; Joe, 1994). Yet, American Indian culture traditionally stigmatizes mental health problems. Combined with their lack of awareness and availability of psychological, social, or economic resources, their situation leaves them at risk for high stress levels (Kramer, 1992).

Samoans and American Indians have adopted new foods after migration to urban settings. These dietary changes, along with their less active lifestyles, have had adverse health consequences. Both groups, particularly American Indians, have maintained some aspects of their cultural heritage but have had a tendency to adopt Western behaviors that were least healthy (Hodge, 1994). To both Samoans and American Indians, food has been an essential component to any gathering, whether it involves the family, the church, or a community celebration. The traditional Samoan diet has consisted of fish, taro, and banana over beef and potatoes (Ishikawa, 1978), but since migration, Samoans have had regular access to foods traditionally available only during celebrations and have been exposed to more processed American food. Similarly, American Indians' natural diet has consisted of low-fat and high-fiber foods, but more typically today, they eat convenience food or federally sponsored "surplus" foods, which have a high content of fat and sugar (Hodge, 1994). Samoans have maintained the quantity *and* quality of their diet after migration despite their tendency to lead more sedentary lifestyles, which has left them at risk for obesity (Janes, 1990b). Thus, these two groups' risk for the development of chronic diseases resides mostly with behaviorally related factors. The next step was to design a culturally sensitive program to educate and motivate Samoan and American Indian women to change their lifestyles.

History of the Program

The Center for Healthy Aging (CHA), formerly Senior Health and Peer Counseling (SHPC), is a Santa Monica-based community organization that focuses on mental health as well as health promotion and disease prevention among seniors. Over the years, the CHA has worked with the local Samoan and American Indian communities in several capacities. In the Samoan community, they pioneered a peer-counseling program to counsel families and assist them in recovering from the civil unrest in 1992. In the American Indian community, the CHA established a relationship with the American Indian Clinic (AIC) by providing breast cancer screening through their Breast Cancer and Cervical Cancer Program (BCCCP). As a result of these programs, the CHA noticed a similarity in these two communities' health problems, including obesity, hypertension, diabetes, vision problems, high stress levels, and inactive lifestyles, among others. The CHA then made a strategic decision to expand its involvement in helping build capacity in underserved areas in Los Angeles County. It partnered with organizations of the two communities and collaboratively designed a program proposal to start a health promotion communication program for older women.

With funding from the California Wellness Foundation in 1994, these communities became the targets of the CAWH program, which program aimed to bring low-cost community involvement in promoting health and to deliver culturally sensitive education about health. It focused on women because of (a) the need for more research-based information on women and minorities' health problems, (b) the tendency of women to use more health services, and (c) the cultural practice of women taking care of the families in both cultures. The underlying assumptions were that women would share the health information with their families and would have the autonomy in health-related decisions and actions.

In each community, the program encountered challenges as it took the first implementation step, which was to set up advisory councils. In the Samoan community, the advisory council included community leaders as well as local Samoan church ministers and their wives, which proved to be a difficult mix. For example, one of the first meetings took several hours to select a program symbol and translate the name into an effective phrase in Samoan. The CHA realized that this larger group would be most useful during more landmark moments in carrying out the program and that a smaller workgroup would be necessary for most of the tasks. The CHA handled this situation delicately by sending out letters to all ministers and their wives informing them that they would be consulted on major issues and outreach. Although the program needed the Samoan ministers' approval and support in accordance with the traditional hierarchical Samoan political structure, they also needed to keep a more efficient pace in developing and implementing the program. The remaining smaller workgroup involved one Samoan leader; the Samoan RN/health educator, who led most of the program segments; the principal investigator; project director; and evaluation manager who more effectively implemented the program.

Other complications arose with the AIC in Bellflower. The clinic had internal budgetary problems, which, in turn, resulted in financial management issues for the program. Because these administrative issues were partly external to the program, the solution was to lessen the administrative role of the AIC in delivering the program. This was accomplished on two fronts. A well-respected, American Indian researcher who worked at the AIC part-time led the American Indian advisory council. She had less financial stake in the internal AIC budget, but her consulting role at the clinic allowed a comfortable working relationship between the AIC and the CHA to continue. Second, the locations for the American Indian women's program shifted from only at the AIC to throughout Los Angeles County. Although some classes were still held at the AIC, dispersing the program into Los Angeles better reflected the program participants' dispersed residences. In a sense, these new locations brought the CAWH into their "community."

The next step in both communities included obtaining more input from lay community members about what health topics they wanted to learn about in their program. To achieve this input, the CHA conducted focus groups. Community leaders assisted in recruiting women for the focus groups that met in community centers, churches, and the AIC clinic. Two important outcomes arose from these groups. First, the older women discussed the health issues that were of concern to them, including managing their weight, proper nutrition, stressors, financial problems, worries over their families (especially children), and employment problems. Many of their concerns revolved around risk factors for chronic diseases, which supported the program's interest in presenting topics on these same risk factors, including managing stress and incorporating leisure time activities, for example. A second important outcome of these focus groups was the revelation of sensitive issues that differed for each group. For example, among the Samoans, cancer was noted as being a traditionally taboo topic as well as any sexual concerns. Among the American Indians, alcohol abuse stood apart from other topics as being the most sensitive. Paradoxically, discussions about these and other "tradition-sensitive" topics were relatively open and free in the context of the focus groups where women became comfortable in a group setting. As a consequence, program planners were able to understand the depth of the issues underlying these topics while at the same time learn how to carefully incorporate them as topics in the actual program's curricula.

In sum, the history of the planning of the CAWH program evolved on two fronts into its final form: the more political community-organizational level, which included each group's advisory council, and the more lay community-member level, which included potential program attendees, themselves. The underlying dynamic to the program's evolution revolved around culturally appropriate and politically sensitive communication between an outside agency (the CHA) and both communities' leaders and members. As will be seen later in this chapter, this communication dynamic continued to operate during program implementation and on into the implications of the program's findings.

The Communication Process

Sources and Program Planning

Following the work with focus groups in each community, the next steps involved developing health curricula, marketing the program, and beginning outreach efforts to potential participants. Although the focus groups explored each community's perception of the program's goals as well as how to market and recruit women to attend the program in each community (U.S. Department of Health and Human Services, 1992), it was important to get the program known. To kick off the CAWH program in both communities, the advisory councils planned events that would publicize the program. In the Samoan community, the most natural setting was at their annual Flag Day celebration in August, which celebrates the raising of the U.S. Flag in their native American Samoan Island on April 17, 1900 (Pouesi, 1994). Samoan attendees picked up information about the program from a booth, which also offered free weight, blood pressure, blood sugar, and eye screenings. Also in this booth, Samoan physicians, nurses, and traditional healers talked about the importance of the program. In the American Indian community, the advisory council invited a well-known, popular Native American woman, Cecilia Firethunder, to speak about menopause. To them, part of her appeal was her ability to talk about an otherwise serious topic lightly. She spoke about menopause—a topic usually not discussed *even among women*—in a humorous but compelling manner *among both men and women.*

The next step was to recruit women to attend the program. In the American Indian community, the CHA attended local powwows and announced the program on Native American radio stations. Recruiters paid particular attention to *not* recruiting nonnatives who were attracted to American Indian culture. Had this group of nonnatives been included, Native Americans would not have attended. The program also used the radio in the Samoan community, but the primary mode of outreach was one-to-one through kin and church networks. Both Samoans and American Indians have histories of oral transmission of knowledge (Kramer, 1997; Levy-Storms, 1998). This was largely because the Samoan program required a larger time commitment than the American Indian program and because of the limited Samoan targeted media. The difference in commitment required of each program becomes apparent in reviewing each program's structure.

From the respective advisory councils and focus groups, it became clear that each community wanted a different structure for its program. The Samoans proposed an 8-week program that met twice a week for 5 hours and included traditional foods for lunch and snacks. Thus, the Samoan program became an 8-week comprehensive program (totaling 80 hours of classroom time for each group) covering a wide range of chronic health-related topics. The Samoans met primarily at two local community-based organizations: the Office of Samoan Affairs and the Samoan Federation of America. These organizations were located less than 3 miles from each another. The American Indians preferred to meet hourly on a topic-by-topic, drop-in basis at a wide variety of locations (totaling 1 hour for every class). Thus, the American Indian program became a series of independent classes that focused on a particular topic for that month with the exception of two segments: weight management and arthritis. These two topics spanned 4 to 12 weeks (totaling 12 hours) because they were a series.

Media/Medium

The curriculum in both communities included health topics such as nutrition, weight management, exercise, hypertension, stress, diabetes, leisure time, physician skills, menopause, breast and cervical cancer, and substance abuse. This curriculum provided a structure of individual and group activities, topics to be covered, the length of time allocated for each activity, and the order of presentation of the topics for each health area. The description of the program primarily describes the Samoan program's curriculum because the American Indian program was loosely based on the same substantive content but much less so on the same structure and time frame because of the differences between each community program's delivery structure.

Message/Content

To ensure that the curriculum was culturally acceptable and interesting, the health educator from the CHA developed it with the assistance of indigenous health professionals. For example, a Samoan nurse worked closely with the health educator to ensure that the terms in the curriculum were meaningful in the Samoan language or could be explained using a combination of Samoan words. Once completed, Samoan community leaders translated the curriculum into Samoan, because most of the target group was monolingual in Samoan. This was necessary because no health education materials existed for Samoans. For example, the health educator called the Red Cross on the Samoan Islands about possible educational materials, and all they had to offer were brochures in English or *Spanish*. A similar but abbreviated version of the Samoan curriculum was adapted for the American Indian women in English. Among American Indians there exist at least 150 different native languages (Kramer, 1992), although in Los Angeles almost all are fluent in English.

Program Implementation

The communication process in each group's program was similar. Indigenous health educators (source) orally presented (channel) the curriculum's preventive health material (message) to women aged 40 and over (receiver). The idea of using health educators was novel in both communities, because they both have histories of traditional healers and remedies. The health educators emphasized how to use the program's preventive health material to complement their traditional healing methods—not to replace them. They accomplished this, in part, by suggesting when to contact a Western health provider and when to contact a traditional healer, depending on the nature of the illness. Traditional healers attended the program only insofar as any of the program participants happened to be traditional healers. The program targeted women aged 40 years and older because of the program's emphasis on prevention.

Part of the American Indian program's communication goals was to teach the nonnative lead agency how to present appropriate programs to the Native American community. In doing so, the nonnative health educator slowly took

over more of the direct education. During the initial programs, she participated as an observer while a Native American woman led the class, allowing the
participants to become more comfortable with her. In addition, she simultaneously attended numerous non-program-related Native American events,
such as powwows, to increase her visibility and acceptance in the general Native
American community. When she actually began teaching classes, she had already been accepted as a part of this program. However, she, as a nonnative,
avoided teaching on tobacco or alcohol because these are sensitive issues within
traditional American Indian culture. For example, tobacco has had traditional,
sacred uses, and it would have been inappropriate for a nonnative to discuss it.
That a nonnative was able to deliver the program at all was a major success.

As part of the program's design, women filled out surveys assessing their
knowledge, attitudes, and practices of each of the health topics. Like the curriculum, the Samoan survey was translated and included pre- and posttests. Initially, surveys were completed at the beginning of each class, but the women felt
that it set a class tone of "research" rather than learning and enjoyment. We responded by shifting all pretests to the 1st and 8th class of the program and
posttests to the 10th and 16th weeks to reduce testing days. Posttests were only
for knowledge and attitude questions because the duration between the tests
was too short to detect long-lasting behavioral changes. Because of the stag-
gered schedule, some women missed part of the tests. Occasionally, tests were
overlooked altogether in the press of finishing an 8-week program. Consequently, the pretest/posttest results were only for those women who completed
both tests. The Samoan women, themselves, collected other physiological data.
During the classes, the Samoan women learned how to take their own blood
pressure, blood sugar levels, and weigh themselves. They regularly recorded
this information during the beginning of each class. In fact, the women enjoyed
their new skills so much that they often weighed themselves and checked their
blood pressures several times *in one class session!*

The original American Indian women's survey was similar to the Samoans,
at least until program attendees actually filled it out. They expressed outrage at
the survey's "request" for their names and addresses. Furthermore, the survey
was too long for them to fill out in the short class time given, because many had
to catch prearranged, scheduled transportation. In response, a Native American advisory council member suggested a more culturally consonant way of
gathering data. The program implemented a shortened survey form that was
designed around a circle or wheel with the four cardinal directions: North,
South, East, and West. Native American culture believes in a symbolic circle of
life that symbolizes harmony and balance (Joe, 1994). Three questions went in

each direction in accordance with what each direction traditionally represented. For example, questions about their background were placed in the East, which represents beginnings. A Native American program administrator read the questions while the women wrote their responses on the wheel *at the beginning of each class session.*[1] In addition, the questions no longer included their names or addresses. Their concerns with the original survey and the program's response exemplified the overcoming of one of the major challenges among the American Indians: developing trust within their community by immediately and appropriately addressing their concerns. Trust in the Samoan community was gained via the participation of local leaders; a similar hierarchy of leadership was not available in Los Angeles' diverse Native American community.

Communication Effects/Impact

Individual Level

One original goal of the health communication program was to increase by 20% preventive health knowledge, attitudes, and practices as well as improve self-reported overall health status among program participants. This goal reflected the California Wellness Foundation's evaluation criteria, although it later proved to be unrealistic both in terms of the program's timeline and the difficulty of bringing Western programs into minority communities. This issue will be discussed further later in the chapter. Changes in preventive health knowledge and attitudes were assessed only in the Samoan community as discussed earlier. Results showed that the program succeeded in reaching its goal among some areas of the Samoan women's knowledge and attitudes. Both groups' baseline health knowledge, attitudes, and practices also show some important patterns.

Samoan Women. The results are organized overall in two sets of tables referring to chronic health and general health knowledge, attitudes, and practices. Table 11.1 presents the change in pre- and posttest knowledge of hypertension, diabetes, and cancer among the Samoan women. Overall, the greatest improvement over baseline occurred in the hypertension and cancer-related questions where almost all women retained the new class material. However, within each area, knowledge levels at pretest and improvement over pretest at posttest varied. The highest proportions of increase over baseline were among those who reported to

Table 11.1 Hypertension, Diabetes, Cancer: Knowledge and Attitudes Among Samoan Women Only (in percentages)

Knowledge of . . .	Pretest Response	Posttest Response	Percentage Increase Over Baseline[a]
Hypertension			
Cigarette smoking can lead to high blood pressure ($n = 19$).	42	84	42*
High salt intake can contribute to high blood pressure ($n = 18$).	72	94	22
Medication can lower high blood pressure ($n = 18$).	83	94	11
Diabetes			
Diabetes can cause blurred vision ($n = 24$).	79	96	17
More women get diabetes than men ($n = 23$).	35	43	8
Cancer			
Breast cancer is the most common cancer among women ($n = 24$).	92	100	8
Women aged 50 and over should have a mammogram yearly ($n = 24$).	29	67	38*
Smoking causes most deaths from lung cancer ($n = 19$).	63	95	32
Regular screenings help prevent cancer ($n = 26$).	88	100	12

Attitudes Toward . . .	Pretest Response	Posttest Response	Percentage Increase Over Baseline[a]
Hypertension			
Very concerned about avoiding salt ($n = 18$).	33	44	10
Diabetes			
Very concerned about avoiding sugar ($n = 18$).	22	44	22
Cancer			
Plan to have a mammogram in the future ($n = 25$).	64	84	20

a. Significance of increase over pretest was assessed by using McNemar's test with a continuity correction to adjust for using a continuous distribution to evaluate a discrete distribution.
*$p < .05$; **$p < .01$; ***$p < 001$.

know about the relationship of cigarette smoking and salt to high blood pressure, the screening recommendations for women aged 50 and over, and the relationship between smoking and cancer. Many questions with less improvement over baseline had the highest baseline levels, which left less room for improvement, except the question relating gender to diabetes, which was already low at baseline. Thus, knowledge is changeable in this group setting. Posttests were often several weeks after the actual class, so these results suggest that retention was more than short-term.

Table 11.1 also shows the change over baseline among Samoan women in their attitudes relating to hypertension, diabetes, and cancer. Most striking from the results is the relatively small improvements in attitudes in comparison to knowledge. The program had aimed for greater changes in light of the high rates of hypertension among Samoans. Although not statistically significant, there was improvement in attitudes about diabetes and cancer. The relatively high proportion at baseline and subsequent increase over baseline in those planning to get a mammogram were unexpected but positive findings. Possibly, mammograms, which are relatively infrequent, limited commitment procedures, are easier to change attitudes about than lifestyle issues such as sugar and salt consumption or, specifically among Samoans, the consumption of coconut oil. For example, during one class, the health educator discussed oils and cooking and eventually the use of coconut cream. The women's reaction was not just dissent but outrage. In their strong opinion, coconut cream and coconut oil represented "natural" Samoan foods, which have traditionally been considered "healthy." Their overwhelming reaction to this information caused the Samoan health educator to change her presentation by not using the word *unhealthy* to describe how coconut cream and coconut oil were bad for their health to a recommendation that they "use less" of it. In this way, the class was able to recompose itself and comfortably move on to the next topic.

Table 11.2 presents knowledge of Samoan women on more general health areas, including obesity, nutrition, exercise, substance use, and health service use. Most concerning of the results was the low improvement over baseline regarding knowledge about *reducing* fat intake given the propensity of Samoan women to be obese (McGarvey, 1991). For example, despite using the food pyramid as a visual, Samoan woman did *not* improve over baseline in knowing that the fat and oils group sits at the top of the pyramid. Knowledge about fat intake was also among the lowest at baseline, which suggests that these women not only knew little about their fat intake at baseline but also were less receptive to new information in the area. By far, the largest, only statistically significant improvement occurred in a nutrition-related question on fiber content of beans.

Table 11.2 General Health: Knowledge and Attitudes Among Samoans Only (percentages)

General Health Concepts	Pretest Response	Posttest Response	Percentage Increase Over Baseline[a]
A high-fat diet can lead to obesity ($n = 15$).	87	100	13
Eating less fat definitely helps one lose weight ($n = 18$).	11	22	11
Beans are high in fiber ($n = 15$).	27	73	46*
"Fat and oils group" is at the top of the food pyramid ($n = 14$).	64	57	−7
Exercise can increase energy levels ($n = 17$).	94	100	6
Tobacco can be addictive[b] ($n = 20$).	65	80	15
Heavy alcohol drinking can contribute to liver disease ($n = 25$).	84	96	12
Routine checkups are an important part of good health ($n = 26$).	85	100	15

Attitudes	Pretest Response	Posttest Response	Percentage Increase Over Baseline[a]
Self-reported good to excellent health status ($n = 12$).	33	49	16
Self-reported overweight ($n = 21$).	31	31	0

a. Significance of increase over pretest was assessed by using McNemar's Test with a continuity correction to adjust for using a continuous distribution to evaluate a discrete distribution.
b. This question implies that *nicotine* is addictive but does not use the word because few women would have known that nicotine is added to tobacco.
*$p < .05$; **$p < .01$; ***$p < .001$.

For the remaining general health areas, knowledge levels were high at baseline and improved to a maximum 100% or close to a maximum at posttest.

General health attitudes presented in the continuation of Table 11.2 include self-reported health and weight status. Both areas had similarly low proportions at baseline. Most notable was the low proportion of Samoan women reporting themselves to be overweight (e.g., 31%) in light of previously mentioned propensity for them to become obese. These results of general attitude levels were similar to chronic attitude levels in Table 11.1 in that they were also low at baseline with only modest changes at posttest.

In summarizing the chronic and general health knowledge and attitudes, the Samoan women's program showed the most influence in changing their knowledge levels and a more modest effect on attitudes. These results raise the question, Is individual-focused communication sufficient enough for significant change? The aim was that the participants' knowledge, attitudes, and practices would change and that they, in turn, would influence others in their networks. The program assumed that women have the autonomy of health-related decisions. However, in light of the results, maybe the networks should be the focus in future interventions. This will be taken up again in the discussion section of the chapter.

Samoan and American Indian Women. The next series of tables present data on the chronic and general health knowledge, attitudes, and practices of both the American Indian and Samoan women. The discussion of the results focuses on the American Indian women first then compares them with the Samoan women because the American Indian women's program collected only baseline (i.e., pretest) data. Table 11.3 shows that there were mixed levels of knowledge at baseline, with each group favoring higher levels in different areas. Still, most knowledge levels among both groups of women were fairly high (i.e., in the 60%-90% range). The only statistically significant comparison in knowledge levels between the two groups occurred in the hypertension areas: American Indian women knew more at baseline than Samoan women about how smoking and exercise affect high blood pressure ($p < .05$). It is troublesome that a higher proportion of American Indian women reported to have diabetes than Samoan women, but knowledge levels among American Indian women were lower than Samoan women in terms of risk factors and management techniques for diabetes.

In the attitudinal realm for hypertension and cancer, Table 11.4 shows that the results between the American Indian and Samoan women had different priorities. American Indian women were almost twice as concerned about avoiding salt *($p < .05$)*. The Samoan women, on the other hand, had a high rate of interest in cancer screening compared with a low concern with salt, at least descriptively, because the sample size for the American Indian was not large enough to statistically compare them.

Turning to these women's chronic health practices, Table 11.4 indicates that similar proportions of American Indian and Samoan women in this program

Table 11.3 Hypertension, Diabetes, Cancer: Baseline Knowledge Only[a] (pretest percentages)

Knowledge of . . .	American Indian		Samoan	
	N	Pretest	N	Pretest
Hypertension				
Exercising helps lower high blood pressure.	40	93	55	75*
Medication can lower high blood pressure.	41	88	54	70
Cigarette smoking can lead to high blood pressure.	69	87	52	44*
Losing weight helps lower high blood pressure.	40	85	N/A[b]	N/A
High cholesterol leads to high blood pressure.	40	80	N/A	N/A
Heart disease affects women less than men.	41	51	N/A	N/A
Diabetes				
Are you diabetic?[c]	67	34	54	26
Diabetes can cause blurred vision.	68	87	39	82
Exercise helps control diabetes.	77	73	40	85
Managing stress is important in preventing diabetes.	67	66	39	69
Numbness or tingling in hands and feet may be a symptom of diabetes.	68	63	39	72
More women get diabetes than men.	68	25	37	38
Cancer				
Most deaths from lung cancer are caused by smoking.	26	77	40	63
Breast cancer is the most common cancer among women.	3	33	38	86
Regular screenings help prevent cancer.	N/A	N/A[d]	40	88

a. Statistical comparison is based on the two-sample test for proportions.
b. N/A = not available.
c. This question was asked differently for each group. American Indian women self-reported; whereas, Samoan women reported if a doctor ever told them that they had diabetes.
d. This item was dropped for the American Indian women because only one respondent answered.
*$p < .05$; **$p < .01$; ***$p < .001$.

Table 11.4 Hypertension and Cancer: Attitudes and Practices Baseline Only[a] (pretest percentages)

Attitudes toward . . .	American Indian		Samoan	
	N	Pretest	N	Pretest
Hypertension				
Concerned about avoiding salt.	27	59	54	26*
Cancer				
Plan to have a Pap test in the future.	3	33	33	64
Plan to have a mammogram in the future.	3	33	37	68

Practices relating to . . .	N	Pretest (%)	N	Pretest (%)
Hypertension				
Salt food often.	39	22	55	29
Cancer				
Had mammogram.	3	67	23	56
Had Pap smear.	3	67	41	63
Made changes to avoid cancer.	2	50	38	66

a. Statistical comparison is based on the two-sample test for proportions.
*$p < .05$; **$p < .01$; ***$p < .001$.

reported salting their food often. Breast and cervical cancer screening rates for both groups were similar, although they were still below desirable rates (American Cancer Society, 1997).

American Indian and Samoan women's general health knowledge levels regarding health service use, nutrition, and substance use were generally good, with a few notable exceptions (Table 11.5). In terms of health services use, a higher proportion of the American Indian women reported that they had a regular health care location compared with the Samoan women, which is an observation to note, but the difference was not statistically significant. This difference may be attributed, in part, to the role of the Indian Health Service in providing a regular source of care to American Indian women or to the consequence of recent migration among some Samoans and their lack of familiarity in where to seek regular medical care. One statistically significant difference

Table 11.5 General Health: Knowledge Baseline Only[a]
(pretest percentages)

General Health Knowledge	American Indian		Samoan	
	N	Pretest	N	Pretest
Routine checkups are an important part of good health.	39	97	40	90
Is there one place you usually go when you are sick or need advice about your health?	39	74	43	56
"Fat and oils group" is at the top of the food pyramid.	41	32	48	58*
The overuse of alcohol is preventable.	41	95	N/A[b]	N/A
Using alcohol to relieve stress is one sign of abuse.	41	85	38	47**

a. Statistical comparison is based on the two-sample test for proportions.
b. N/A = not available.
$*p < .05; **p < .01; ***p < .001$.

included the almost half of the American Indian women compared with the Samoan women who reported that fat sits at the top of the food pyramid ($p < .05$). Another statistically significant difference was the higher proportion of American Indian women compared with the Samoan women who reported to know that using alcohol to relieve stress is one sign of abuse ($p < .05$). These results suggest important trends among program attendees: the possibility of differential access to health care and limited knowledge of major "consumer-friendly" nutrition information. Thus, the FDA's (Food and Drug Administration) marketing knowledge of the amount of fat to include in one's diet relative to other food groups may not be as effective among such women as it is in the general population. This is especially important among Samoans who have been described as possibly "the world's heaviest subpopulation" (Pawson & Janes, 1982).

Some general health attitudes were similar for American Indian and Samoan women, including similar proportions who self-reported "good to excellent" health status and almost all thinking that bringing a list of questions to the doctor's office is a good idea (Table 11.6). Samoan women were more likely to report stress and concern over alcohol use. Although they were statistically sig-

Table 11.6 General Health: Attitudes Baseline Only[a]
(pretest percentages)

General Health Attitudes	American Indian		Samoan	
	N	Pretest	N	Pretest
"Good to excellent" self-reported health status.	317	56	46	50
See self as overweight.	13	92	53	38**
Bringing list of questions to doctor is a good idea.	39	85	36	94
Had severe stress in past year.	30	37	52	58
Worry over family member's alcohol use.	39	49	36	81*
Ever felt you should cut down on drinking?	38	26	38	95***

a. Statistical comparison is based on the two-sample test for proportions.
*p < .05; **p < .01; ***p < .001.

nificantly less likely to see themselves as overweight ($p < .01$), it is, in general, a greater problem for them. Samoan women's attitudes toward their weight is of concern because the average weight of women in the program was over 200 pounds with an average height just over 5 feet. Weight and height data were not available for the American Indian women. Obesity is also a problem in their community, but it has been less investigated with specifically older American Indian women (Story et al., 1994). That more than twice the number of American Indian women compared with Samoan women reported seeing themselves as overweight supports the need for more research on older American Indian women. The statistically significant higher proportion of Samoan women compared with the American Indian women who reported to feel that they should cut down on their drinking ($p < .001$) is perplexing, because alcohol abuse is much more common among the American Indians (Hodge, 1994). Likewise, more Samoan women than American Indian women reported to worry over a family member's alcohol use ($p < .05$). Less is known about Samoans and alcohol use, but these findings call for more research about how it affects older Samoan women's stress levels.

Table 11.7 General Health: Practices Baseline Only[a]
(pretest/postest percentages)

General Health Practices	American Indian		Samoan	
	N	Pretest	N	Pretest
Often trim the fat from red meat.	27	67	54	33**
Often eat baked goods such as pies, ice cream, cookies, sweet rolls, and doughnuts.	29	66	55	9***
Often eat whole grains or brown rice.	29	45	54	9***
Never use fat in cooking./Never use coconut cream.	40	43	55	16
Smoke cigarettes now.	28	21	40	18
Five or more drinks of beer, wine, or liquor at least once this past month?	39	13	38	5
Often practice relaxation exercises.	31	32	50	26
Check prescription for expiration date.	38	71	40	100**

a. Statistical comparison is based on the two-sample test for proportions.
*p < .05; **p < .01; ***p < .001.

General health practices in Table 11.7 encompass the areas of nutrition, substance abuse, stress management, and medication use. The data show that the American Indian women were more likely than Samoan women to trim the fat from red meat (p < .01) and eat whole grains (p < .001), but the American Indian women were also more likely to eat sweets (p < .001). Similar proportions of both groups reported to smoke cigarettes now, but the proportion of American Indian women who reported alcohol consumption in the past month was almost 3 times higher than the proportion of Samoan women, which is important as a trend but not statistically significant. The highest proportions of both groups occurred in their checking the prescription medications for their expiration date, with Samoan women more likely to do so than American Indian women (p < .01). Last, similar proportions of American Indian and Samoan women reported often practicing relaxation exercises, but both groups of women could certainly improve.

In summarizing the chronic and general health knowledge, attitudes, and practices of the American Indian and Samoan women, several trends emerge.

Within the chronic health areas, both within and between groups, program attendees differed in their knowledge levels at baseline. American Indian women had better knowledge of risk factors and management techniques for hypertension than did Samoan women. Attitudes toward risk factors for hypertension reflected each group's knowledge levels, with American Indians having higher levels than Samoans. The findings in terms of both groups' chronic health practices support that knowledge and attitudes do not necessarily predict behaviors because both groups had similar levels of chronic health practices, despite having different knowledge and attitudinal levels.

General health knowledge, attitudes, and practice levels among these two groups reveal similar and different trends between the two groups. Both groups reported similar levels of health management via routine checkups, health status, and smoking habits, which reflect areas of knowledge, attitudes, and practices, respectively. Neither group had particularly high knowledge levels of regular access to health care or of understanding nutrition recommendations. In terms of attitudes, each group had *worse* levels in areas *most* relevant to them: Samoans did not see themselves as overweight, and American Indians did not see themselves as needing to cut down on alcohol consumption. Unlike the chronic health attitudes, their general health attitudes were reflected in their general health practices in that Samoans had poorer nutrition-related behavior compared with the American Indians, and the American Indians had higher levels of alcohol consumption. Given both groups' reported levels of stress, they could use improvement in the area of relaxation exercises.

Implications for
Communication Interventions and Research

Successful communication requires feedback from the receiver to the source and vice versa. This case study presents two main stages of successful communication: at the program's commencement and later in its implementation. Although initially this communication dynamic was primarily between the CHA and the respective advisory councils and community organizations, it quickly evolved into a dynamic between the health educators and the program attendees themselves. To review the overall implications of the CAWH program, both stages of communication dynamics will be discussed.

Community Organization/Leader Level

An earlier point in the chapter referenced the difficulty of bringing a Western health promotion program into these two communities. The CAWH program was able to overcome many of the initial challenges in both communities by responding to community-level feedback. Part of the response involved extensive planning and adapting of the original program to each community's needs. Beyond using advice from local community organizations, the program took an additional step of attaining "ethnic approval." The term *ethnic approval* refers to an approach that involves gaining the endorsement of the ethnic group's leaders (Chen, 1993). This program achieved ethnic approval on several fronts. First, at the level of peer groups, focus groups included a mix of community women and community leader women. For example, among Samoans, community leader women may have included a chief, minister, or deacon's wife. She may also have been a women's group president in her church. Second, meetings were called with community organizations to incorporate their ideas on program planning. Third, in the Samoan community, additional meetings invited church ministers from throughout the Samoan community in Los Angeles County to offer their suggestions on outreach strategies and program planning.

Multilevel "approval" also occurred on a pragmatic level for both groups of women. For example, in each community, there were transportation barriers. Like Samoans, the older American Indian women had transportation problems because they lacked cars and often depended on working children for mobility. Other research has noted transportation problems among urban-dwelling American Indians (Kramer, 1991). The program arranged for vans to bring the women to the classes at various community churches and clinics. The vans came from different community organizations such as the churches. The drivers of the vans were either church employees or community leaders. Communication between program attendees and potential program attendees as well as church announcements helped spread the word about the availability of the vans. Thus, obtaining ethnic approval resulted in how to organize efforts within each community to deliver the program and actually get the women to the program. That a program reached women in both communities was a major success in and of itself.

Individual Level

Data from the surveys in each community provided individual-level feedback about where the program attendees' knowledge, attitude, and practice levels stood in relation to the topics presented. Data were presented first as pretest/posttest for the Samoan women only and then as pretest for both the American Indians and Samoans. The trends in these data have different implications for each group at the individual level.

First, among the Samoan women only, the data present the actual change in knowledge and attitude levels of program attendees during 4-week intervals between pre- and posttests. Only these pretest/posttest data are able to give insight into the effectiveness of the program from a communication perspective. The overall finding that the most significant changes occurred in the knowledge levels and not in the attitudes of Samoan program attendees raises questions regarding individual-focused versus network-focused communication interventions. The underlying issue is what communication strategies might work better at attitude and behavior change in naturally highly communal/networked cultures. This issue becomes more salient in a discussion of Samoan culture's traditional emphasis and dependence on their networks, which easily extends in relevance to communication interventions in other migrant and ethnic communities.

Modern health education foci include an emphasis on the community as both the facilitator and resource for health promotion (Green, 1984). One can easily see the "top-down" aspect of this approach because individuals cannot be expected to change their behavior without assistance from larger community forces and resources. However, on considering multicultural health promotion issues where communities may be networked, one can begin to see the "bottom-up" aspect embedded in this approach. However, much remains to be understood about how to tap into multicultural community networks. Part of the difficulty of tapping into such networks is developing effective ways to activate networks to influence individuals. For example, in this program, the data show how some of the Samoan women's knowledge and attitude levels changed but less so with the latter. So these data show how program attendees may have moved through the stages of behavior change from, for example, the precontemplator to the contemplator stage (Boutwell, 1994). However, these earlier stages of behavior change are less influenced by networks than are the later stages of behavior change (Rogers, 1995). Future communication interventions, then, need to target not only the individuals within communities but also the networks in communities if behavior change is the ultimate goal. In practice, this involves gaining an understanding of the cultural organization of the community, first, then designing a communication program that targets networks within it. Communities have different levels of resources (e.g., individual, group, and organizational) that need to be tapped to promote effective communication and behavior change.

The implications from the pretest/posttest findings among Samoans are also supported by the baseline-only findings from both the American Indian and Samoan women. Those data show how *preexisting health practices* did not always reflect *preexisting knowledge and attitudes.* This knowledge-attitude-practice incongruity is not surprising; McGuire's (1989) behavior change process notes that the stages of behavior change are not necessarily linear, which is supported by other theoretical perspectives (Rogers, 1995). The knowledge-attitude-practice incongruity also implies that other forces might have influenced these women, which effectively motivate them to do the behaviors without really knowing why or thinking about the potential impact on their health. These forces can influence both ways. For example, the fact that the data show some areas of poor health practices for both groups brings attention to the possible influence of non-health-promoting forces at any level within the community. Although these baseline-only findings do not show communication effectiveness, per se, they do support the importance of targeting networks in future communication interventions, because networks theoretically have the most influence on behavioral change. With a network approach, however, one must be cognizant of the possibility that networks will have negative influences on behavior.

There is an important limitation of the baseline-only data, particularly for the American Indian women and their traditional cultural organization relative to Samoan cultural organization. Because this chapter is closing with an emphasis on targeting networks instead of individuals in future communication interventions, it cannot ignore the differences between these two cultural groups. That is, although Samoan culture tends to be uniform, American Indian culture is completely different. American Indian culture includes a wide range of tribes, and although any one tribe may be networked on a traditional reservation, all of the program attendees in this study were urban dwelling. Thus, they came from a diverse number of tribal affiliations. Consequently, one cannot assume that urban-dwelling American Indians are naturally networked as one may expect of reservation-dwelling American Indians, although others have noted the effectiveness of peer group outreach among them (Kramer,

1991). In any case, American Indian women may have received an individual-focused communication program differently, if the pretest/posttest data had been available.

One remaining important point involves the message of the health promotion program. This issue transcends multicultural communities in that it notes the importance of communicating how one area of health influences other areas. For example, regardless of whether the data were baseline or pretest/posttest in both communities, women who attended the program had insufficient understanding about how their health behaviors are *linked to one another and to their health status*. This program tried to address this issue by developing a curriculum that encompassed a wide spectrum of health promotion issues by including both chronic and general health areas. This approach should be used in future programs rather than focusing on only one or two areas at a time.

These data are the remaining link between the two programs (which began as one program) in two very different cultures. Although at face value these data provide some comparable information about the knowledge, health practices, and health status of two communities with different cultures, they also serve to point out several themes in the findings. In general, with regard to the baseline data only, low proportions suggest areas that could be targeted in the future. Although both groups need more understanding of risk factors for diabetes, most areas differ between them. For example, Samoans would benefit most in future programs from understanding more about their risk for obesity, factors that contribute to it, and effective ways to lose weight. Although the attendance for the cancer segment was low among the American Indian women, research on cancer issues among American Indians show how cancer control efforts have been under way in this population (Burhansstipanov, 1993). With regard to the pretest/posttest data among the Samoans, the finding that some areas improved more than others suggests that some content areas were not communicated in a culturally appropriate manner (e.g., the food pyramid) and others not emphasized enough (i.e., fat and obesity relationship).

There are more specific implications of the findings. First, in the knowledge area, overall, the women have more of a grasp on practical knowledge of chronic diseases (e.g., treatment) and less of a grasp on preventive concepts. This trend appears in the diabetes area among both groups and in the cancer area among the American Indian women only and calls attention to the need for more emphasis on prevention. This is especially important among Samoans because of their traditional cultural lack of any concept of prevention (Olsen & Frank-Stromborg, 1993). Furthermore, it is important that program participants can learn skills in managing and preventing chronic diseases, which increases the likelihood of long-term behavioral changes (Goldsmith Cwikel, 1994). Another important lesson exists with the need for more emphasis in future programs on how the same behaviors affect the courses of several chronic diseases. This emphasis will enable a better understanding among program participants of how chronic diseases link to one another. Last, from the beginning, this program recognized the importance of traditional healing practices. It sought to teach the women how Western and traditional healing health practices can be complementary rather than competing, although this remains a very sensitive topic among American Indians who consider traditional healing discussions sacred. In the complementary approach to teaching both traditional and Western healing practices, it is especially important for non-Western societies to respect the fact that how societies organize and deliver health care depends to a large degree on their beliefs in health and illness (Joe, 1994). This is an important lesson for future programs in ethnically diverse communities. By considering the lessons learned from this program, future health promotion interventions can make a community a classroom where traditional and Western ideas are exchanged and where participants feel empowered to know when and how to use what approach to promote health and prevent illness.

Note

1. Thus, the American Indian women's results should be considered "pretest" responses because they filled out the surveys before the class.

References

American Cancer Society, California Division, and Public Health Institute, California Cancer Registry. (1997). *California facts & figures-1996*. Oakland: American Cancer Society, California Division.

Boutwell, W. B. (1994). Theory-based approaches for improving biomedical communications. *Journal of Biocommunication, 21(1)*, 2-6.

Burhansstipanov, L. (1993). National Cancer Institute's Native American cancer research projects. *Alaska Medicine, 35(4)*, 248-254.

Chen, M. S., Jr. (1993). Cardiovascular health among Asian Americans/Pacific Islanders: An examination of health status and intervention approaches. *American Journal of Health Promotion, 7(3)*, 199-207.

Chovan, M. J., & Chovan, W. (1985). Stressful events and coping responses among older adults in two sociocultural groups. *Journal of Psychology, 119*(3), 253-260.

Crews, D. E. (1989). Multivariate prediction of total and cardiovascular mortality in an obese Polynesian population. *American Journal of Public Health, 79*(8), 982-986.

Crews, D. E., & MacKeen, P. C. (1982). Mortality related to cardiovascular disease and diabetes mellitus in a modernizing population. *Social Science &Medicine, 16*, 175-181.

Department of Health Services. (1992). *Final draft: 1991-1992 Los Angeles County alcohol and drug master plan.* Los Angeles: Alcohol and Drug Program Administration.

Farmer, G. C., Barnett, P. S., & Bouchard, R. (1993). *Cervical cancer survey: Urban American Indian women* (Final report to NCI for Research Grant 5 R01 CA49553). Bethesda, MD: National Cancer Institute.

Fitzgerald, M. H., & Howard, A. (1990). Aspects of social organization in three Samoan communities. *Pacific Studies, 14*(11), 31-53.

Goldsmith Cwikel, J. (1994). After epidemiological research: What next? Community action for health promotion. *Public Health Reviews, 22*, 375-394.

Green, L. W. (1984). Health education models. In J. D. Matarazzo, S. M. Weiss, J. A. Herd, N. E. Miller, & S. M. Weiss (Eds.), *Behavioral health: A handbook of health enhancement and disease prevention* (pp. 181-198). New York: John Wiley.

Hanna, J. M., Fitzgerald, M. H., Pearson, J. D., Howard, A., & Hanna, J. M. (1991). Selective migration from Samoa: A longitudinal study of pre-migration differences in social and psychological characteristics. *Social Biology, 37*, 204-214.

Hodge, F. (1994). Contemporary U.S. Indian health care. In D. Champagne (Ed.), *The Native North American almanac: A reference work on Native North Americans in the United States and Canada* (pp. 811-820). Detroit, MI: Gale Research.

Hornor, E. R. (1995). *California cities, towns, & counties: Basic data profiles for all municipalities & counties* (ISSN 0891-2718). Palo Alto, CA: Information Publications.

Indian Health Service. (1992). *Trends in Indian health.* Rockville, MD: Department of Health and Human Services.

Ishikawa, W. H. (1978). *The elder Samoan.* San Diego, CA: Center on Aging.

Janes, C. R. (1990a). Migration, changing gender roles and stress: The Samoan case. *Medical Anthropology, 12*, 217-246.

Janes, C. R. (1990b). *Migration, social change, and health: A Samoan community in urban California.* Stanford, CA: Stanford University Press.

Janes, C. R., & Pawson, I. G. (1986). Migration and biocultural adaptation: Samoans in California. *Social Science and Medicine, 22*(8), 821-834.

Joe, J. R. (1994). Traditional Indian health practices and cultural views. In D. Champagne (Ed.), *The Native North American almanac: A reference work on Native North Americans in the United States and Canada* (pp. 801-811). Detroit, MI: Gale Research.

John, R. (1991). The state of research on American Indian elders' health, income security, and social support networks. In Gerontological Society of America (Ed.),

Minority elders: Longevity, economics, and health, building a public policy base (pp. 38-50). Washington, DC: Gerontological Society of America.

Kincaid, L., & Yum, J. O. (1987). A comparative study of Korean, Filipino, and Samoan immigrants to Hawaii: Socioeconomic consequences. *Human Organization, 46*(1), 70-77.

Kramer, B. J. (1991). Urban American Indian aging. *Journal of Cross-Cultural Gerontology, 6,* 205-217.

Kramer, B. J. (1992). Cross-cultural medicine a decade later: Health and aging of urban American Indians. *Western Journal of Medicine, 157*(Special Issue), 281-285.

Kramer, B. J. (1997). Chronic disease in American Indian populations. In K. S. Markides & M. R. Miranda (Eds.), *Minorities, aging, and health* (pp. 181-202). Thousand Oaks, CA: Sage.

Levy-Storms, L. (1998). *The influence of communication networks on the diffusion of mammography screening among older Pacific Islander women.* Unpublished Doctoral Dissertation, University of California, Los Angeles.

McGarvey, S. T. (1979). Blood pressure of Samoan migrants and sedentes. *American Journal of Physical Anthropology, 48*(3), 417-418.

McGarvey, S. T. (1991). Obesity in Samoans and a perspective on its etiology in Polynesians. *American Journal of Clinical Nutrition, 53,* 1586S-1594S.

McGarvey, S. T., & Baker, P. T. (1979). The effects of modernization and migration on Samoan blood pressure. *Human Biology, 51*(4), 461-479.

McGuire, W. J. (1989). Theoretical foundations of campaigns. In R. E. Rice & C. K. Atkin (Eds.), *Public communication campaigns* (pp. 43-65). Newbury Park, CA: Sage.

Olsen, S. J., & Frank-Stromborg, M. (1993). Cancer prevention and early detection in ethnically diverse populations. *Seminars in Oncology Nursing, 9*(3), 198-209.

Paksoy, N., Bouchardy, C., & Parkin, D. M. (1991). Cancer incidence in Western Samoa. *International Journal of Epidemiology, 20*(3), 634-641.

Pawson, I. G., & Janes, C. (1982). Biocultural risks in longevity: Samoans in California. *Social Science and Medicine, 16,* 183-190.

Pearson, J. D., James, G. D., & Brown, D. E. (1993). Stress and changing lifestyles in the Pacific: Physiological stress responses of Samoans in rural and urban settings. *American Journal of Human Biology, 5,* 49-60.

Pouesi, D. (1994). *An illustrated history of Samoans in California.* Carson, CA: Kin Publications.

Rogers, E. M. (1995). *Diffusion of innovations* (4th ed.). New York: Free Press.

Story, M., Hauck, F. R., Broussard, B. A., White, L. L., Resnick, M. D., & Blum, R. W. (1994, June). Weight perceptions and weight control practices in American Indian and Alaska Native adolescents. *Archives of Pediatric Adolescent Medicine, 148,* 567-571.

Tanjasiri, S. P., Wallace, S. P., & Shibata, K. (1995). Picture imperfect: Hidden problems among Asian Pacific Islander elderly. *Gerontologist, 35*(6), 753-760.

U. S.Bureau of the Census. (1992). *1990 populations, Table 5, CP.* Washington, DC: Government Printing Office.

U.S. Bureau of the Census. (1993). *Statistical abstract of the United States: 1993.* Washington, DC: Government Printing Office.

U.S. Department of Health and Human Services. (1992). *Making health communications programs work: A planner's guide.* Bethesda, MD: Public Health Service and the National Institutes of Health.

Wykle, M., & Kaskel, B. (1991). Increasing the longevity of minority older adults through improved health status. In Gerontological Society of America (Ed.), *Minority elders: Longevity, economics, and health, building a public policy base* (pp. 24-31). Washington, DC: Gerontological Society of America.

12

Health Communication Campaign Design

Lessons From the California Wellness Guide *Distribution Project*

Robert A. Bell
Rina Alcalay

M inority status and poverty are associated with poorer health and quality of life in America (Puryear, 1992; Seccombe, Clarke, & Coward, 1994; U.S. Department of Health and Human Services [DHHS], 1991). In particular, the poorer health status of blacks and Hispanics has been well established (Alcalay, Sabogal, & Gribble, 1992; Council of Scientific Affairs, 1991; Ferraro

AUTHORS' NOTE: The authors are indebted to Susan M. King and Dr. W. James Popham of IOX Assessment Associates and to Dr. Gary Nelson of The California Wellness Foundation for making data from the WIC *Wellness Guide* Distribution Project evaluation available to us. The authors are also grateful to The California Wellness Foundation for providing financial support for the secondary analyses on which this case study is based.

281

& Farmer, 1996; Ginzberg, 1991; Powell, 1991; Rice & Winn, 1990; Russell, 1992; Veal, 1996). The substantial health inequalities that have been found between blacks and Hispanics on the one hand, and non-Hispanic whites on the other, are most likely due to the lower social economic status (SES) of these two minority groups (Cooper, 1993; House et al., 1994; Sanders-Phillips, 1996).

Certainly, improvements in areas such as education, income, and housing would eventually advance the health status of minorities and poorer non-Hispanic whites (Ginzberg, 1991), but there is an urgent need for health promotion interventions designed to improve the current situation of disadvantaged populations (Alcalay, 1992). Such interventions should teach individuals about more healthful behaviors, motivate them to adopt healthier lifestyles, and inform them of the availability of health and social services that will enable them to access needed care and resources. Such interventions will succeed only if they address the unique needs of distinct populations in ways that are true to the cultural values, practices, and traditions of those groups.

This case study focuses on a wellness promotion intervention, the California *Wellness Guide* Distribution (WGD) Project, which represents an effort to provide poor women in the state's Women, Infants, and Children (WIC) program with basic information on a diverse range of personal and social issues related to health and well-being. We will focus on the impact of this intervention on three distinct client populations: blacks, Hispanics, and non-Hispanic whites, paying particular attention to the mediating role played by acculturation on the impact of the intervention for Hispanic clients. At the heart of this intervention was *The Wellness Guide* and its Spanish-language version, *La Guía del Bienestar* (California Department of Mental Health, 1993a, 1993b), which are illustrated booklets linked with a telephone referral service through which information about local health and social services can be obtained. In the summer of 1993, approximately 100,000 WIC clients received a copy of the *Guide* or *Guía*. In essence, the intervention represents a concerted effort to teach members of the targeted populations how to access extant health and human services and to inform them of things they could do on their own to improve their situation.

The Communication Process

The *Guide* was intended to be both culturally sensitive and suitable for distribution to all households in California, objectives that are difficult to achieve simultaneously. The print medium of communication was chosen because a printed resource can be retained and consulted in the future as wellness issues arise. Printed sources of information can also be highly credible when presented in culturally appropriate ways (Marín & Marín, 1990). In this section, we will describe how the *Guide* was developed, its content and design, its adaptation for Spanish-speaking audiences, and its distribution.

Development of Health Promotion Materials

Development of the Wellness Guide

The process by which the *Guide* and *Guía* were developed is outlined in Table 12.1 and detailed at length by Schwab et al. (1992). From 1987 through 1992, the California Department of Mental Health provided funding to the UC Berkeley School of Public Health to develop English and Spanish-language versions of a wellness guide for enhancing physical and mental well-being. The California Wellness Foundation (TCWF) provided subsequent funding for a revision of the *Guide* and *Guía.*

Initial efforts to devise the *Guide* employed a traditional, *expert-based model* of development (Schwab et al., 1992). During 1986 and 1987, potential topics to be included were identified through consultation with a variety of health experts and by perusing public health research. Sample pages were then prepared and presented for evaluation and comment to local focus groups composed of members of the target audience. Their judgments were extremely harsh. The materials were criticized for being unnecessarily complicated and out-of-touch with the everyday situations in which the evaluators lived, the solutions advanced were judged to be naive and condescending, and some of the materials were even found to be offensive. Older evaluators, for instance, were upset about how the elderly were portrayed. Others felt that the description of some problems tended to blame victims.

Clearly, a new strategy was required. In 1988, the *Guide* development team adopted a new, *community-based approach* in its revision efforts to take full advantage of "local knowledge" available at the community level. New drafts were based primarily on extensive discussions with focus groups composed of more than 300 residents representing the demographic diversity of California. Data from these groups were supplemented with individual interviews of members of target audiences. Great efforts were made to involve residents of California

Table 12.1 A Chronology of the Development of the *Guide* and *Guía*

Date	Issue	Product and Evaluation Process	Outcomes
1986-1987	**Identification of wellness issues** *Goal:* To develop a guide on well-being that could be distributed to all households in the State of California.	Traditional, expert-based model was employed. A total of 42 wellness topics were identified by consulting with experts and by reviewing published research. Topics were organized chronologically, based on life cycle stages. Sample pages for several of these topics were prepared.	The sample materials were evaluated very negatively by members of the target audience. Materials were perceived as being too complex, some of the problem statements were considered to be irrelevant to these people's everyday lives, and some depictions were offensive.
		Focus groups, including low-income individuals, examined these sample pages and commented on them. Some focus groups were conducted at centers in low-income communities. Evaluation examined the appropriateness and clarity of materials and the quality of solutions.	Expert-based model rejected in favor of a participatory approach to formative research.
1988	**Obtaining community input** *Goal:* To develop a revised version of the *Guide* that would be suitable to a culturally diverse population.	Sample pages were revised, new topics were added, and more appropriate illustrations were developed, culminating in new drafts.	The feedback obtained was used to develop a new draft of the *Guide,* which was then subjected to further evaluation via focus groups. Some of the prior groups were consulted again during this process, but new groups were also formed.
		Focus groups were formed, representing the diversity of the state. Groups were created in Los Angeles, the San Francisco Bay Area, the Central Valley, and Northern California, based on	By the end of this year, 308 persons representative of the general state population had participated in the development and evaluation process.

	Revision to be based on a community participatory approach that makes use of "local knowledge."	Recommendations from a multicultural panel of consultants. Focus groups were conducted by trained graduate students, who led discussions on the relevance of concepts, the usefulness of the information provided, and the overall design of the *Guide*.	
1989	**Spanish-language adaptation** *Goal:* Develop a Spanish-language adaptation of the *Guide*.	*La Guía del Bienestar* was developed. This booklet's topical content was identical to that in the *Guide* but contained more culturally suitable examples, concepts, and idioms. Adaptation was based on input from 59 researchers, community-based reviewers, and technical advisers.	Adaptation deemed to be culturally sensitive and linguistically appropriate for Hispanic readers of low acculturation.
1988–1992	**Resource referral** *Goal:* Develop a standardized taxonomy for listing social, human, and health services that would be adopted by all 21 Yellow Pages directory publishers in the state.	Given that California has tens of thousands of local and state human service agencies, nonprofit organizations, and self-help groups, how can a resource intended to be distributed to all state residents make program referrals? A Community Services Task Force was established to develop a standardized taxonomy of services. The task force was composed of representatives from various organizations and networks. Criteria	New taxonomy introduced into telephone directories beginning in October 1989. By end of 1991, the taxonomy was used in most Yellow Pages directories in the state. This made it possible for the *Guide/Guía* to report Yellow Pages topics under which relevant community resources could be found.

(continued)

Table 12.1 Continued

Date	Issue	Product and Evaluation Process	Outcomes
		were developed for selecting organizations and agencies to be listed in the *Guide/Guía*. Established and evaluated practicality of potential categories of services.	
1988–1990	**State review** *Goal*: Obtain state approval of the *Guide*.	Despite questions about the ability of referenced state- and federal–funded health and welfare services to absorb additional demands for services and benefits, these services were listed in the *Guide* and *Guía*.	Approval was obtained in 1989, contingent on minor corrections. Final state approval was obtained in early 1990.
		Community organizations known to be challenging the policies of the federal or state governments were not referenced in the *Guide* and *Guía* (e.g., Planned Parenthood and the Sierra Club).	
		Informal reviews were obtained from a sample of county directors of the primary welfare and health agencies of the state. Corrections were made based on these comments prior to submitting the materials to the Department of Mental Health for official review and approval.	

SOURCE: Table adapted from Schwab et al. (1992).

from all regions of the state. The purpose of these group discussions and interviews was to examine the cultural relevance of concepts to be included in the *Guide*, the usefulness and credibility of various kinds and sources of information, the design of the *Guide*, and the cultural appropriateness of the examples used. An iterative development process was employed, with feedback leading to the formulation of new drafts of the *Guide* that were then resubmitted for fresh evaluation. Thus, community input was obtained at both the preproduction and production stages (Palmer, 1981) of the project's formative evaluation activities. The product of these deliberations was the *Wellness Guide*, an 80-page glossy booklet.

Content and Design of the Wellness Guide

The content of the *Guide* is organized largely from a life span perspective. A detailed outline of its contents is provided in Table 12.2. The first chapter, titled "The Beginning Years," covers topics related to pregnancy, infancy, child care, and parenting. The next chapter, "Teenagers," includes materials on physical development, social maturation, and future planning. "Staying Well" describes the need for and value of a variety of health promotion behaviors. Other issues covered include sex, physical and mental disabilities, substance abuse, and dying and death. "Growing Older" canvasses the issues and concerns that often confront us in middle age, including aging, involvement, and caring for elderly relatives. The final chapter, "Basic Needs" discusses issues such as food, housing, work, money, medical care, immigration, rights, and emergencies. It is evident from the nature and range of topics covered that the WGD Project staff conceived of "wellness" as "not simply an absence of disease, but a process tending towards lifestyles and environments conducive to preventing disease" (Schwab et al., 1992, p. 29).

Each topic in the *Guide* is covered in a standardized, two-page spread that includes a summary of main points, a "things you can do" checklist, and a "where to find help" box that provides phone numbers to relevant local and state services. The language level is basic enough to be accessible to the more disadvantaged segments of the California population. A variety of strategies were employed to make the *Guide* an inviting resource. For instance, rhetorical questions are used throughout to induce thinking (e.g., "Is it time to change your diet?") and to get people to recall past significant events (e.g., "Do you remember being a child? What was it like? What would you change for your kids?"). Testimonials of social models (Bandura, 1986) who have successfully adopted the recommendations proffered are presented in many of the spreads.

Table 12.2 Content of the *Guide*

Chapter	Sections
"The Beginning Years"	Pregnancy, Birth, Babies, Being a Parent, Child Care, School, Just for Kids
"Teenagers"	It's Your Body, Family and Friends, Looking Ahead
"Staying Well"	Coping With Stress, Eating Well, Exercise and Relaxation, Sex and Health, Disability, Mental Distress, Alcohol and Drugs, Violence, The Environment, Dying and Death
"Growing Older"	The Middle Years, Every Body Ages, Staying Involved, Care for the Elderly
"Basic Needs"	Food, Housing, Work, Money, Medical Care, Immigration, Know Your Rights, Emergencies

Checklists are included that help the reader to determine if he or she is experiencing stress, should go back to work after child birth, has a drug or alcohol problem, has adequately stocked up on disaster supplies, and so forth. A budgeting worksheet is provided to help the client devise a household strategy for living within means. The visual appearance of each spread is enhanced through the use of color, the inclusion of many graphics, a variety of font sizes and styles, drop caps, short paragraphs, icons, drawings, and cartoons that highlight the ways in which various ethnic groups deal with specific problems. The most significant visual element, however, is the extensive use of photographs; by our count, a total of 83 photos are incorporated into the *Guide*, an average of more than one per page. Sample pages from the *Guide* are reproduced in black and white in Figures 12.1 and 12.2.

Development of the Guía

The *Guía*, a Spanish adaptation of the *Guide*, was developed through a second review in 1989 that garnered additional input through focus groups com-

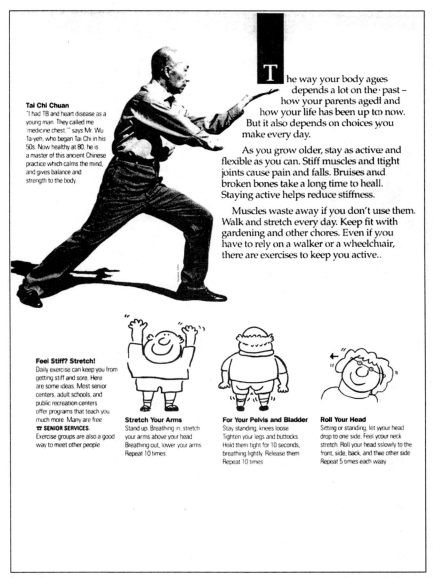

Tai Chi Chuan
"I had TB and heart disease as a young man. They called me 'medicine chest,'" says Mr. Wu Ta-yeh, who began Tai Chi in his 50s. Now healthy at 80, he is a master of this ancient Chinese practice which calms the mind, and gives balance and strength to the body.

T he way your body ages depends a lot on the past – how your parents aged and how your life has been up to now. But it also depends on choices you make every day.

As you grow older, stay as active and flexible as you can. Stiff muscles and tight joints cause pain and falls. Bruises and broken bones take a long time to heal. Staying active helps reduce stiffness.

Muscles waste away if you don't use them. Walk and stretch every day. Keep fit with gardening and other chores. Even if you have to rely on a walker or a wheelchair, there are exercises to keep you active..

Feel Stiff? Stretch!
Daily exercise can keep you from getting stiff and sore. Here are some ideas. Most senior centers, adult schools, and public recreation centers offer programs that teach you much more. Many are free ☎ **SENIOR SERVICES**. Exercise groups are also a good way to meet other people.

Stretch Your Arms
Stand up. Breathing in, stretch your arms above your head. Breathing out, lower your arms. Repeat 10 times.

For Your Pelvis and Bladder
Stay standing, knees loose. Tighten your legs and buttocks. Hold them tight for 10 seconds, breathing lightly. Release them. Repeat 10 times.

Roll Your Head
Sitting or standing, let your head drop to one side. Feel your neck stretch. Roll your head slowly to the front, side, back, and the other side. Repeat 5 times each way.

Figure 12.1. Sample Spread From the *Wellness Guide,* "Every Body Ages" Section
SOURCE: The California Department of Mental Health (1993b, p. 54); photos by Suzanne Arms (p. 289) and Kathy Sloane (p. 290).

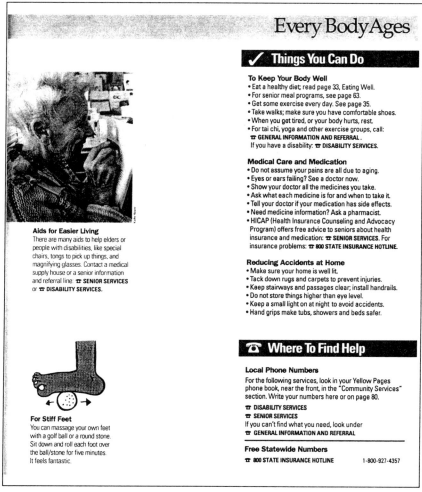

Every Body Ages

✓ Things You Can Do

To Keep Your Body Well
• Eat a healthy diet; read page 33, Eating Well.
• For senior meal programs, see page 63.
• Get some exercise every day. See page 35.
• Take walks; make sure you have comfortable shoes.
• When you get tired, or your body hurts, rest.
• For tai chi, yoga and other exercise groups, call:
  ☎ GENERAL INFORMATION AND REFERRAL .
  If you have a disability: ☎ DISABILITY SERVICES.

Medical Care and Medication
• Do not assume your pains are all due to aging.
• Eyes or ears failing? See a doctor now.
• Show your doctor all the medicines you take.
• Ask what each medicine is for and when to take it.
• Tell your doctor if your medication has side effects.
• Need medicine information? Ask a pharmacist.
• HICAP (Health Insurance Counseling and Advocacy
  Program) offers free advice to seniors about health
  insurance and medication: ☎ SENIOR SERVICES. For
  insurance problems: ☎ 800 STATE INSURANCE HOTLINE.

Reducing Accidents at Home
• Make sure your home is well lit.
• Tack down rugs and carpets to prevent injuries.
• Keep stairways and passages clear; install handrails.
• Do not store things higher than eye level.
• Keep a small light on at night to avoid accidents.
• Hand grips make tubs, showers and beds safer.

Aids for Easier Living
There are many aids to help elders or
people with disabilities, like special
chairs, tongs to pick up things, and
magnifying glasses. Contact a medical
supply house or a senior information
and referral line: ☎ SENIOR SERVICES
or ☎ DISABILITY SERVICES.

☎ Where To Find Help

Local Phone Numbers
For the following services, look in your Yellow Pages
phone book, near the front, in the "Community Services"
section. Write your numbers here or on page 80.
  ☎ DISABILITY SERVICES
  ☎ SENIOR SERVICES
If you can't find what you need, look under
  ☎ GENERAL INFORMATION AND REFERRAL

Free Statewide Numbers
  ☎ 800 STATE INSURANCE HOTLINE   1-800-927-4357

For Stiff Feet
You can massage your own feet
with a golf ball or a round stone.
Sit down and roll each foot over
the ball/stone for five minutes.
It feels fantastic.

Figure 12.1. Continued

posed of members of the Hispanic community and through consultations with
bilingual health experts. These activities led to a conviction that for the *Guide*
to be effective with Hispanics it would need to be adapted, not simply translated. Although the outline of the *Guía* and *Guide* are identical, changes in concepts, idioms, and examples were made to better reflect Hispanic culture and
the several forms of Spanish spoken in California. A few examples illustrate the
kind of adaptations made:

- The *Guide* addresses the importance of making infants feel safe, whereas the *Guía* emphasizes security, warmth, and love (*cariño*).

- The *Guide* depicts exercise as something you should do because it is "good for you," whereas the *Guía* characterizes exercise as something that is "fun." In the *Guide*, walking and hiking are presented as valuable forms of healthful physical activity; in contrast, the *Guía* offers swimming, singing, dancing, and gardening as enjoyable exemplars of exercise.

- The *Guide* encourages the stressed reader to consider obtaining help from outside sources, but the *Guía* emphasizes more personal strategies for stress management.

- The *Guide* observes that children can experience stress, a statement that was deleted from the *Guía* because it could be interpreted as an attack on the parenting abilities of the Hispanic reader.

- In its coverage of death and dying, the *Guide* encourages the mourning reader to cope with bereavement by turning to loved ones, clergy, grief counselors, and support groups for help. The *Guía*, however, stresses the value of friends and family when coping with grief; reliance on outside sources of support is not specifically promoted. The *Guía* also notes that each culture has its own traditions for managing grief and that mourning is a valuable ritual that can help people contend with their anguish.

Distribution of the Guide and Guía

With funding from The California Wellness Foundation, the *Guide* and *Guía* were distributed in 1993 to an estimated 100,000 WIC clients. Approximately 20% of recipients received their copy of the *Guide* or *Guía* in individual nutrition counseling sessions with WIC clinic staff. For the remaining recipients, the publications were distributed in groups during clients' regularly scheduled nutrition classes. Approximately 52% of treatment clinic clients received the English-language *Guide*, 46% took a copy of the Spanish-language *Guía*, and 2% were unsure of whether they had taken the *Guide* or *Guía*.

The staff members responsible for *Guide/Guía* distribution received prior training by the WGD Project staff on how the materials should be distributed and explained and how the *Guide* and *Guía* could be best used by clients. WIC staff members were instructed to spend no less than 7 minutes explaining these materials to clients individually, and approximately 10 to 25 minutes when distribution took place in groups. In practice, introduction of the materials was typically accomplished in only 6 to 10 minutes. Over 91% of clients reported that a WIC staff member had explained use of the publication to them. When asked to evaluate the quality of these instructions, 77% said that the explanations of *Guide/Guía* use were "very well" done, 18% said they had received "so-so" instructions, and only 5% said that the explanations were "not very well" conducted.

Evaluation Research Strategy

The California Wellness Foundation contracted with IOX Assessment Associates of Los Angeles to carry out an independent evaluation of the effectiveness of the WGD Project. The effects of the *Guide* on WIC recipients was evaluated by IOX during 1993 and 1994; the IOX/TCWF evaluation is described at length by King and Popham (1994). The initial assessment did not explore ethnic or racial differences in the impact of the *Guide*. We were invited by a representative of TCWF to determine through secondary data analyses if the effectiveness of the intervention varied as a function of race and ethnicity. These secondary analyses focused on the three subgroups with large enough sample sizes to make statistical comparisons possible: blacks, Hispanics, and non-Hispanic whites (Alcalay & Bell, 1996; Bell & Alcalay, 1997).

Theoretical Framework

The original evaluation was carried out in a largely atheoretical manner. In our analyses, we imposed theory and research on the "knowledge gap" on the data to guide our questions and interpretations. At times, the knowledge gap construct has been employed to denote variations in knowledge among groups at different SES levels. Such an approach leads to questions about *main effect* differences in knowledge among groups. Other scholars, however, have used "knowledge gap" for the hypothesis that people of lower SES acquire information on publicized issues more slowly than do individuals with higher education and income (Tichenor, Donohue, & Olien, 1970); this conceptualization of knowledge gaps leads to questions about the *interaction* between socioeconomic status and exposure to an intervention on learning. For clarity, we have consistently reserved the phrase "knowledge gap" in our work to refer to the main effect prediction of differences in the knowledge and skills among different ethnic groups. We prefer the phrase "differential learning rate" for representing the interaction hypothesis of variations in the rate of learning among these groups as a result of exposure to the *Guide.*

An important implication of such a differential impact is that interventions intended to narrow the gap in knowledge between information "haves" and "have-nots" could actually increase it (Cook et al., 1975; Tichenor et al., 1970). Research has not been very kind to this hypothesis. In fact, a number of investigations have demonstrated that information campaigns can actually *decrease* gaps in knowledge between low- and high-SES groups (e.g., Ettema, Brown, & Luepker, 1983; Friemuth, 1990; Gaziano, 1983; Shingi & Mody, 1976; Tichenor, Rodenkirchen, Olien, & Donohue, 1973). In response to such investigations, it has been suggested that SES may be a less important factor in information acquisition than the perceived utility, salience, and appeal of the information (Chew & Palmer, 1994; Ettema & Kline, 1977; Viswanath, Kahn, Finnegan, & Hertog, 1993).

Evaluation Design

An experimental model of evaluation was used (Flay & Cook, 1989). Thirty-six WIC clinics participated in the evaluation; 24 were *treatment* clinics at which the *Guide* and *Guía* were distributed, and 12 functioned as *control* clinics. Approximately 40 respondents were randomly selected at each clinic by the IOX evaluation team. These clinics were selected from a sampling population of 134 clinics that had more than 60 clients (there were a total of 374 clinics in the state at the time of the evaluation). Clinics were selected based on a probability sampling procedure, in which the chance of a site's inclusion in the study was proportional to the size of its client base, after stratifying by region (north, middle, and south California) and ethnicity. (Technical details are provided by King and Popham, 1994.)

Data were collected by means of a questionnaire administered in each of three waves: *predistribution* (May-July 1993), *postdistribution* (July-December 1993), and *delayed postdistribution* (January-March 1994) (King & Popham, 1994). At each wave, respondents completed the instrument described below. However, due to a lack of resources, fewer clinics were sampled for the first and third wave. In particular, a substantially reduced sample size at delayed postdistribution made statistical comparisons of the three ethnic groups infeasible. As a result, our analyses have focused on the first two waves, creating what is essentially a simple pretest/posttest design. The treatment group sample sizes for pre-, post-, and delayed postdistribution were, respectively, $n = 816$, 994, and 362; control group sample sizes for the three data collection waves were $n = 373, 895$, and 310, respectively.

Evaluation Instrument

Each client-participant completed a questionnaire administered either individually or in a group distribution session. Participants had the option of completing either an English or Spanish version of the instrument, with assistance given to those individuals with weak reading and writing skills. The questionnaire included measures of participating clients' *knowledge confidence, actual knowledge, information-seeking confidence* and *competence;* self-reported *wellness-related behaviors;* and *self-efficacy.*

Knowledge and Information Seeking

Each client reacted to five hypothetical scenarios, as follows: (a) Your children need free medical care; (b) a friend confides in you that he or she has a serious drug problem; (c) you and your family have been spending too much money over the past few months; (d) a friend has been denied government benefits that the friend feels are deserved; and (e) a friend thinks that he or she is entitled to a tax refund. Only the first four scenarios were covered in the *Guide/ Guía;* the tax refund situation was included as a control scenario. For each scenario, respondents indicated if they would know what to do in the situation (knowledge confidence variables) and if they would know how to obtain additional information (information-seeking confidence variables). When they responded in the affirmative, they were asked to describe what they would do and how they would acquire needed information. Each of these open-ended responses was coded for whether or not they contained at least one strategy presented in the *Guide*—that is, whether the response was "guide appropriate"— to derive measures of actual knowledge and information-seeking abilities. Thus, actual knowledge was assessed only for the subset of respondents who said they would know how to manage the situation (i.e., knowledge-confident clients), and information-seeking abilities were assessed only for those respondents who thought they knew how to get additional information (i.e., information/acquisition-confident clients).

Self-Reported Behavioral Outcomes

Clients responded to several questions about the impact of the *Guide* on their behavior. Specifically, each participating client was asked if she had retained her copy of the *Guide,* read the publication, reported doing anything differently because of the *Guide,* anticipated using the *Guide* in the future, or called any of the phone numbers in the *Guide* due to the advice in the publication.

Self-Efficacy

Responses were also obtained to Likert-type statements written to assess various constructs related to self-efficacy. Our factor analyses of these items identified two distinct components of efficacy, which we labeled *assistance-seeking efficacy* and *helplessness.* The assistance-seeking efficacy items pertain to one's self-evaluated ability to obtain assistance from others for dealing with physical, mental, family finance, and legal problems. The helplessness items each describe an inability to respond to environmental exigencies. These two factors parallel the distinction between internal and external control that has long been made in the literature on health locus of control (DeVito, Bogdano-wicz, & Reznikoff, 1982; Strickland, 1978; Wallston & Wallston, 1978).

Communication Effects

Overall Impact of the Intervention

Initial analyses (King & Popham, 1994) revealed that *Guide* recipients were consistently more knowledgeable on the issues covered in the booklet than were control clinics clients. Furthermore, the benefits of the *Guide* were evident both 2 to 4 months after the intervention (Wave 2) and 6 to 8 months out (Wave 3). These intervention effects were observed regardless of whether the materials were distributed individually or within a group context.

What did the clients' do with their copies of the *Guide* after distribution? Approximately 86% said they had retained their copies at immediate post-distribution; this figure dropped somewhat to 74% 6 to 8 months after the intervention. Of course, the booklet can do no good if it is not read and acted on. Fortunately, 84% reported having read the *Guide,* and 20% said they had made changes in behavior due to the materials. The most common outcomes were "seeking additional information" on issues examined in the booklet (39% of recipients), "lifestyle changes" (26%), "seeking of a service or product" (17%), and "providing guidance" to another person (6%). Only 6% or recipients claimed to have made phone calls to a social or health service because of suggestions in the *Guide,* but a more impressive 73% anticipated that they would use the resource in the future.

Finally, our reanalyses of the data revealed that prior to distribution of the *Guide,* control site respondents actually scored slightly higher on self-efficacy and somewhat lower on powerlessness than did treatment site clients. However, after distribution of the materials, there was no difference in powerlessness and a significant difference in self-efficacy favoring *Guide* recipients. The effect for efficacy can be attributed to an increase in efficacy scores among clients exposed to the intervention.

Ethnic Group Differences

Our first endeavor was to reexamine the IOX/TCWF evaluation data to determine (a) if there were any differences among blacks, Hispanics, and non-Hispanic whites on the knowledge, behavior, and efficacy criterion measures and (b) if the impact of the intervention varied across the three ethnic groups. A detailed report of these analyses is reported in Alcalay and Bell (1996); we will focus on major findings here. Our analyses used *ethnicity* (black, Hispanic, and non-Hispanic white) and *treatment* (treatment clinic vs. control clinic) as categorical independent variables. A main effect for ethnicity would suggest a knowledge gap, as defined earlier; a main effect for treatment that favors *Guide* recipients would evidence an intervention effect; and a significant Ethnicity × Treatment interaction would indicate that the outcomes of the intervention were unequal across the three ethnic groups—that is, that there were differential impacts.

On the knowledge measures, there were significant main effects for ethnicity for the medical, financial, government benefits, and tax refund (control) situations; blacks and non-Hispanic whites consistently reported more knowledge confidence than did Hispanic clients. However, we found no evidence that the benefits of the WGD Project on knowledge confidence reported by King and Popham (1994) differed across the three ethnic groups. We followed up these analyses by examining the guide appropriateness of knowledge-confident clients' responses to the questions about what, specifically, they would do in each of the hypothetical scenarios. Even though these analyses excluded all individuals who did not know how to respond to the situations, Hispanics still gave poorer quality (less guide-appropriate) responses than did the other clients. Once again, there was no indication that the impact of the intervention on guide appropriateness of knowledge varied across the three ethnic groups.

On the information acquisition variables, black and non-Hispanic white clients were significantly more confident in their abilities to acquire additional information than were Hispanic clients for all of the scenarios examined. There was no evidence that the magnitude of the positive effects found for the intervention on information acquisition confidence varied across ethnicity. When we examined the guide appropriateness of clients' information acquisition strategies, we found significant ethnic group differences for two of the five scenarios. For the medical scenario, Hispanic and non-Hispanic whites were more likely to give a guide-consistent strategy for acquiring additional information than were black clients. On the government benefits scenario, black and non-Hispanic white clients gave more appropriate information acquisition strategies.

For the behavioral measures, ethnicity was not associated with *Guide* recipients' retention of their copies of the booklet, with reports of having read it, with reports of having made changes in behavior as a result of it, or with anticipations of future use. The only significant difference was for the question, "Have you ever called any number in the phone book because of suggestions in the *Guide?*" Blacks and non-Hispanic whites were about twice as likely to have responded affirmatively than Hispanics. Nationwide, hotline services have often reported that a disproportionately low number of calls are received from Hispanics. This underuse of phone-based information resources may reflect the cultural value of *personalismo,* which is expressed in a preference for interpersonal networks in problem-solving (Marín, 1990).

Substantial differences were found on the measures of self-efficacy and powerlessness. Once again, the pattern was one in which black and non-Hispanic white clients did not differ from one another but experienced considerably more self-efficacy and less powerlessness than did Hispanic clients. Perhaps more interesting was the finding that the intervention enhanced the general sense of efficacy and lowered feelings of powerlessness only for the Hispanic clients. Thus, there was a differential impact, one that favored Hispanics.

Overall, these analyses indicate that ethnicity did not appear to mediate the impact of the intervention on knowledge gains and improvements in information acquisition abilities. The effects of the intervention on self-efficacy and powerlessness did differ across the ethnic groups, however, with Hispanic clients showing the most improvement as a result of *Guide/Guía* exposure. Sadly, substantial and fairly consistent knowledge gaps were documented. Despite an occasional exception, the overall pattern of results suggests that the black and non-Hispanic white groups did not differ much from each other but that both of these groups fared much better than the Hispanic client group on the measures of knowledge, information acquisition, self-efficacy, helplessness, and (to a lesser extent) behavior.

We initially thought that this knowledge gap between Hispanics and their black and non-Hispanic white counterparts might have been due to educational differences; the black and non-Hispanic white groups, although not differing from each other in educational attainment, were both better educated than the Hispanic group. However, when the analyses described above were repeated, statistically controlling for education, virtually all of the effects reported persisted. This led us to consider the possibility that the low levels of acculturation of many of the Hispanic clients might have been responsible for their poor showing on the criterion measures.

Acculturation as a Mediator of the Impact of the Intervention on Hispanic Clients

In a second set of analyses, we focused exclusively on the impact of the intervention on Hispanics in an effort to determine if its effectiveness was mediated by level of acculturation (Bell & Alcalay, 1997). No acculturation scales were included in the original IOX/TCWF evaluation, so we needed to improvise. We used language preference as our index of acculturation, placing each respondent into one of two admittedly crude categories: *acculturated* (i.e., English-preference Hispanics) and *lesser acculturated* (Spanish-preference Hispanics). We acknowledge that language preference does not capture all aspects of acculturation (Marín, 1992), but preferred language has been shown to be a valid shorthand operationalization of it (Marín & Marín, 1991; Marín, Sabogal, Marín, Otero-Sabogal, & Pérez-Stable, 1987). In fact, language use has typically accounted for the largest proportion of variance in acculturation (Félix-Ortiz, Newcomb, & Myers, 1994; Ramirez, Cousins, Santos, & Supik, 1986). A preference for Spanish was expressed by approximately 75% of the 590 predistribution Hispanic clients and 72% of the 665 postdistribution Hispanic respondents.

Using this classification strategy, a considerable knowledge gap was found between acculturated and lesser-acculturated Hispanic respondents. The acculturated group had more confidence in their knowledge for all of the scenarios, both before and after the intervention. Furthermore, knowledge-confident acculturated respondents were more likely to give guide-appropriate responses than were knowledge-confident, lesser-acculturated clients. Hence, the greater confidence of the acculturated group reflected an objectively better understanding of options for managing the exigencies described in the scenarios. Acculturated Hispanics also felt more confident in their information acquisition abilities than did their lesser-acculturated counterparts for three scenarios. However, acculturated, information-confident respondents were not more likely to provide guide-appropriate information acquisition strategies than were information-confident, low-acculturated respondents. Consistent with their greater wellness knowledge and information acquisition confidence, acculturated Hispanics scored higher on the efficacy scale and lower on the helplessness measure than did lesser-acculturated respondents.

More critical is the question of whether or not the impact of the intervention was greater for the more acculturated clients, as would be predicted by the differential rate of learning hypothesis. We found no support for this hypothesis. Treatment respondents did consistently better on the outcome measures than did control respondents, with no evidence of larger gains in improvement for acculturated WIC clients. In fact, we found that the *Guía* actually enhanced the efficacy of Spanish-language-preference respondents more so than did the *Guide* for acculturated respondents, suggesting that those clients with the greatest needs may have actually benefited most from the intervention. Nor was the (self-reported) behavioral impact of the *Guide/Guía* constrained by lower levels of acculturation. English-preference respondents, in comparison with Spanish-preference respondents, were about equally likely to have retained their copy of the *Guide/Guía* (84.2% vs. 83.7%), to have changed their behavior due to studying the *Guide/Guía* (20.6% vs. 17.4%), and to have called a phone number in the *Guide/Guía* because of suggestions in the publications (5.5% vs. 4.4%).

These findings suggest that there are substantial knowledge gaps between acculturated and lesser-acculturated Hispanic clients on wellness-related issues but that acculturation did not interfere with the educational objectives of the intervention. Thus, low acculturation need not be a barrier to health education, provided that materials are adapted to the linguistic and cultural needs of the target audience. More generally, these analyses demonstrated that simple comparisons across the three ethnic groups did not tell the entire story of the WGD Project's outcomes, for the disadvantaged position found for Hispanics could largely be attributed to the segment of lesser-acculturated clients within the Hispanic sample.

Implications for Communication Interventions and Research

The story of the development of the *Guide* underscores the importance of extensive pretesting as a requisite for success in health promotion education. For example, the initial versions of the *Guide* simply did not jibe with the lives and experiences of the people it was intended to help. The section on drug abuse, for instance, did not address motivations for drug use, an omission that weakened the credibility of the materials. The *Guide* began to resonate with its intended beneficiaries only when its developers abandoned the "expert-based" model and took full advantage of the knowledge and expertise of the citizens of local communities. Such a community-based approach to campaign development is generally acknowledged as important (Atkin & Freimuth, 1989), but campaigns often do not seriously adopt such a tack. Furthermore, by connecting the *Guide* to community resources via the telephone referral system, the benefits of such involvement could continue both throughout and beyond the duration of the project.

The persistence of the effects of the *Guide* on WIC clients' awareness—effects that were still detectable more than half a year after distribution of the materials—is especially noteworthy when one considers the truly modest nature of the intervention and limitations in its evaluation. For instance, interpersonal channels of influence were not used extensively to promote reliance on the materials. Second, the intervention did not make use of multiple, mutually reinforcing channels of communication. With the exception of the brief introduction of the *Guide* given to each client at the time of distribution, the WGD Project was essentially a print media campaign. It is a truism among health communication experts that campaigns are most effective when they use multiple channels of communication rather than a single channel. Third, no concerted effort was made to reinforce attention to and use of the *Guide* over time. Even so, the large majority of clients took it upon themselves to read the materials, and most indicated that the information affected their behavior in some ways. Fourth, the assessments of knowledge and information acquisition confidence and quality were based on single-item measures, which suffer inherently from a restriction of range and low reliabilities (Nunnally, 1978). Despite these rather imprecise operationalizations, consistent intervention effects were detectable.

The design of the WGD Project evaluation does not provide a strong basis for making inferences about the behavioral effects of the *Guide* and *Guía*. The questions about behavioral impact incorporated into the questionnaire were based on self-reports, not observation. It is possible that clients' claims of having made behavioral changes reflect, at least to some extent, social desirability concerns. Even if such concerns were not present, insufficient information was collected to understand fully just how meaningful the behavioral changes might have been. For instance, although nearly 2 of 5 clients reported that they obtained additional information on topics covered in the *Guide,* and a small percentage said that they contacted a health or social services organization as a result of the booklet, it is not known how many of these individuals acted on the information they acquired. Likewise, some clients reported making "lifestyle changes," but such changes could have ranged from modest efforts to improve health (e.g., switching from whole milk to low-fat milk) to more significant efforts (e.g., smoking cessation). On the basis of the data collected, we are hesitant to make any claims about effects that extend beyond the intervention's success in enhancing knowledge and information acquisition skills. To be fair, it would be unrealistic to expect a single publication, by itself, to alter behaviors in any substantial way. Health communication practitioners agree that behavioral changes typically necessitate more extensive and ongoing interpersonal contacts than those incorporated into the WGD Project (Backer, Rogers, & Sopory, 1992). Without ongoing interpersonal channels of influence, it is less likely that a client attempting to change her behavior would receive the social reinforcement that is necessary to make such changes an enduring part of her personality and lifestyle (Bandura, 1989).

We find it reassuring that most of the intervention's outcomes were found for all three client populations examined. To be sure, there were substantial knowledge gaps between Hispanics and their black and non-Hispanic white fellow clients, with lesser-acculturated Hispanic women showing especially low levels of baseline knowledge, information acquisition abilities, and efficacy. Even so, with the exception of efficacy and powerlessness, there was little indication that any one of these three groups benefited more from the materials than did the others. Nor did the lesser-acculturated Hispanic client group differ from their English-preference counterparts in knowledge gains from pre- to postdistribution assessments. In fact, the finding that Spanish-preference Hispanics were the ones whose sense of efficacy was most improved by the intervention is especially heartening. In some ways, the finding of greater benefit for Spanish-preference clients makes good sense. These individuals, after all, probably have lower baseline levels of knowledge about the American system of health and social services. As a result of their newness to the American culture, they may lack a basic understanding of how to access the health and social service system and how to use it to advance their life situations.

In speculating about why this intervention had such a positive and lasting impact on clients' knowledge, several possibilities merit consideration. First, given their self-selection into the WIC program, the clients were by definition highly motivated to improve their lives. No printed information source, however well prepared, can be expected to improve the knowledge of a person lacking such motivation. Second, it is possible that distribution of the *Guide* within the context of the WIC program increased the perceived relevance of the materials. WIC program activities could have underscored the importance of the issues raised in the *Guide,* even without explicitly mentioning the booklet. We cannot rule out the possibility that the intervention's benefits might not have been realized if the materials had been distributed in other ways or in other venues. It is also possible that those clients who received the *Guide* may have learned from reading it how to make better use of the WIC staff's professional expertise, which could result in postdistribution improvements on the criterion measures for *Guide* recipients. Examining this possibility would have required inclusion in the evaluation design of a second treatment group consisting of ethnically diverse, poor women not enrolled in WIC or any other health services program.

We believe that the health promotion materials themselves deserve much of the credit for the intervention's impact. The *Guide* and *Guía* are truly impressive products that exhibit a high degree of thought, planning, and professional craftsmanship. In particular, the design of the materials creates a sense of novelty that has been found by health communication professionals to be effective in gaining attention (Parrott, 1995). In addition, an upbeat tone is used throughout the *Guide.* The focus is on how the reader's health and life can be improved—not on what dire consequences might occur if the recommendations advanced are ignored. In other words, the *Guide* makes use of positive-affect messages (Monahan, 1995), not high-threat fear appeals. Although we agree that fear can be a very effective motivator, use of fear is probably not the best choice for target audiences with low levels of self-efficacy (Witte, 1995). Positive messages may also be more effective when attempting to market preventive behaviors (Backer et al., 1992), which was the primary focus of the *Guide.*

These findings have several implications for the design of health promotion interventions. Most notably, they suggest that such materials can be very effective in increasing awareness when developed judiciously and with extensive and continuous input from members of the target audiences. Language and culture are not inherent barriers to health promotion campaign effectiveness when appropriate materials are used (Dervin, 1989). Second, the results suggest that it is possible to develop a single resource that rings true to a diverse range of individuals and to adapt that resource for other language groups. This is an important finding because resources simply do not exist to design unique materials "from scratch" for every ethnic and cultural group that is a part of the target audience.

These results also provide yet another data point calling into question the validity of the "differential rate of learning" version of the knowledge gap hypothesis. The notion that the most disadvantaged members of our society learn less (or learn at a slower rate) in response to disseminated information is contrary to the finding that the lesser-acculturated Hispanic WIC clients seemed to benefit from the intervention as much as, and perhaps more than, other clients. We find objectionable attempts to attribute low-acculturated people's health knowledge and skill deficits to their isolation from the mainstream or to fatalistic and passive personalities. Materials that are culturally sensitive and relevant to the lives of the most disadvantaged members of our society can apparently overcome cultural, linguistic, and educational barriers to health promotion. At this point it must be acknowledged that we can only speculate that the intervention's positive outcomes for lesser-acculturated Hispanics was due to the cultural adaptation of the *Guide* and not just to its translation. Attributing the benefits to adaptation would require a comparison of the effects of a simple translation of the *Guide* with the culturally adapted *Guía*.

We have been encouraged by the results of the WGD Project. This intervention suggests that one publication, when extensively pretested, revised on the basis of formative research, and appropriately adapted can be helpful to a diverse set of social groups. In a state with a population as ethnically diverse as California's, this is an important find.

References

Alcalay, R. (1992). Using health promotion to intervene against community health problems. *Minority health issues for an emerging majority: Proceedings from the 4th National Forum on Cardiovascular Health, Pulmonary Disorders, and Blood Resources.* Washington, DC: National Heart, Lung, and Blood Institute and the National Medical Association.

Alcalay, R., & Bell, R. A. (1996). Ethnicity and health knowledge gaps: Impact of the California *Wellness Guide* on poor African American, Hispanic, and non-Hispanic white women. *Health Communication, 8,* 303-329.

Alcalay, R., Sabogal, F., & Gribble, J. (1992). Profile of Latino health and implications for health education. *International Quarterly of Community Health Education 12,* 151-162.

Atkin, C. K., & Freimuth, V. (1989). Formative evaluation research in campaign design. In R. E. Rice & C. K. Atkin (Eds.), *Public communication campaigns* (2nd ed., pp. 131-150). Newbury Park, CA: Sage.

Backer, T. E., Rogers, E. M., & Sopory, P. (1992). *Designing health communication campaigns: What works?* Newbury Park, CA: Sage.

Bandura, A. (1986). *Social foundations of thought and action.* Englewood Cliffs, NJ: Prentice Hall.

Bandura, A. (1989). Theoretical foundations of campaigns. In R. E. Rice & C. K. Atkin (Eds.), *Public communication campaigns* (2nd ed., pp. 43-65). Newbury Park, CA: Sage.

Bell, R. A., & Alcalay, R. (1997). The impact of the Wellness *Guide/Guía* on Hispanic women's well-being-related knowledge, efficacy beliefs, and behaviors: The mediating role of acculturation. *Health Education and Behavior, 24,* 326-343.

California Department of Mental Health. (1993a). *La Guía del Bienestar.* Sacramento, CA: Author.

California Department of Mental Health. (1993b). *The Wellness Guide.* Sacramento, CA: Author.

Chew, F., & Palmer, S. (1994). Interest, the knowledge gap, and television programming. *Journal of Broadcasting and Electronic Media, 38,* 271-287.

Cook, T. D., Appleton, H., Conner, R. F., Shaffer, A., Tamkin, G. A., & Weber, S. J. (1975). *Sesame Street revisited.* New York: Russell Sage.

Cooper, R. S. (1993). Health and the social status of blacks in the United States. *Annals of Epidemiology, 3,* 137-144.

Council of Scientific Affairs. (1991, January 9). Hispanic health in the United States. *JAMA, 265,* 248-252.

Dervin, B. (1989). Audience as listener and learner, teacher and confidante: The sensemaking approach. In R. Rice & C. Atkin (Eds.), *Public communication campaigns* (2nd ed.). Newbury Park, CA: Sage.

DeVito, A. J., Bogdanowicz, J., & Reznikoff, M. (1982). Actual and intended health-related information seeking and health locus of control. *Journal of Personality Assessment, 46,* 63-69.

Ettema, J. S., Brown, J. W., & Luepker, R. V. (1983). Knowledge gap effects in a health information campaign. *Public Opinion Quarterly, 47,* 516-527.

Ettema, J. S., & Kline, F. G. (1977). Deficits, differences and ceilings: Contingent conditions for understanding the knowledge gap. *Communication Research, 4,* 179-202.

Félix-Ortiz, M., Newcomb, M. D., & Myers, H. (1994). A multidimensional measure of cultural identity for Latino and Latina adolescents. *Hispanic Journal of Behavioral Sciences, 16,* 99-115.

Ferraro, K. F., & Farmer, M. M. (1996). Double jeopardy to health hypothesis for African Americans: Analysis and critique. *Journal of Health and Social Behavior, 37,* 27-43.

Flay, B. R., & Cook, T. D. (1989). Three models for summative evaluation of prevention campaigns with a mass media component. In R. E. Rice & C. K. Atkin (Eds.), *Public communication campaigns* (2nd ed., pp. 175-200). Newbury Park, CA: Sage.

Friemuth, V. S. (1990). The chronically uninformed: Closing the knowledge gap in health. In E. B. Ray & L. Donohew (Eds.), *Communication and health: Systems and applications* (pp. 171-186). Hillsdale, NJ: Lawrence Erlbaum.

Gaziano, C. (1983). The knowledge gap: An analytical review of media effects. *Communication Research, 10,* 447-486.

Ginzberg, E. (1991). Access to health care for Hispanics. *Journal of the American Medical Association, 265,* 238-241.

House, J. S., Lepkowski, J. M., Kinney, A. M., Mero, R. P., Kessler, R. C., & Herzog, A. R. (1994). The social stratification of aging and health. *Journal of Health and Social Behavior, 35,* 213-234.

King, S. M., & Popham, W. J. (1994). *An evaluation of the WIC Wellness Guide Distribution Project.* Report Submitted to The California Wellness Foundation. Los Angeles, CA: IOX Assessment Associates.

Marín, G. (1990, December). *Culturally-appropriate interventions in health promotion: Why and how.* Paper presented at the First International Workshop of Experts on Drug Abuse Prevention, Santa Pola, Alicante, Spain.

Marín, G. (1992). Issues in the measurement of acculturation among Hispanics. In K. F. Geisinger (Ed.), *Psychological testing of Hispanics* (pp. 235-251). Washington, DC: American Psychological Association.

Marín, G., & Marín, B. V. (1990). Perceived credibility of channels and sources of AIDS information among Hispanics. *AIDS Education and Prevention, 12,* 153-164.

Marín, G., & Marín, B. V. (1991). *Research with Hispanic populations.* Newbury Park, CA: Sage.

Marín, G., Sabogal, F., Marín, B. V., Otero-Sabogal, R., & Pérez-Stable, E. (1987). Development of a short acculturation scale for Hispanics. *Hispanic Journal of Behavioral Sciences, 9,* 183-205.

Monahan, J. L. (1995). Thinking positively: Using positive affect when designing health messages. In E. Maibach & R. L. Parrott (Eds.), *Designing health messages: Approaches from communication theory and public health practice* (pp. 81-98). Thousand Oaks, CA: Sage.

Nunnally, J. C. (1978). *Psychometric theory.* New York: McGraw-Hill,

Palmer, E. (1981). Shaping persuasive messages with formative research. In R. E. Rice & W. J. Paisley (Eds.), *Public communication campaigns* (pp. 227-238). Beverly Hills, CA: Sage.

Parrott, R. L. (1995). Motivation to attend to health messages: Presentation of content and linguistic considerations. In E. Maibach & R. L. Parrott (Eds.), *Designing health messages: Approaches from communication theory and public health practice* (pp. 7-23). Thousand Oaks, CA: Sage.

Powell, D. L. (1991). Health care crisis in the black community: Challenges, prospects and the black nurse. *National Journal of Black Nurses Association, 5,* 3-10.

Puryear, P. (1992). Better health policy starts with knowledge of communities. *Minority health issues for an emerging majority: Proceedings from the 4th National Forum on Cardiovascular Health, Pulmonary Disorders, and Blood Resources* (p. 52). Washington, DC: National Heart, Lung, and Blood Institute/National Medical Association.

Ramirez, A. G., Cousins, J. H., Santos, Y., & Supik, J. D. (1986). A media-based acculturation scale for Mexican-Americans: Application to public health education programs. *Family and Community Health, 9*(3), 63-71.

Rice, M. F., & Winn, M. (1990). Black health care in American: A political perspective. *Journal of the National Medical Association, 82,* 429-437.

Russell, K. (1992). Strengthening black and minority community coalitions for health policy action. *National Journal of Black Nurses Association, 6,* 42-47.

Sanders-Phillips, K. (1996). Correlates of health promotion behaviors in low-income Black women and Latinas. *American Journal of Preventive Medicine, 12,* 450-458.

Schwab, M., Newhauser, L., Margen, S., Syme, L., Ogar, D., Roppel, C., & Elite, A. (1992). The *Wellness Guide:* Towards a new model for community participation in health promotion. *Health Promotion International, 11,* 27-36.

Seccombe, K., Clarke, L. L., & Coward, R. T. (1994). Discrepancies in employer-sponsored health insurance among Hispanics, blacks and whites: The effects of sociodemographic and employment factors. *Inquiry, 31,* 221-229.

Shingi, P. M., & Mody, B. (1976). The communication effects gap: A field experiment on television and agricultural ignorance in India. *Communication Research, 3,* 171-190.

Strickland, B. R. (1978). Internal-external expectancies and health-related behaviors. *Journal of Consulting and Clinical Psychology, 46,* 1192-1211.

Tichenor, P. J., Donohue, G. A., & Olien, G. N. (1970). Mass media flow and differential growth in knowledge. *Public Opinion Quarterly, 34,* 158-170.

Tichenor, P. J., Rodenkirchen, J. M., Olien, C. N., & Donohue, G. A. (1973). Community issues, conflict and public affairs knowledge. In P. Clarke (Ed.), *New models for mass communication research* (pp. 45-79). Beverly Hills, CA: Sage.

U.S. Department of Health and Human Services. (1991). *Healthy people 2000: National Health promotion and disease prevention objectives* (DHHS Publication No. PHS 91-50212). Washington, DC: Government Printing Office.

Veal, Y. S. (1996). Health care in the African-American community: A chronology of successes, an examination of realities, and a hope for remedies. *Journal of the National Medical Association, 88*(5), 265-267.

Viswanath, K., Kahn, E., Finnegan, J., Hertog, J., & others. (1993). Motivation and the knowledge gap: Effects of a campaign to reduce diet-related cancer risk. *Communication Research, 20,* 546-563.

Wallston, B. S., & Wallston, K. A. (1978). Locus of control and health: A review of literature. *Health Education Monographs, 6,* 107-117.

Witte, K. (1995). Generating effective risk messages: How scary should your risk communication be? *Communication Yearbook, 18,* 229-254.

PART III

EVALUATION OF HEALTH COMMUNICATION IN MULTICULTURAL POPULATIONS

13

Evaluation of Multicultural Health Communication

Snehendu B. Kar
Rina Alcalay
with Shana Alex

Evaluation is too serious a matter to be done by someone who has never been a client in a program.

—Halcolm's Evaluation Laws, cited by Patton (1980, p. 15)

"As used by philosophers, 'methodology' is often indistinguishable from epistemology (theory of knowledge) or philosophy of science. In this sense, the subject matter of methodology consists—very roughly speaking—of the most basic questions that can be raised concerning the pursuit of truth" (Kaplan, 1964, p. 20). In this chapter, we review key questions/issues in the evaluation of health communication process from a multicultural perspective. A detailed discussion of program evaluation designs and methods is beyond the scope of this volume; several excellent volumes on evaluation methods and designs meet that need (Judd, Smith, & Kidder, 1991; Patton, 1990; Rossi & Freeman, 1993; Schutt, 1996). The purpose here is to review additional issues

311

that are key to a meaningful evaluation of communication processes and outcomes in multicultural populations.

Dual Dimensions of Indicators

One of the central problems in health communication evaluation is that, although the goal of health communication is to improve the health status of the
community, the health status of a population is affected by forces within the socioeconomic system (macro system) that can be more powerful than a specific
health communication or prevention intervention. In addition, improvement
in the health status of a population often takes years, if not decades. Therefore,
changes in health status alone would not be valid indicators of the effectiveness
of health communication programs. Indicators of cognitive changes (knowledge and attitudes) alone are not fully adequate either because of the frequently
observed lack of or weak relationship between health-related knowledge and
attitudes and behavior (see the discussion of the *health behavior model* in
Chapter 3). Input indicators (e.g., dollars and efforts spent) are equally inadequate because rarely can we establish a direct link between inputs and health
outcomes.

The critical questions, therefore, are these: What are the appropriate domains and indicators for evaluating health promotion communication processes, and how do we identify them? Scholars in the social indicator movement have long emphasized the importance of using two categories of
indicators to measure quality of life: *subjective indicators* (e.g., psychological well-being, helplessness) and *objective indicators* (e.g., functional limitations, life events; see Alexander & Willems, 1981; Andrews, 1989; Land &
Spilerman, 1975). Several volumes contain reviews and discussions of categories of health promotion indicators for evaluation of health promotion effects (Abelin, Brzezinski, & Carstairs, 1987; Kar, 1989). During the past decades, health promotion evaluation frameworks have expanded beyond
depending on indicators of *individual* health promotion actions alone
and have included indicators of *societal or community* level health promotion actions (Abelin et al., 1987; Andrews, 1989; Green & Lewis, 1986; Kar,
1989).

Several authors also have reviewed the state of the art in health promotion
indicators on a 2 × 3 matrix; indicators of *individual actions,* and *societal actions*
as two separate but complementary categories actions and each directed at
three levels of health outcomes proposed by the World Health Organization:

physical health, mental health, and *societal health* (Kar, 1989). A project sponsored by the Centers for Disease Control and the Kellogg Foundation allowed us to carry out multinational research to identify health promotion indicators appropriate in different settings. The outcome of that project is presented in a volume titled *Health Promotion Indicators and Action* (Kar, 1989).

Using a simplified Delphi technique, over 300 public health experts from 41 nations identified *individual* and *societal actions* for *physical, social, and mental health promotion* on a 2 × 3 matrix as described above. The first round of surveys identified over 2,668 indicators covering a wide range, some clearly beyond the scope of public health programs in action (e.g., spiritual liberation, poverty level, drugs for cure of life-threatening illness, supply of doctors in rural areas). We excluded these and others that require technological innovations and interventions beyond the scope of health programs. The subsequent two rounds of Delphi surveys enabled us to identify indicators that 50% or more experts elected as most appropriate outcome measures.

Table 13.1 shows the ranking of indicators by individual and societal actions for physical health promotion. The data show two interesting areas of consensus among the experts. Ranking indicators include both cognitive (knowledge and attitude 55%), and behavioral (recommended practice 77%, timely use of services 68%) indicators at the individual level of program impact. Ranking of societal-level indicators, on the other hand, focuses on actions by the program/ health care providers. Provision of resources for basic health needs (access to services) and health education/information (access to communication) were the two top ranking indicators chosen (77% and 73%, respectively).

This and other studies referred to above suggest that for the purposes of designing and implementing effective communication, it is essential to include rigorous formative and summative evaluations as two components of the overall evaluation system. Usually, emphasis is placed on a summative evaluation, which, although highly desirable (at least from the funding agency perspective), does not help an ongoing program. Summative evaluation can help future programs and improve our collective knowledge of what works and what does not. It does not enhance the effectiveness of a program in action. Formative evaluation is the essential mechanism for monitoring and generating information for improving an ongoing program. The role of formative (process) evaluation is particularly important in multicultural communication interventions because it often attempts to reach groups about whom we have very little prior research or direct knowledge. These groups include recent immigrants, members of a distant culture (e.g., American Indians), non-English-speaking minorities (e.g., Asian and Latinos), and high-risk subcultures (e.g., homeless youths).

Table 13.1 Ranking of Physical Health Indicators in Order of Percentage of Experts Who Placed the Indicator Among the Top Five

Individual Actions		Societal Actions	
Action	Percentage of Experts	Action	Percentage of Experts
Recommended personal health promotion actions	77	Provide resources to meet basic physical needs	77
Timely use of services	68	Provide health education information network	73
Correct knowledge/attitude	55	Make services available	71
Practice proper skills	52	Provide environmental health protection measure	68
Seek information/knowledge	51	Make services accessible/ acceptable	56
Participate in community health promotion program	51	Provide adequate training of health care providers	51
Recommended clinic visits	40	Provide community health actions	38
Use recommended products	39	Appropriate legislation	36
Planned parenthood	30	Adequate resources	28
Use personal protectives	30	Provide incentives for health promotion	21
Participate in social/political actions for health	11	Provide recreation	15

SOURCE: Kar (1989, pp. 86-87).

Communication experts interviewed in one study (Backer, Rogers, & Sopory, 1992) were unanimous that one of the main reasons communication campaigns fail is that the message does not reach the audience; that is, the language and/or the meaning is not understood by the audience. Asked about the most common reasons that communication campaigns do not achieve "hoped-for results," Juan Flavier, an internationally recognized pioneer in rural reconstruction and family planning movement in the Philippines, sums up the problem in these words: "The language is not culturally correct and does not fit in the targeted social context. The audience fails to identify with it and thus it has little impact" (quoted in Backer et al., 1992, p. 79). It is therefore important to know the language and cultural context of the targeted group before an intervention and to build in a carefully planned formative (process) evaluation that includes indicators of appropriateness and effectiveness of the communication process. Consequently, evaluation and indicators of health communication effects should use a systems approach that includes a dual-dimension framework composed of two complementary dimensions: (a) individual cognitive and behavioral indicators (those at risk) and (b) program-level process indicators that affect access to and the effectiveness of the intervention. On the basis of the analyses presented in this volume and limited literature on this topic, we identify additional issues that must be considered in developing a meaningful evaluation framework from a multicultural perspective.

Hierarchy of Communication Effects

At the individual level, effects of health promotion interventions are often measured by various categories of indicators, ranging from exposure to communication as the least effective to maintenance of desired behavior change as the most effective. The "Hierarchy of Effect" framework by Backer et al. (1992, p. 5) presented in Table 13.2 (column 1) is a valuable conceptual tool for designing evaluations of communication effects on the audience or those at risk.

In the case of multicultural communication, our analyses suggest that additional factors affect both the health communication process (program level) and health communication effects on the audience (individual level). Within the mainstream (or aggregate) population, a macro system domain of determinants of health outcomes includes education, income, gender, relative deprivation (specifically poverty), past experience with providers, and lack of access to health services. Additional factors that affect health promotion and communication in multicultural communities (MCs) include language barrier, acculturation, ethnic identity and experience, cultural attributes directly affecting health (see the cross-cultural health behavior matrix in Chapter 14), inter-ethnic relationships, cultural competency of communicators, and cultural

Table 13.2 Domain and Hierarchy Matrix of Communication Effects

Domain 1	Domain 2	Domain 3
Hierarchy of Effects: Individual Level (Backer, Roger, & Sopory, 1992)	*Communicator/Program Effects: Cultural Competency*	*Community Effects*
1. Audience *exposure*	1. Language competency or bilingual interpreter use	1. Community interest
2. Audience *awareness*	2. Cultural competency	2. Community awareness & trust
3. Audience's being *informed*	3. Participatory program planning with multi-cultural communities	3. Leadership involvement & support
4. Audience's being *persuaded*	4. Use of "cultural capital" (e.g., ethnic community network)	4. Community willingness to invest resources/ volunteers
5. Audience's *intent* to act	5. Coalitions with community-based organizations	5. Community norms change
6. Actual *change* in audience's behavior	6. Partnership for program implementation	6. Community adoption of preventive behaviors
7. Maintenance of audience's behavior	7. Institutionalized participatory planning & evaluation	7. *Community empowerment and ownership of program by the community and organizations*

distance between health care providers (including health communicators) and their clients. These issues are discussed in greater depth in Chapters 1, 5, and 14. We integrate our findings with the "hierarchy effect" by Backer et al. (1992) and propose a combined "domain and hierarchy matrix," which we believe helps in designing evaluations of health communication in MCs.

It is important to note that the items in Domains 2 and 3 in Table 13.2 are the concepts central to multicultural interventions that we have extracted from our review; these items are not necessarily in a strict hierarchy as is the case with items in the first column. Our analysis concludes that a meaningful evaluation of a communication program's effects, and most certainly a formative evaluation, must go beyond measuring effects on the audience alone (Domain 1) and include evaluation at the program/communicator level as well. At the same time, as of this writing there is a lack of consensus, except on two items, about what constitutes reliable indicators of effectiveness at the program/communicator level. The two items on which there appears to be a consensus are (a) the importance of *cultural competency* of the communicators and (b) *community participation* in the program.

A Multicultural Evaluation Model

During the past decade, several community-based risk reduction campaigns have dealt with multicultural populations. Examples include Partnership for Drug Free America sponsored by the National Institute of Drug Abuse (NIDA), and AIDS/HIV prevention programs targeted at high-risk groups (Backer et al., 1992; Morisky & Ebin, Chapter 9 in this volume; Orlandi, Weston, & Epstein, 1992). One innovative model proposed for enhancing cultural competency in evaluation of substance abuse prevention in intercultural settings is the "linkage approach to program evaluation planning and implementation" (Orlandi et al., 1992). This model provides a useful framework and suggests specific steps that can be taken to enhance cultural competency in evaluation. It identifies two approaches to multicultural evaluation: (a) approaches that rely on those who are culturally competent but may or may not have program evaluation expertise as shown in the first box in Figure 13.1 (this involves program evaluation by culturally competent persons only) and (b) approaches that rely on those who have program evaluation expertise but may or may not have multicultural competency. Orlandi acknowledges that his model is a variation of the linkage model developed by Havelock (1971) and proposes to bring these two types of expertise together to constitute the "linkage" (Box 4 in Figure 13.1). The key to the success of this approach is "flexibility, strategic planning, and the practical use of available resources" (Orlandi et al., 1992, p. 18). It stipulates: "It is critical to the success of this approach that each area of expertise is accorded equal significance and that the collaboration's effectiveness is dependent on equal input and representation from each area" (p. 17). Consequently, the model includes a process through which the number of persons who are "bicompetent" is increased over time.

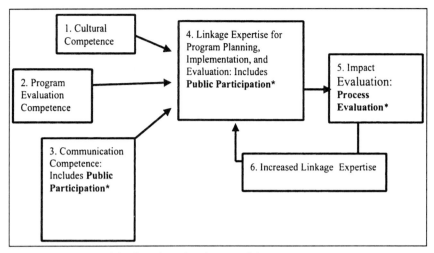

Figure 13.1. A Multicultural Evaluation Model
SOURCE: Adapted from Orlandi et al. (1992).
*Items include participation of ethnic community representatives and public empowerment.

Our analysis supports the basic premise of this model; however, we conclude that this model should be expanded to meet special needs of multicultural communication evaluation. We present our supporting arguments, followed by our suggested changes. First, in a recent volume, nationally recognized experts have repeatedly underscored the need for culturally appropriate research and evaluation using an interdisciplinary approach and with community input (Kar, 1999). Second, there is a growing interest among researchers in the health and human services field in "participatory action research" and empowerment strategy; both require active participation of communities in program planning and evaluation (discussed in detail in Chapter 1; Kar, Chickering, & Sze, 1999). Finally, the Community Health Improvement Process (CHIP) model proposed by the Institute of Medicine (IOM, 1997), discussed later, is firmly based on the theory and pragmatic merit of participatory research; community participation is an indispensable requirement of this CHIP model.

These trends lead us to conclude that multicultural communication evaluation must include meaningful involvement and empowerment of the "audience" or the community as an equal partner—that it should not be driven solely by external "experts." The model proposed by Orlandi et al. (1992)

depends on two types of experts (Boxes 1 & 2, Figure 13.1), but it does not include the audience or the public in evaluation; hence, it is not fully participatory. This approach may be more appropriate for summative evaluation than
for formative evaluation. In the true spirit of participatory research and evaluation, this model should be expanded to include two additional categories of
persons: (a) those with expertise in health communication and (b) representatives of the ethnic communities, including opinion leaders, who can bring their
valuable experience in local communication networks and health-related beliefs, values, attitudes, and practices in designing an effective evaluation plan.
Consequently, we add a third category of expertise (Box 3, Figure 13.1). This
third category is distinctly different from the first category in Box 1, which may
include persons who are culturally competent with a specific minority group
(e.g., African Americans) group but who may be unfamiliar with other cultures
of the community (e.g., Latinos, Asian Americans, homeless youth) or health
communication issues affecting multicultural and underserved communities.
Our analysis concludes that design and evaluation of effective communication
interventions among multiethnic communities, especially among groups
about whom very little or no research is available, must depend heavily on use
of (a) formative evaluation, (b) participatory action research and evaluation,
and (c) qualitative methods to augment quantitative methods and summative
evaluation. Also, true to the spirit the new model of public health, communication evaluation should include the "public" as a partner in the planning, implementation, and evaluation of communication campaigns (Boxes in Figure 13.1
marked by asterisks). Participation of the public is critically important, especially in designing and evaluating programs for ethnic groups about whom we
know very little as of this date. Finally, all communication should enhance public competency and self-efficiency; consequently, empowerment of the public
should be within the criteria of community empowerment.

Finally, cultural competency of the communicator would be an important
domain of process evaluation. In Chapter 4, we elaborate a three-step cultural
competency framework (cultural understanding, acceptance, and reciprocal
relationship). Meaningful indicators of cultural competency would have to
extend much beyond bilingual skills; indeed, we suggest that language skill is
necessary but not sufficient for effective multicultural competency. Additional
domains of indicators for cultural competency evaluation would be (a) a
sound understanding of how the culture in question affects health behavior
and health status of its members (see Table 4.2) and (b) the three levels of cultural competency discussed in detail in Chapter 4.

Qualitative Evaluation: Choice of Paradigms

The following story, which the writer heard decades ago in India (source since forgotten), illustrates the undercurrents of the battle between the proponents of quantitative versus qualitative methods in social research and program evaluation.

A missionary goes to an Indian village with the intent to save the untouchables or Harijans.[1] He pronounces to his eager listeners that Christianity is a much better religion than Hinduism and in it lies their salvation. He supports his claim by proclaiming that as a Christian they all will be God's children equal in His eyes, that they should not have to suffer the humiliation they now endure as untouchables, that Christianity treats everyone equally, that they may have any job or marry anyone without having to worry about their caste, and above all their children would never be untouchables. Very powerful incentives and persuasive arguments indeed. The missionary exhorts them to convert to Christianity—to his brand of course. But the missionary soon runs into a problem. Having been notified of the missionary's subversive activities, the village chief priest, a Brahman no doubt, confronts the missionary. A battle of turf ensues. The priest lashes out at the missionary for his arrogance and falsehood. The priest asserts that Hinduism is obviously superior to Christianity, that it came from a far advanced civilization that matured thousands of years ago when the ancestors of Christians were savages and nomads; it endured for thousands of years before Christianity was born and thrived despite repeated assaults from foreign occupations; its *Vedas* and *Puranas* (metaphysical and spiritual texts) are time-tested and were dictated by the God to sages who spoke with God directly long before Christ was born; and the Harijans are simply paying the price for their past deeds (Karma), a step that is necessary to regain God's blessings. The priest was especially enraged that the missionary was serving a neocolonial plot to export everything Western—religion, McDonalds, Coca Cola, blue jeans, rock music, and so on—to corrupt Indian culture and exploit its poor masses. The priest asked the missionary to leave the Harijans alone in God's name. The missionary was not ready concede a defeat, and soon the two of them engaged in an exhausting and heated debate each endlessly repeating their respective arguments. Now, true believers, no matter how much factual information or persuasive arguments are presented that challenge their beliefs, always hold on to their own faith; indeed, they become more aggressive defenders of it. Our missionary and the priest were no different. Finally, realizing that he cannot win, the missionary extends an olive branch to the priest and says, "Brother, let us at least agree on one thing—we are both God's messengers; we are both doing God's works earnestly and as best as we can. But the difference between us is that you are doing it your way—and I am doing it HIS way."

The concern about methodological prejudice or the reign of the dominant paradigm (quantitative methods), in social research in general and program evaluation in particular, is succinctly stated by Patton (1980) in his now classic book *Qualitative Evaluation Methods*. Qualitative methods are best defined by the following quote:

> Qualitative measurement has to do with the kinds of data or information that are collected. Qualitative data consist of *detailed descriptions* of situations, events, people, interactions, and observed behaviors; *direct quotations* from people about their experiences, attitudes, beliefs, and thoughts; and excerpts or entire passages from documents, direct quotations, and case documentation of qualitative measurement are raw data from the empirical world. The data are collected as open-ended narrative *without* attempting to fit program activities or peoples' experiences into predetermined, standardized categories such as the response choices that comprise typical questionnaires or tests. (Patton, 1980, p. 22)

The ideological and academic debate about the relative superiority of quantitative methods and qualitative methods has no place in a use-focused evaluation plan. Besides, the debate has sifted from relative superiority of quantitative versus qualitative methods to a new paradigm, which Patton calls a "paradigm of choices"—that is, a recognition that different methods are appropriate for different situations (Patton, 1990). Those interested in qualitative method, data gathering, and analysis in greater depth would benefit from Patton's volume. We wish to raise key issues that affect evaluation of multicultural communication.

Role of an Evaluator

Research may be undertaken for the sake of knowledge per se, but an evaluation is always done to serve practical needs. Both are purposive. Basic research seeks truth for the sake of knowledge, but a program evaluation seeks answers to practical questions such as these: How well is the program doing? How can we improve it to achieve the predetermined program goals? How effective has the program been? The primary role of an evaluator in a use-focused evaluation is to operationalize the questions that decision makers need to answer and match the methods best suited to answer these questions (Denzin, 1978;

Havelock, 1971; Patton, 1990). The purpose of a program evaluation is to serve the needs of the program and its decision makers; the evaluator should not inject his or her own ideology and preference of methods to test how well they serve evaluation needs. To serve his or her role well, "Today's evaluator must be sophisticated about matching research methods to the nuances of particular evaluation questions and the idiosyncrasies of specific decision maker needs" (Patton, 1980, p. 17).

Paucity of Multicultural Research

Qualitative methods have a special role in multicultural research and programs evaluation. Our research-based knowledge, especially in social sciences, tends to progress in gradual steps, beginning with accumulation of descriptive knowledge, moving to testing a hypothesis based on prior knowledge, and finally to theory building, verification, and application. One cannot test hypotheses about a phenomenon or a causal relationship in the absence of prior knowledge, which must be used to construct a meaningful hypothesis. Multicultural research is still in its formative phase; it requires creative applications of both qualitative and quantitative methods to explore and describe issues and phenomena in multicultural social realities. Testing hypothesis using experimental or quasi-experimental designs, conducting large-scale sample surveys, and using quantitative surveys to generalize findings require methods that are cross-culturally valid. Adequate prior knowledge about issues under investigation in specific ethnic groups is also needed—for example, what religious beliefs and traditional healing practices affect adoption of modern preventive practices among immigrants from El Salvador? Or who are the most trusted health communicators among the Hmongs, or Vietnamese immigrants? The problem with conducting these types of studies in multicultural communities is that we are still at the formative stage of multicultural research. We have very little research on major ethnic groups and none on others. There is a consensus among the authors of this volume and others who have worked with health issues and substance abuse in ethnic minorities that current lack of reliable and systematic information on major ethnic groups is perhaps the most significant barrier to research-based interventions in multicultural communities (Kar, 1999).

This lack of reliable and research-based knowledge about health-related behavior and communication patterns among major ethnic minorities, especially first-generation immigrants from distant cultures, and the lack of knowledge about the cultural dynamics of multicultural communities makes it most difficult, if not impossible, to justify large surveys or hypothesis-testing study designs. We need a series of exploratory studies to generate working knowledge about specific ethnic groups on which informed health communication programs can be based; until that happens, used of "rigorous quantitative methods" to evaluate communication impacts would be placing the cart before the horse.

One of Halcolm's Evaluation Laws warns us that "an evaluation not worth doing is not worth doing well" (Patton, 1980, p. 15). Evaluation of modern communication media effects on a specific health behavior among Vietnamese "boat people" in the absence of any knowledge of their health-related beliefs and communication patterns would be violating Halcolm's law cited above. Qualitative methods augmented by quantitative methods if needed would be most appropriate in analogous situations.

Evaluation Design

Researchers, for good reasons, generally prefer a rigorous design that allows hypotheses testing using statistically sound, validated instruments, control or comparison groups, and sophisticated statistical analyses. These are *sine qua non* of a study aimed at testing hypothesis and generalizing findings. But there are situations in which such a design is neither feasible not warranted.

One example will illustrate this point. Professor Harry Kitano, an eminent sociologist well-known for his pioneering studies of Japanese Americans, likes to tell those who will listen one of his unforgettable experience. Years ago, he submitted a proposal to a very prestigious federal research granting agency; the aim was to study the impact of the Japanese Americans' experience in internment camps and its effect on them. The proposal was turned down with a question from the reviewers: "Where is the control group?" We all should remember that inglorious time in our history when all Japanese Americans, law-abiding citizens of the United States, including children and ill elderly, were interned during World War II. Where can one find a control group among Japanese Americans for this study? But this experience exemplifies how blind adherence to a rigid demand for an "ideal" design may kill a legitimate project. The implication is that design should match the problem and purpose, not the other way around. For communication planning and evaluation in multicultural populations, one must be flexible enough to use ethnographic methods that generate rich and detailed process-oriented data that can be most valuable to planners and decision makers; these include use of in-depth and small-sample case studies, key informants, oral histories, cultural artifacts, and careful participant observations.

Measurement Tools and Scales

Standardized questionnaires and measurement scales (tools) are important for obtaining reliable measurements and comparisons of knowledge, beliefs, values, intentions, and behavior within and between groups. Indeed, one of the problems we have with multicultural populations is that there are no standardized measures of health risks and related behavior from these groups. Yet using tools standardized for the dominant majority to study another ethnic groups does not solve any problem. Intercultural experience teaches us that a faithful translation of a questionnaire from one language to another does not solve the problem; one must ensure that the same concepts are communicated and are relevant in that culture as well (cultural equivalence).

One example will illustrate a fundamental problem in communication; that is, one may correctly translate a concept or words into another and yet may not communicate. The late Professor Andie Knutson, a respected health psychologist, at the University of California, Berkeley was directing a pioneering cross-cultural study on beliefs about human life in the mid-1960s. One of the questions was, "When does a new human life begin?" The graduate students in public health and social sciences were his first cohorts of study sample. The American students had no problem answering the question, although their responses varied widely (about one third said at conception, about a third during gestation—most of them said during the first trimester—and another third said at birth—so much for our biology education!). A couple of years later, the study was expanded by one of the authors of this volume to include a sample in India. We began with a sample that was highly proficient in English but also translated the questionnaire into the local language. Respondents had a choice of questionnaire—in English or in his or her native language. The first round of responses was quite startling. Over one third did not respond or said "don't know" to the question when does a new human life begin. On probing, it became clear that those responding believed firmly in "reincarnation"—that life or *Atma* or *Jeevan* is eternal and may be reborn in different bodies or incarnations, but it is never created or destroyed. It is a fundamental belief among the devoted Hindus that human life is an extension of the "Ultimate God and it is indestructible" (in Sanskrit, *Atma Parameshwara*). The problem here is not in language or translation but in overlooking a fundamental belief that is intrinsic to that culture.

We identify several barriers in using standardized tools beyond the language barrier. These include differences in (a) underlying meaning of the basic concepts (e.g., life, death, birth, disease), (b) cultural relevance of the concept (e.g., what can one do about it?), (c) social desirability of expression of personal or intimate information (e.g., domestic abuse—one does not wash dirty laundry in public), (d) appropriateness in giving information about family and friends to strangers (interviewers), and (e) certain types of response sets (e.g., never use the word *no* or say "I don't agree" to a person of higher status or never contradict an elderly family member). The first appropriate step is a judicious use of qualitative method.

Access to Study Population

A major question in research related to multicultural communication and evaluation is how to access a study population. Cultural distance between researchers and intended respondents; language barriers; prevalent mistrust; fear of possible harm due to participation, especially among high-risk groups (e.g., substance abuser, undocumented immigrant, teens afraid of adults who may speak with their parents); and lack of perceived and often real relevance of the particular research in their day-to-day survival needs are major problems. Many minority and poor communities have been subjected to waves of researchers who descend on them with clipboards and long questionnaires, ask many questions, including very personal and often objectionable questions (notwithstanding human subject approval), and then disappear forever. To them, these studies are at best, unwelcome nuisances.

Other problems also exist. We mention two that we had experiences with in Los Angeles to illustrate the structural problems we face in multiethnic field study. In the first study, we wanted a sample of Asian Indians parents and youths in California. No known textbook method was any help to us in designing a representative probability sample, especially among the parents. One could not do a random population sample; they are too few for that. One could not oversample because there is no master list of Asian Indians from which to draw a sample. We could not draw a sample from last names in phone directories because Indian last names cover almost the entire range of Anglo-Saxon, Latin, Islamic, and more identifiable Indian last names. We could not select geographic areas and do door-to-door interviews because unlike many minority groups, highly educated and affluent Asian Indians do not cluster in specific geographic localities. They are invisible and scattered but not necessarily assimilated. How does one draw a representative probability sample in such a case? We had to use multiple sources to disseminate requests to participate, use convenient samples and snowball techniques, and provide incentives to the respondents to mail responses to us. The limitations of these techniques are well-known; what is not well-known to proposal reviewers is the impracticality of implementing some of the standard sampling methods routinely used in surveys with the dominant majority non-Hispanic whites.

The second was aimed at empowering Latina women to promote coverage of recommended immunizations of their children in poor and underserved Los Angeles communities. Our intended sample was Latina mothers with a child born in the past 2 years and residing in zip codes that fell below poverty level. We knew that many of them do not have a telephone and that the population is highly transient. So we decided to increase the size of our initial contacts to three times more than the number of completed interviewees planned. We obtained birth records (last names of the mothers and phone numbers) from county hospitals where more than 95% of the babies are born. Our phone contacts revealed something we have never expected; we could contact less than 5% of the mothers on the list.

These two examples from two extreme groups—Asian Indians, who according to the 1990 census are the nation's most educated and affluent ethnic group; and Latina mothers, who are among the most impoverished—pose equally difficult challenges for large-scale sample surveys. We cite these examples to make one important point: Because of the unique problems of access to study populations, studies of multicultural populations often must use methods suitable for localized and in-depth studies using qualitative methods and augment these with quantitative methods when possible.

Participatory Research and Evaluation: The CHIP Model

Within the United States, there is a consensus among scholars, planners, and professionals that our continued emphasis on a sophisticated and expensive tertiary care paradigm is described in detail in the landmark document titled *Healthy People 2000: National Health Promotion and Disease Prevention Objectives* (U.S. Department of Health and Human Services, 1991; see Chapters 2 and 3 in this volume). As discussed further in Chapter 1, the distinctive features of this new consensus and health promotion and disease prevention (HPDP) health paradigm, in contrast to the medical paradigm, are that (a) its goal is prevention of disease and promotion of positive health rather than treatment of the sick; (b) its unit of intervention is the public (the community), not individual patients; and (c) its strategy is to facilitate lifestyle and societal changes necessary for reduction of risks and promotion of health for communities as a whole. The public health model focuses on promoting and sustaining desired changes through effective partnerships among health planners, providers, and the public. Within this new paradigm of HPDP, health communication emerges as a vital component with vastly expanded roles extending far beyond the traditional emphasis on communication and education for patient compliance or for timely use of health services.

The new paradigm (HPDP) requires effective use of communication interventions for achieving program goals and additional objectives, including (a) empowerment of communities at risk, (b) advocacy on behalf of underserved groups for affecting policy and services, (c) coalition and consensus building for social actions for better health, and (d) education and reeducation of millions of health professionals of our nation to prepare them to be more responsive to the changing needs of the communities. This is admittedly a formidable challenge, but the challenge of developing effective health promotion and communication strategies is far greater in multicultural and disadvantaged communities for reasons explained. Within this context, participatory research and evaluation have a central role.

The importance of participatory research has gained considerable support among health researchers and professionals; this approach could not be truer in multicultural research and evaluation, for reasons discussed elsewhere (Chapters 1 and 5; see also Kar, Pascual, & Chickering, 1999). We focus here on the legitimate concern about limitation of research and evaluation driven exclusively by external experts. This concern is deep enough that the Institute of Medicine (IOM), the highest health-related research unit of the National Academy of Science, has proposed a participatory model of Community Health Improvement Process (CHIP; see Figure 13.2) (IOM, 1997, p. 7). The concept that many social agencies share responsibility in a healthy population acts as the basic foundation of CHIP. Although the report recognized that assigning responsibility to many agencies could allow the accountability for actions taken to disintegrate, IOM still insisted that each agency would have to devise accountability measures to deter this possible problem.

The CHIP model includes two cycles that constantly interact with each other: (a) the problem identification and prioritization cycle and (b) analysis and implementation cycle (see Figure 13.2). As the first to occur, the problem identification and prioritization cycle begins with the formation of a community health coalition to perform a needs assessment of the targeted population. Therefore, the ensuing health promotion will address health issues that have been identified by the community itself as important to them. During the

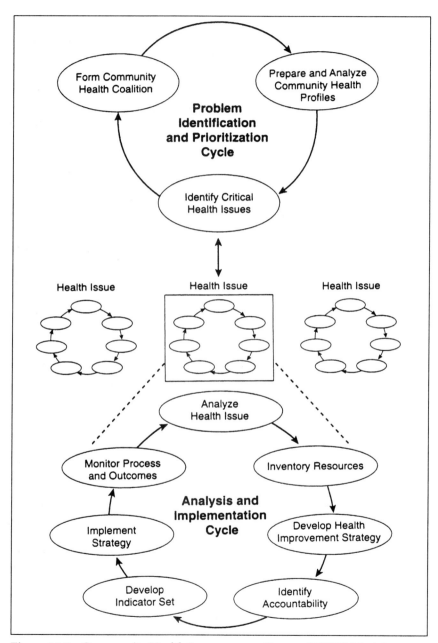

Figure 13.2. Community Health Improvement Process (CHIP) Model
SOURCE: Institute of Medicine (1997, p. 7).

second cycle, health practitioners and the community act as equal partners both working together throughout each step. Note that this cycle includes the "monitor process and outcomes" step, emphasizing the importance of continual evaluation. This model exemplifies the lessons learned from our own research, as well as from the case studies in this volume: In multicultural communities, when disparate interests must act in concordance for the benefit of the community, all participants must bring their expertise and experience to the program for it to be effective.

Empowerment Evaluation

Finally, taking a community empowerment approach (see discussion on empowerment in Chapter 5) to its logical conclusion, the practice of *empowerment evaluation* has gained in usage since the early 1990s (Fetterman, Kaftarian, & Wandersman, 1996). Fetterman et al. (1996) define empowerment evaluation as, "the use of evaluation concepts, techniques, and findings to foster improvement and self-determination" (p. 4), meaning that the evaluation process itself does not necessarily have to be the sole domain of the researchers, as it has been in the past. Instead, community participants should also be included in the evaluation process, which not only contributes to their own empowerment but also gives the health practitioners and professionals valuable insights into the effectiveness of the program as perceived by its beneficiaries (Kar, Pascual, & Chickering, 1999; Manderson & Mark, 1997).

Note

1. The Hindu caste system is a closed system; once born in a caste, you die in the same caste. Historically, it determines major domains of peoples' lives, including occupation and marriage. It classifies people in four castes: Brahman—the highest priestly caste; Kshatriya—the kings, rulers, and warriors; Vaishya—the professionals, merchants, and the like; and Shudra—those who do semiskilled or unskilled jobs. The untouchables are even below the fourfold caste system and do the most unwanted jobs (e.g., collect garbage, clean toilets, remove sewage, etc.). They are the most dispossessed and live under humiliating conditions. Gandhi called them "Harijans"—or children of God to remove the social stigma attached to the label "untouchable." The situation has changed considerably since Indian independence, especially in occupational mobility across castes. But the caste system still has a major control over marriage decisions.

References

Abelin, T., Brzezinski, Z. J., & Carstairs, V. D. L. (Eds.). (1987). *Measurement in health promotion and protection.* Albany, NY: World Health Organization, WHO Publications Center USA.

Alexander, J. L., & Willems, E. P. (1981). Quality of life: Some measurement requirements. *Archives of Physical and Medical Rehabilitation, 62,* 261-265.

Andrews, J. (1989). *Poverty and poor health among elderly Hispanic Americans.* Baltimore, MD: Commonwealth Fund Commission on Elderly People Living Alone.

Backer, T. E., Rogers, E. M., & Sopory, P. (1992). *Designing health communication campaigns: What works?* Newbury Park, CA: Sage.

Denzin, N. K. (1978). The logic of naturalistic inquiry. In N. K. Denzin (Comp.), *Sociological methods: A source book.* New York: McGraw-Hill

Fetterman, D. M., Kaftarian, S. J., & Wandersman, A. (Eds.). (1996). *Empowerment evaluation: Knowledge and tools for self-assessment and accountability.* Thousand Oaks, CA: Sage.

Green, L. W., & Lewis, F. M. (1986). *Measurement and evaluation in health education and health promotion.* Palo Alto, CA: Mayfield.

Havelock, R. (1971). *Planning for innovation through dissemination and utilization of knowledge.* Ann Arbor: University of Michigan, Institute for Social Research.

Institute of Medicine. (1997). *Improving health in the community: A role of performance monitoring.* Washington, DC: National Academy Press.

Judd, C. M., Smith, E. R., & Kidder, L. H. (1991). *Research methods in social relations* (6th ed.). Fort Worth, TX: Holt, Rinehart & Winston.

Kaplan, A. (1964). *The conduct of inquiry: Methodology for behavioral science.* Scranton, PA: Chandler.

Kar, S. B. (Ed.). (1989). *Health promotion indicators and action.* New York: Springer.

Kar, S. B. (Ed.). (1999). *Substance abuse prevention: A multicultural perspective.* Amityville, NY: Baywood.

Kar, S. B., Chickering, K. L., & Sze, F. (1999). Summary and implications. In S. B. Kar (Ed.), *Substance abuse prevention: A multicultural perspective.* Amityville, NY: Baywood.

Kar, S. B., Pascual, C. A., & Chickering, K. L. (1999). Empowerment of women for health promotion: A meta-analysis. *Social Science & Medicine, 49,* 1431-1460.

Land, K. C., & Spilerman, S. (Eds.). (1975). *Social indicator models.* New York: Russell Sage.

Manderson, L., & Mark, T. (1997). Empowering women: Participatory research in women's health and development projects. *Health Care for Women International, 18*(1), 17-30.

Orlandi, M. A., Weston, R., & Epstein, L. G. (Eds.). (1992). *Cultural competence for evaluators: A guide for alcohol and other drug abuse prevention practitioners working with ethnic/racial communities.* Rockville, MD: U.S. Department of Health and Human Services, Office for Substance Abuse Prevention.

Patton, M. Q. (1980). *Qualitative evaluation methods.* Beverly Hills, CA: Sage.

Patton, M. Q. (1990). *Qualitative evaluation and research methods* (2nd ed.). Newbury Park, CA: Sage.

Rossi, P. H., & Freeman, H. E. (1993). *Evaluation: A systematic approach* (5th ed.). Newbury Park, CA: Sage.

Schutt, R. K. (1996). *Investigating the social world: The process and practice of research.* Thousand Oaks, CA: Pine Forge.

U.S. Department of Health and Human Services. (1991). *Healthy people 2000: National health promotion and disease prevention objectives* (DHHS Publication No. PHS 91-50212). Washington, DC: Government Printing Office.

14

Lessons Learned and Implications

Snehendu B. Kar
Rina Alcalay
with Shana Alex

This concluding chapter has two complementary aims. The first is to review the lessons learned from the analyses of communication studies and case studies presented in this volume and to interpret the key observations within the context of the theories and models of communication. The focus is on identification of cultural, social, and behavioral factors and how they affect positive and negative outcomes of health communications in ethnic minorities in multicultural communities. We draw the implications from our review of interventions that produce dramatic results in culturally diverse populations (nations) and the role of communication interventions in the outcomes—for example, cardiovascular risk reduction in North Karelia (Puska et al., 1996), dramatic reduction of infant mortality in Indian villages by one third in less than 1 year (Bang et al., 1990), the success of family planning programs in rural Asian and Latin American nations (Piotrow, Kincaid, Rimon, & Rinehart, 1997; Rogers, 1973), and the relative success of school-based tobacco and substance abuse prevention interventions (Backer, Rogers, & Sopory, 1992; Chou et al., 1998; Pentz, 1994). Conversely, why is it that, despite intensive efforts by sophisticated teams of scientists and health professionals over several years, the outcomes of programs are modest? For example, the outcomes of the intensive and expensive Multiple Risk Factor Intervention Trial (MRFIT) project (Gotto, 1997), the school-based drug abuse resistance education (DARE) project (Ennett, Tobler, Ringwalt, & Flewelling, 1994), and the Stanford project (Farquhar et al. 1994; Maccoby & Altman, 1988) all showed initial success but ended up with sobering effects over the long term.

The second aim is to discuss the issues and processes that determine the effective implementation of health promotion interventions in a highly distressed multicultural community. This segment will be based on our ongoing health promotion and disease prevention project in South Central Los Angeles. This project, now in its third year, offers us firsthand experience in working in a highly diverse (no single ethnic group is in the majority), rapidly changing, economically distressed, and traumatized community. Our experience in this community allowed us to understand important social processes, which can be very valuable in working effectively in multicultural communities. This review is presented in three sections: (a) communication studies including health communication campaigns, (b) health communication in multicultural groups, and (c) empowerment case studies across the world.

Communication Studies:
Media Effects on the Dominant Majority (MEDM)

Communication researchers have been concerned with the effects of modern media and messages on the public ever since mass media became a pervasive force of our culture. These studies focus on two complementary domains: (a) the effects of mass media on the public and (b) the nature of interactions between mass media and interpersonal communications in shaping public opinion, attitudes, and behavior. Several major efforts have been undertaken to addresses this issue through extensive reviews of the effects of media exposure (see Chapters 1, 3, and 4). These reviews fall into four categories:

1. The study of the effects of television on behavior, particularly the impact of exposure to violence on aggression and the impact of media campaigns on political choices

2. The study of the impact of advertising and marketing strategies on sales and product promotion

3. The study of diffusion of innovations in several domains, including adoption of medical, agricultural, and health innovations

4. The review of communication campaigns targeted at health and human services programs

The last category includes programs designed to reduce specific health risks in schools and communities, community development and organization, and empowerment and will be discussed later in further detail. All these types of studies, however, tend to focus on the media effects on the majority (MEDM) and do not pay attention to relative differences by major ethnic groups. These reviews almost always refer to media effects on the white population at the aggregate level; they do not deal with the extent to which and what media affect the increasing proportion of ethnically diverse populations.

Health Communication Campaigns

The question remains: What generalizations can we draw about the effects of mainstream media on culturally diverse populations? The literature is silent on this question. The communication theories, studies, and reviews published to date do not deal with and hence do not shed any light on how modern media and messages affect health-related beliefs and behavior in multicultural communities. For that reason, in this volume we have made a special effort to include some of the pioneering health communication interventions aimed at ethnic minorities and hard-to-reach high-risk groups (e.g., homeless youths, American Indian and Samoan elderly). Admittedly, ours is not a definitive study, and given the current gap in our collective knowledge, it is not possible to draw sound generalizations about media effects on health behavior among multicultural and high-risk groups. However, on the basis of our analysis and the cases presented, we draw several important implications for policy deliberations, research, interventions, and evaluation.

During the last four decades, major public health campaigns have used intensive media coverage to promote adoption of preventive behavior against leading causes of deaths and disabilities across the world. Lessons learned from them are presented by several authors elsewhere (see Backer et al. 1992; Kar & Alex, 1999; Piotrow et al., 1997; Rice & Atkin, 1989; Rogers, 1973). Space would not permit a full review of the content covered in these volumes, and it would be redundant to do so. Backer et al. (1992) have presented an excellent summary of generalizations from health communication campaigns; they present 27 generalizations and an additional 7 that specifically refer to substance abuse prevention in high-risk youths. Our review of these and other generalizations derived from the materials in this volume leads us to conclude that effective health communication campaigns should meet the following 10 conditions. It is important to note that these generalizations are based on studies that used a MEDM paradigm, not on the multicultural experiences presented in the following section.

Health communication campaigns are likely to be effective when the following are true:

1. The goal meets an existing need or priority of the population concerned (and it does not clash with the culture and deeply held values).
2. The campaign uses a participatory needs assessment, planning, implementation, and formative evaluation.
3. The goal is modest, attainable, and sustainable over a defined time period.
4. The strategy is based on sound theories of human behavior and communication, as well as on lessons from similar programs.
5. The campaign effectively combines mass media with interpersonal communication, including local leaders, role models, and local ethnic media.
6. The campaign focuses on specific behavior and tangible outcomes, preferably on short-term positive achievements.
7. The campaign builds on existing behavior, promotes behavioral skills, and provides normative support and reinforcement to maintain the desired behavior.
8. The message contains feasible solutions to perceived threats and is simple, clear, understandable, positive, interesting, and repetitive.
9. The campaign develops partnerships and coalitions with government and local organizations for resource mobilization and program support.
10. The campaign includes systematic evaluation and feedback with active participation of the public.

Health Communication in Multicultural Groups

Communication studies focuses on impacts at the aggregate level, but this MEDM perspective does not examine the relative effects of media and messages on different ethnic groups or on gender. Indeed, two major findings of our analysis presented in this volume are these: (a) No systematic comparative study of the psychosocial determinants of health risk behavior with representative samples of five major ethnic groups exists as of today (African Americans, American Indians, Asian Americans, Latinos, and non-Hispanic whites); (b) we know very little about health-related behavior and their determinants among many minorities, especially recent immigrants (Flack et al., 1995; Kar, Jimenez, Campbell, & Sze, 1998; Penn, Kar, Kramer, Skimmer, & Zambrana, 1995; Takeuchi, Sue, & Yeh, 1995). Waves of immigration have increased America's foreign-born population from 10.4 million in 1900 to 19.8 million in 1990, according to U.S. census data (U.S. Bureau of the Census, 1993). More recent estimates show that the foreign-born population has increased to 25.8 million in 1997 (U.S. Bureau of the Census, 1998). These immigrants were socialized in their native cultures, which are significantly different from our American society in terms of language; values, beliefs, and practices related to health, illness, and healing practices; and communication and interpersonal relations.

Theories and research reviewed earlier tell us that communication campaigns alone, however robust and perfect in design, cannot significantly change health risk behavior (usually they are most effective in changing awareness and knowledge). Although the health communication campaigns cited earlier are pioneering and exemplary (e.g., the North Karelia Project, the Stanford Five Community Project, Minnesota Heart Disease Prevention, MRFIT), they deal with homogeneous populations and consequently shed no light on multicultural responses to these interventions. In addition, health risk behaviors are often deeply rooted in culturally conditioned beliefs, values, knowledge, attitudes, and practices (BVKAP). The effects of communication on behavior are at the least mediated, if not determined, by these cultural elements. Consequently, we must look at lessons from both the case studies in this volume and our own meta-analysis of community empowerment to derive the following lessons concerning multicultural communities: (a) the definition of multiculturalism, (b) a cross-cultural framework for health behavior, (c) mainstream media and how it interacts with minorities, (d) microcommunication using local community ethnic networks, (e) that threats to children act as a unifying force within multicultural communities, (f) that mothers are often willing to work as partners in prevention, (g) that local health promoters (LHPs) can be extremely effective, and (h) that cultural competency and collaboration remains important.

Multiculturalism

The "melting pot" metaphor (hypothesis) has continued to influence our social policy; it is based on the assumption that people in the United States as a whole subscribe to a common culture, values, norms language, and so on and that ethnic minorities in general are eager to assimilate or "melt" into the mainstream dominant U.S. culture. In recent years, this melting pot metaphor has been replaced by a new metaphor of the "rainbow" coalition, according to which, groups with rich cultural traditions tend to retain many of their culturally rooted values and practices. Metropolitan areas are increasingly becoming multicultural communities (MCs); in many MCs, there is no ethnic majority (e.g., South Central Los Angeles). The 1990 census data show that 15 of the largest metropolitan areas of our nation have become multicultural; that is, non-Hispanic whites are no longer in the majority and, collectively, minorities are in the majority (American Demographics, 1991). In addition, these ethnic minorities in general are increasing at much faster rates than the population as a whole. With the reform of immigration laws in 1965, Americans of Asian and Hispanic heritage began to increase rapidly. Indeed, between 1980 and 1990, while the overall population of the United States increased by 9.8%, Asian Americans increased by 107.8% and the Hispanics by 53% (U.S. Bureau of the Census, 1990). The U.S. Bureau of the Census (1996) projects that by the year 2050, the percentage of non-Hispanic whites in America will be reduced to 52.8%.

The demographic portrait further diversifies because of waves of immigrants from countries suffering traumatic political developments and the American policy to accept refugees (from Vietnam, Cambodia, Laos, Korea, China, and several Central and South American nations). Many of these immigrant groups have had no direct exposure to the way of life in the United States and often do not speak English. Their health-related knowledge, beliefs, behaviors, and preferred modalities of treatment and prevention are often very different from those in the Western societies. Compared with national averages, these groups also suffer from higher rates of poverty and increased health risks.

These trends have led to a greater diversification of U.S. communities within each ethnic category. One eminent sociologist and a strong proponent of the assimilationist position recently summed up the current consensus in his book aptly titled *We Are All Multiculturalists Now* (Glazer, 1997).

To make matters worse, most health care providers tend to be English speaking and socialized in modern medical systems; consequently, they are unable to communicate effectively with unfamiliar ethnic groups. In addition, prevailing stereotypes and myths about ethnic minorities often adversely affect communication and rapport between health professionals and minority groups. For instance, Asian Americans are often stereotyped as the "model minority" who are seen as hard working, successful, well adjusted, and without any major problem and, therefore, they do not need special attention (Kar et al., 1998). That stereotype is far from the truth, yet such stereotyping can adversely affect the types and quality of care provided to them. From the health communication standpoint, we must ask, In what ways are these various cultural groups similar or different from one another, in terms of sociocultural factors that affect their health behavior and health communication?

Our experiences during the past decades teach us that appropriate consideration of our cultural diversity is both necessary and desirable in planning effective social programs, particularly in those domains where significant ethnic differences are still evident (e.g., health, education, employment). Multicultural and disadvantaged urban communities consist of high-risk groups with special needs. In recognition of the needs of special populations, the landmark document *Healthy People 2000*, which defined our national strategy for disease prevention and health promotion, states, "Special population groups often need targeted preventive efforts, and such efforts require understanding the needs and the disparities experienced by these groups. General solutions cannot always be used to solve specific problems" (DHHS, 1991, p. 29).

There is no standard model of effective health promotion and disease prevention intervention, and even if there was one, it is not likely to be effective among all ethnic groups. Our foremost challenge is to develop innovative strategies for health promotion and risk reduction in distressed and multicultural communities. Effective health promotion and disease prevention strategies in such a multicultural community must be based on the important *felt needs* of the community and on what Tagore defined as "a bond of relation" between various ethnic groups and heath care professionals (Chakravarty, 1961).

Health Behavior and Communication:
A Cross-Cultural Framework

Healthy People 2000 (DHHS, 1991) formally acknowledges that our national objectives will not be met unless we accept the fact that health risks and needs vary significantly by social class, ethnicity, and special high-risk groups (they often overlap); these differences are significantly affected by the cultural, socio-economic, environmental, and lifestyle factors unique to these groups. Indeed, the report's major goal is to reduce ethnic and racial differences in health status (DHHS, 1991). Yet many medical and social science communities hold on to a "standard model" of health behavior, which states that a set of common socio-cultural factors affects health behavior and outcomes among all people in the United States, and therefore, what is true for non-Hispanic whites is also true for everyone else. Literature on culture and health, experiences of frontline health care providers, and evidence from communities do not support this contention.

Mainstream Media and Minorities

We define "mainstream media" as the major national TV networks and English language media, both printed and electronic. As stated before, reliable data on mainstream media use and their effect on minority groups are not available. We examine two sources of data that are available. First, the Nielsen rating of Spanish language TV programs. The Nielsen rating results presented in Chapters 1 and 4 clearly show that Latinos predominantly prefer prime-time programs broadcast by Hispanic TV network; this suggests that major mainstream TV network shows have significantly lower popularity among Latino populations. Comparable data on TV viewing by Asian Americans is not available.

Our second source provides a better insight about the role of media in health information dissemination across major ethnic groups. A recent survey by the Los Angeles County Department of Health Services (LACDHS, 1994) asked a sample of respondents from different ethnic groups to name the sources from which they seek and receive health-related information. Table 1.3 (in Chapter 1) shows interesting ethnic differences in media use and health information sources. Whites least frequently and Hispanics most frequently obtain health-related information from TV programs. We do not know whether Hispanics obtain health information from Hispanic networks or mainstream TV stations. Given the Nielsen data, it is at least likely that Hispanic programs are a major source for them. African Americans, more than any other ethnic group, obtain health information from doctors; in contrast, Asian Americans mention doctors least often as a source of health information. Hispanics, more than any other group, depend on family and friends for health information; African Americans mention these sources least frequently. Of all groups, Asian Americans use newspapers most frequently, African Americans least frequently. It is important to note here that at least 76 local newspapers exist in Los Angeles alone, the majority of which are dedicated to specific ethnic communities.

With the data from Table 1.3 (Chapter 1) in mind, a question arises: How effective is mainstream media at reaching multicultural audiences? No conclusive answer exists. Therefore, health practitioners must shed the firmly held belief that only mainstream media, particularly television commercial spots, remain the most desirable method by which to target their communities. Along with this concern, two other factors have emerged as major detriments to focusing on mainstream advertising for health promotion programs. The sheer cost of most advertising of this nature—compounded because the message must be repeated to increase effectiveness—places mainstream media out of the reach of many health promotion programs. Also, mainstream media itself has fragmented drastically in recent years; even if the funds existed, it would be difficult for a program to target its audience among the vast choices of channels and information outlets.

Microcommunication Using Local Community Ethnic Networks

Our analysis suggests that we must go beyond the study of mainstream media effects on the aggregate population and look into local communication networks (LCNs) specific to multicultural communities. Recent data from reliable sources show some encouraging health trends among high-risk populations. For the first time, the National Center for Health Statistics (NCHS) in 1998 reported that AIDS is no longer among the top 10 causes of death; age-adjusted HIV death rates fell from the 8th to the 14th leading cause of death. At the aggregate level, from 1996 to 1997, in one single year there was an unprecedented 47% decline in death due to HIV infection (NCHS, 1998).

A note of caution is warranted here. Although the HIV deaths have declined, the annual number of new infections has not declined; in addition, minorities have a higher prevalence of the disease, as well as less access to medical services. Highly effective antiretroviral therapy is prolonging the lives of those infected, but there is also an increase in the practice of preventive behavior among high-risk population (NCHS, 1998). The same source reports that teenage pregnancy, infant mortality, and homicide rates have also fallen significantly. At the same time, significant ethnic differences exist in these risk factors. According to the Alan Guttmacher Institute, two key factors have contributed to teen pregnancy decline: (a) fewer teens are having sex, and (a) more adolescents are using contraceptives (Tew, 1998). Data from the Youth Risk Behavior Surveillance System (Tew, 1998) show significant ethnic differences in teen pregnancy rates, frequency sexual of intercourse, age of initiation of sexual intercourse, multiple sexual partners, use of condoms, and discussion of AIDS/HIV infection with a parent or another adult.

These and other findings presented in this volume suggest that there are positive changes in the horizon and that these changes are happening among high-risk groups in local settings. Somehow, LCNs are reaching some segments of high-risk populations. To understand the role of mass and interpersonal communication in these developments, we must go beyond aggregate analysis of media effect and examine the dominant patterns of "microcommunication systems," by ethnicity, gender, and age. Traditional population surveys, or studies of captive audience (e.g., in schools, at worksites), will not reveal these local processes. More effective usage of LCNs would help reduce current inequalities in communication needs across ethnic groups. A closer examination of these developments would reveal the processes, including health communication, that played significant roles. We must ask, Along with effective communication media, what other forces and factors may affect the goal of a health communication campaign in a multicultural community?

Threats to Children as a Unifying Force

A major question we face in dealing with a multicultural and distressed community is this: What common causes and concerns may override ethnic diversities and bring together a multicultural and distressed community for unified action for health promotion? We identified two issues that have the power to mobilize: (a) concerns for survival (jobs, job training, and legal/immigration needs) and (b) concerns for well-being of children (Kar et al., 1999). Children and adolescents in multicultural and distressed communities are highly vulnerable to multiple risks resulting from drug abuse, unprotected sex, and violence. Teens are becoming sexually active at younger ages and are increasingly exposed to sexually transmitted diseases, HIV/AIDS risks, and unwanted pregnancy. In addition, children in distressed and multicultural communities are at a greater risk of violence, both at home and in the community. Our experiences from public health practice activities in South Central Los Angeles clearly demonstrate that saving children from harm is one of the most, if not *the* most, important community concerns. Furthermore, although ethnic groups ranked their priorities differently, protecting their children from harms was the highest priority for all ethnic groups; it was the only problem against which all parents were willing to unite for action

Mothers as Partners in Prevention

Primary prevention requires active community participation (World Health Organization [WHO]/UNICEF, 1978). Community participation, in turn, depends on the extent to which a program meets community priorities. The *Ottawa Charter for Health Promotion* (1996) holds that advocacy on behalf of a community should be a major strategy for generating community participation. Several community development models (Freire, 1994; Yunus, 1997) hold that community empowerment, especially empowerment of families and women, remains essential to a successful social program, especially in poor and distressed communities. Major challenges for public health professionals, therefore, are (a) to develop effective methodologies to involve a diverse community in articulating its own priorities, (b) to identify and/or develop consensus regarding a common cause or concern that may unite a diverse community for collective action, and (c) to sustain partnerships with the community and local agencies to address their particular needs.

Four case studies in this volume specifically deal with the role of parents, especially mothers, in community-based prevention efforts in multiethnic populations when supported by bottom-up planning and educational efforts integrated within well-articulated health care service programs. The chapter by Bell and Alcalay (Chapter 12 in this volume) shows a how a wellness guide developed with the active participation of mothers and reinforced by trained professional staff can be an important medium for changing knowledge, attitudes, and actions of at-risk mothers about maternal and child health risk reduction in poor African American and Latina mothers in California. The Healthy Start program in six U.S. cities described by Raykovich, Wells, and Binder (Chapter 7), shows significant impacts of health diaries combined with case management by clinic staff on effective pregnancy management and maternal and child health risk reduction among African American, Latino, and Native American mothers. Glik and Mickalide describe (Chapter 6) the roles that mothers play in childhood injury prevention across ethnic groups. Finally, Chapter 8 analyzes the roles of parent-child communication on drug use prevention in Asian American youths.

Local Health Promoters (LHP)

Peer educators/counselors and heath promoters, trained from local ethnic communities and supported by professional staff, would be an important medium to bridge the cultural gap between at-risk populations and providers of health care. Two case studies in this volume describe the roles and limits of peers as health promoters among two high-risk groups. The HIV/AIDS education project among homeless youths by Russell (Chapter 10) exemplifies how a multistage theater project was able to reach 211 persons from six ethnic groups who were not accessible through other programs. The project showed youths a play titled *The Street Where I Live,* followed by a didactic educational session. Results show several ethnic differences among the data regarding change in knowledge, perceived norms, behavioral intentions, and approval of the program. It is interesting to note that the peer educators themselves gain most from their participation, with a few reporting that they have discussed HIV/AIDS problems with their parents. This finding is especially significant because of the potential for reaching non-English-speaking adult immigrants through their teen children who are relatively more exposed to mainstream culture. Younger Hispanics and African Americans, both from underprivileged ethnic groups, seem to benefit most from peer education programs. Also, the chapter by Morisky and Ebin (Chapter 9) reviews lessons learned from peer education programs for HIV/AIDS prevention in general, and the PEP-LA program based in Los Angeles in particular, analyzing data from an ethnic perspective.

American Indians, however, have historically been neglected by these kinds of studies, mainly because of their smaller numbers relative to the population as a whole. The chapter by Levy-Storms, Wallace, Goldfarb, and Burhansstipanov (Chapter 11) tackles this issue and illustrates how community-based, bottom-up social action program can enhance health promotion among elderly American Indian and Samoan women.

The analyses above suggest two major implications for health communication in multicultural and hard-to-reach populations. First, small-scale, localized, and ongoing face-to-face communication constitutes the core of effective health communication in MCs, because printed and electric media can complement the health messages but cannot directly reach the audience. Second, local communicators selected, trained, and supported by health professionals are more effective than professionals themselves in reaching the population at risk. Consequently, an effective strategy for health communication requires a paradigm shift from use of mainstream media by professionals to a new paradigm that focuses on involving LCNs, empowering local leadership and community members in the process.

Cultural Competency and Collaboration

That cultural competency of health communicators and collaboration between communicators and their audience is the *sine qua non* of an effective program acts is common theme throughout the analytical chapters and multicultural studies presented in this volume. The point we wish to emphasize here is that cultural competency is much more than learning the language of the audience; language competency is a necessary, but not sufficient, condition for intercultural communication. Clearly, it requires much more than learning a different language; indeed, we hold the view that if a communicator is culturally competent, then a language barrier should not be insurmountable. Language barriers can be diminished in many ways: learning the language, recruiting outside interpreters, or cultivating key informants from the community, a method often used by cultural and medical anthropologists.

Much has been written on this topic, and considerable debate exists on how best to enhance cultural competency. We hope that the specific issues raised in Chapter 5 of this volume, the lessons from multicultural case studies presented earlier, and the cross-cultural health behavior matrix will provide some conceptual framework for developing a better understanding of what health professionals and communicators can do to improve cultural competency. Cultural competency includes additional factors: mutual trust, a symbiotic relationship, and a commitment to work together in a way that respects one another's culture. Above all, it involves building trusting relationships, or a "bond of relation" as Tagore describes it, with the community, its leadership, and the community-based organizations (CBOs) dedicated to serving multicultural populations. We identify three levels of cultural competency: (a) cultural understanding, (b) cultural acceptance, and (c) reciprocal relationships. This topic has been discussed in further detail in Chapter 13, regarding the evaluation of programs using cultural competency as an indicator.

Beyond Communication:
Empowerment for Health Promotion

Meta-Analysis of Women's Empowerment Case Studies

Community empowerment as a strategy for health promotion has not received sufficient attention from communication researchers. Necessity drove bold and imaginative minds to initiate grassroots movements and health risk prevention programs in both poorer and richer nations, with remarkable results.

Strong evidence of the effectiveness of mothers and women as leaders and as a powerful force for social change is contained in several case studies from different nations:

1. Rosa Parks and Jo Ann Robinson's bold defiance of segregation in public buses, which triggered massive social action

2. The Mothers Against Drunk Driving (MADD) movement initiated by a mother of a teenage daughter killed by a hit-and-run driver with a prior drunk-driving record, which has become a national grassroots movement with more than 500 local chapters and which serves as a major force pushing to implement laws increasing the minimum drinking age in 44 states

3. The Grumman Bank program in Bangladesh, which empowered impoverished mothers with small financial loans to help generate a second income for their families and thus empowered them while enhancing their status and self-esteem

4. The Madres de la Plaza Mayo (mothers of the main plaza) case in Buenos Aires, Argentina, where middle-aged women drew international attention through their campaign against the ruling military junta on behalf of their disappeared sons and husbands

5. The De Madres a Madres ("from mothers to mothers") program in Houston's inner-city Hispanic community, which empowered volunteer mothers to promote preventive health behavior, including the use of prenatal care

6. The effectiveness of Mothers Clubs in promoting family planning and maternal and child health programs in India, Thailand, and several other Asian nations

7. The grassroots movement by women in rural Gujrat, India, which secured a safe water supply for their families

8. The Peruvian women's leadership roles in grassroots opposition against the forces of imperialism and sexism

9. Marylea Kelly's leadership in organizing the Tri-Valley Citizens Against a Radioactive Environment (CARE), which successfully transformed nuclear weapons research programs and significantly reduced radioactive toxic hazards produced by the University of California Lawrence Livermore facilities

10. Nobel laureate Rigoberta Menchu's bold leadership in effectively organizing the Guatemala resistance movement against military oppression

These case studies from nations with diverse cultural and sociopolitical systems strongly suggest that mothers and women can be a very effective force and allies for community-based health promotion and risk reduction programs when they are empowered, motivated by a goal they highly value, and supported by the larger community.

To examine whether and to what extent that powerless mothers and women can initiate grassroots movements to improve their quality of life, we conducted an intensive search and analysis of case studies from around the world. We focus on mothers and women for three reasons. First, mothers and women in almost all cultures are the primary, if not the only, caregivers in their families. Therefore, when they are adequately empowered and engaged in health promotion strategies, they are likely to exert a strong and sustained positive influence on the health and well-being of family members. Second, mothers and women in all social strata are relatively less powerful than men throughout the globe. Within poor and disadvantaged populations, they are likely to be even more powerless, yet they bear most, if not all, the burden of caring for their children and other family members. Third, there is a global consensus that a greater emphasis be placed on the public health model and the prevention of health risks than on the provision of tertiary clinical care alone. In the public health approach, the public or the community (broadly defined) is conceptualized both as an *active partner* in prevention programs and as the *beneficiary* of them. For these reasons, the importance of women as active partners in effective public health strategy cannot be overemphasized.

Our meta-analysis of 40 important case studies has as its primary objective the examination and identification of (a) the factors that affect women's empowerment and leadership under the most difficult conditions; (b) the methods women use to initiate and sustain their struggle; (c) the role of nonformal empowerment education, communication media, and advocacy in these initiatives; (d) the source and nature of the support and opposition encountered; and (e) the context or sociopolitical environment that affects women's problems as well as the effectiveness of their actions. We examined the strategies used in the empowerment of women and in their struggle to enhance their quality of life in four important domains: (a) basic *human rights* and democracy, (b) *equal rights* for women, (c) *community development and microenterprises* for family economic enhancement, and (4) *health promotion and disease prevention* (hereafter, *health promotion*). We also intend with the ongoing study to identify factors common to these cases as well as those unique to specific categories. To this end, we examined cases from disparate cultures and at different levels of economic development. A better understanding of these factors and processes will, we hope, be useful in the development of policies and programs that seek to benefit women who are relatively disadvantaged and powerless (Kar et al., 1999).

The findings are most educational. A major conclusion, which we include in our proposed model (Figure 14.1), is that *all involvement in social action initiatives—regardless of their specific goals, methods, or outcomes—has strong empowering effects.* These effects are twofold. First, there was an enhancement of the women's subjective well-being; their self-esteem, self-efficacy, and local reputation increased significantly as a result of their involvement in even small-scale self-help initiatives and local programs. Second, as women acquired important technical and organizational skills, their quality of life and social status were significantly enhanced. As the programs expanded, many of the women attained positions of responsibility as supervisors, trainers, and managers of units. Organized and led by women, many of these programs are now considered pioneers in women's empowerment and development and are regarded as sources of inspiration for grassroots and community development movements worldwide.

Several case studies show that the women were initially met with skepticism by established organizations and male members of the community. This was indeed the case for women in the Aollas communes, or community kitchen program, in Santa Maria, Peru (Macera & Oyola, 1997). The quotations below describe the prevailing attitude toward women in Peruvian culture, which stereotypes them as weak, indecisive, dependent on men, socially ineffective, lacking in organizational ability, and unequal to the pressures of leadership.

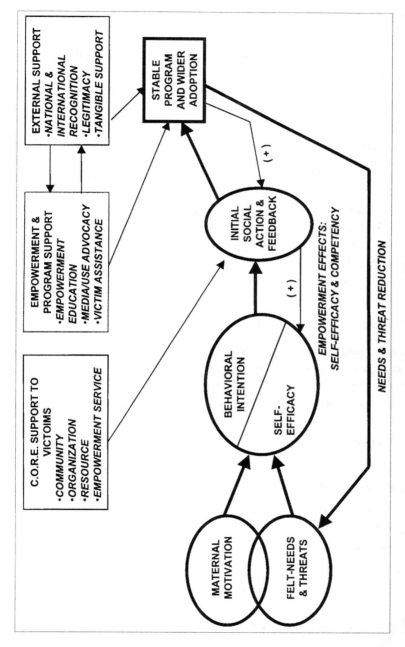

Figure 14.1. Empowerment of Women and Mothers: A Proposed Model

SOURCE: Kar, Pascual, and Chickering (1999).

.ismo exists because men do not want to recognize women as *compañeras;* in-
., women are treated as servants.

The only difference between men and women is that men cannot become pregnant, and women can. Because everything else you can both do—work, earn
money, and raise children.

Through their actions, these women dispelled cultural stereotypes and won
recognition by men as equals. One of the most common findings of our meta-
analysis is the transformation in the attitude of males from one of male chau-
vinism to an acceptance of women as equal partners. This *empowerment effect
of involvement* was observed in all of the case studies. Furthermore, the media,
initially local and subsequently regional and national, played a significant role
in promoting public support for their cause and contributed significantly to
their success. See Table 14.1 in the next section for an in-depth discussion of the
role of media in various empowerment methods.

Media Use, Support, and Advocacy

A major finding of our meta-analysis mentioned in the previous section is
that communication media play significant roles at different phases of a grassroots movement. We identified seven methods most frequently used by these
movements. The acronym **EMPOWER** stands for these methods:

1. Empowerment education and training

2. Media support, use, and advocacy for policy and program support

3. Public information and education for opinion and resource support

4. Organizing associations and unions for collective and group empowerment

5. Work skills and job training for enhancing autonomy and internal locus
   of control

6. Enabling services, support, and microenterprise or essential opportunities and resources

7. Rights protection and promotion through victim protection, legislative
   lobbying, and social action litigation

Table 14.1 Empowerment Methods, by Domain (HPDP vs. non-HPDP)

Method	Frequency of Method Use (%) Health Promotion Disease Prevention (HPDP), n = 15	Non-HPDP, n = 25	Total Cases per Method N = 40
Enabling service and assistance	12 (80.0)	19 (76.0)	31 (77.5)
Rights protection and social action/reform	6 (40.0)	18 (72.0)	24 (60.0)
Public education and participation	9 (60.0)	14 (56.0)	23 (57.5)
Media use, support, and advocacy	8 (53.3)	12 (48.0)	20 (50.0)
Organizing partnerships, associations, cooperatives and coalitions	5 (33.3)	15 (60.0)	20 (50.0)
Empowerment training and leadership development	7 (46.7)	12 (48.0)	19 (47.5)

SOURCE: Revised from Kar and Alex (1999).

Results in Table 14.1 for these seven methods show that communication, both mass media and interpersonal, plays a significant role in generating public awareness and support for their cause.

Modern communication media (television, radio, and newspapers) are used to accomplish two complementary objectives: (a) *media support* for existing programs and (b) *media advocacy* to influence public policy, mobilize public opinion, or generate public pressure. To achieve the first objective, the media are used to draw attention to a particular organization or movement by publicizing a groundbreaking organization, a landmark action, or another newsworthy event. Half of all cases used this method. However, a significant difference was found in the frequency of use of media by cases in industrialized and less industrialized nations (81% and 29%, respectively; chi-square = 10.4;

$df = 1, p < .001$); this is perhaps due to greater access to mass media for social action in industrialized societies. To illustrate, in the United States, the National Organization of Women (NOW) has garnered media support through protests, demonstrations, and speeches by NOW leaders. In New York, in the 1970s, NOW members captured the attention of the media by invading the regional office of Equal Employment Opportunity Commission carrying bundles of classified ads bound with red tape to symbolize the sexual discrimination faced by women in the workplace (Davis, 1991, pp. 15-25, 52-68).

To achieve the second objective of media advocacy—that is, influencing public policy, mobilizing public opinion, or both—the media must be persuaded to relay the organization's message through media campaigns, press conferences, and press releases. For example, Women Against Gun Violence drives home its antigun message through community-based media advocacy programs that draw attention to alarming facts and statistics. The organization also serves as an expert source of information for the media, both local and national, both print and electronic, through interviews, articles, and editorials that articulate issues related to gun violence (A. Reiss-Lane, personal communication, January 8, 1997).

Note that public education and participation, which entails informing and educating the general public, community leaders, and leaders of CBOs that serve affected communities (such as churches, temples, and voluntary and human service agencies) was used by 23 of the 40 cases (57.5%, see Table 14.1). The primary objective with this method is to shape public opinion, generate material support for programs, and bring about desired policy reforms as well as public action and participation. These ends are achieved by means of community-based, face-to-face programs, such as speakers bureaus; the use of local media (public service announcements, newsletters, the Internet, leaflets, and brochures); and the development of ethnic networks, such as advisory councils or boards, designed to enlist public support for specific programs or initiatives. A significant difference was found in the use of this method between cases from industrialized and less industrialized nations (81% vs. 41%; chi-square = 6.15; $p < .013$; Table 14.1); perhaps due to the relatively high cost of such programs, less industrialized nations are unable to use this method as frequently as those in affluent nations.

Synergy Between Empowerment and Media Support

Empowerment serves to imbue communities with the necessary will to create and sustain lasting, positive change, and the media can assist in this process.

Our meta-analysis of case studies of successful grassroots movements led by women around the world shows that effective media support and public education play a vital role in the success of these movements (Kar et al., 1999; Kar, 2000). These case studies reveal that media use and empowerment have a synergic relationship. Effective media use and advocacy empower women and their movements; empowered women in turn are more effective users of media for public education designed to generate public support and to mobilize social capitals necessary for their movements. Next to crisis interventions and trauma relief methods (e.g., enabling services and rights protection measures), media use, public education, and organizing coalitions are the most frequently used methods by the successful movements. Also, as expected, due to higher availability of modern media in richer nations, movements in industrialized nations used modern media more frequently than in less industrialized nations. In industrialized nations, 8 of 10 (81%) of these successful empowerment movements included media use, support, and advocacy (Kar et al., 1999, p. 1448, table 3). Even in poorer nations and populations, media support can significantly change the course of a movement from a stalemate to a success. The Madres de Plaza de Mayo movement in Argentina by semi-illiterate mothers in search of their "disappeared" sons and the Mothers of East Los Angeles who successfully opposed construction of a prison and a waste disposal incinerator in their neighborhood are only two examples of how media support can mobilize public opinion and support for their cause. Our analysis shows that modern media have been effectively used by successful movements for two complementary objectives: (1) media support for existing movement and (2) media advocacy for agenda setting, influencing public policy, and promoting legislative actions (Kar et al., 1999, pp. 1449-1450). In spite of significant differences in sociocultural contexts, political systems, history, and economic pressures, these two movements illuminate how communication systems, especially when the program has allies in the news media, can bolster grassroots movements.

Ten Findings and Propositions for Health Promotion and Communication

The following 10 propositions summarize the key findings of our metaanalysis as they relate to health communication in underserved and ethnically diverse communities. They may serve as guidelines for planning community-based interventions designed to empower disenfranchised populations and enhance their quality of life and health (see Figure 14.1). Although the propositions refer to social actions for empowering women and mothers, they would be equally relevant to empowering other groups. Indeed, many of these same points arose in the case studies presented in this volume.

1. *Maternal motivation to prevent harm to their children is a driving force for social action.* Deep commitment to protect and promote the well-being of children and families often serves as a motivating force for action. We observe this phenomenon in all cases.

2. *A struggle for basic survival needs and human rights is likely to engender wider social support,* even in societies under authoritarian rule and even under military dictatorships, when women lead struggles for minimum survival needs (e.g., a minimum wage, human rights violations).

3. *Struggles led by nonpolitical women and mothers for their children's well-being, safety, and prevention of harm are likely to generate social approval and support.* Case studies suggest that even corrupt officials and gang members respect their own mothers.

4. *Participation and involvement have empowering effects.* Involvement as leaders or participants at any level has empowering effects independent of tangible program outcomes. Initially, involvement in self-help initiatives at the local level enhances self-esteem and self-efficacy. Subsequently, involvement in empowerment programs enhances social status, professional competence and leadership, leading to an improved quality of life for the participants, their families, and their community.

5. *CORE support at the early phase of a local self-care initiative is essential for developing a viable enabling program.* CORE is an acronym: Community support, Organizational support from CBOs, Resource support from local resources (either in cash or kind) for initial efforts, and Empowerment support from various instrumental support and empowerment methods. CORE support may come from citizens, volunteers from neighborhood religious institutions (churches, temples, etc.), or from CBOs.

6. *Enabling services and assistance are essential in allowing victims to resist abuse and sustain their struggles.* Fear of retaliation by abusers often deters victims from seeking help, resisting abuse, or both. Enabling services and assistance help victims deal with traumatic experiences and empower them with the knowledge that they have protection against future abuse. These services enhance the likelihood that the abused will join the struggle against their tormentors.

7. *Training and leadership development programs that have empowering effects on women and mothers significantly influence program outcomes.* This method is critical in enhancing their competency to organize programs for themselves. Nonformal education includes the following: (a) educating and informing the public to generate community approval and support for an initiative (in turn, such approval and support from the immediate community translate into positive public opinion, cash and in-kind instrumental support, and community-based activities); (b) education and training of women and mothers in survival and income-generating skills; and (c) training in organizational and leadership skills.

8. *Media use, support, and advocacy complement program efforts and can significantly enhance their effectiveness.* Media support is defined as the effective use of communication media (both modern and indigenous) to promote an existing initiative or program. Media advocacy is defined as the effective use of modern media to bring public opinion to bear on policy reform and on the better implementation of existing policies and laws.

9. *External recognition and support enhances institutionalization and wider adoption of landmark local initiatives.* Recognition from credible national and international organizations legitimizes a struggle and empowers those involved. It also helps to generate resources, stabilize, and expand the program, and enhance its diffusion.

10. *A nonviolent social action movement for a just cause is likely to gain social approval and, thus, enhance its ultimate effectiveness.* The Gandhian Sarvodaya movement for India's independence, the civil rights movement led by Dr. Martin Luther King, Jr. in the United States, and Argentina's Madres de Plaza de Mayo are but a few of the many remarkable examples that attest to the effectiveness of this method.

The case studies in this volume, our own meta-analysis, and the discussion of the history and theories underlying health promotion communication all point to a new public health paradigm that must be implemented to effectively reach MCs. Using community empowerment and communication methods, a sustainable program must incorporate partnerships with the targeted population to effectively achieve its goals. However, it cannot be enough simply to create a program and unleash it on a targeted population; health practitioners must ensure that the program will have the desired effect. Therefore, comprehensive evaluation must be an integral part of any health promotion program, particularly those in MCs, to expand on the little current knowledge regarding the most effective methods by which to reach this segment of the public.

In Conclusion

Over 150 years ago, Alexis de Tocqueville observed that despite our rugged individualism, Americans' unique sense of personal efficacy combined with our self-interest make us more likely to participate in civic affairs and organizations than other nationals. This cultural character has served us well in our pursuit of democracy and prosperity (Tocqueville, 1961). Since then, many social thinkers and reformers, including Thoreau, Gandhi, Martin Luther King Jr., and Freire, have convincingly argued and demonstrated through their own actions, the importance of empowerment of the poor and underserved communities as an effective means for promoting democracy, self-efficacy, and well-being for all. Inequalities in health status and access to care are threats not only to those in poor health but to the well-being of all people in the United States. Consequently, both for ethnical/deontological and practical/utilitarian reasons (discussed fully in Chapter 1), our national health promotion agenda and objectives for the year 2010 focuses on empowerment of the underserved and reduction of ethnic differences in health status, risk, and access to care. The extent to which health communication and evaluation process may play a critical role to empower multicultural communities and thus enhance our collective competency for risk reduction and health promotion would be the ultimate criterion of its effectiveness.

References

American Demographics. (1991). *American diversity* (Desk reference series, No. 1). Ithaca, NY: American Demographics Magazine.

Backer, T. E., Rogers, E. M., & Sopory, P. (1992). *Designing health communication campaigns: What works?* Newbury Park, CA: Sage.

Bang, A. T., Bang, R. A., Tale, O., Sontakke, P., Solanki, J., Wargantiwar, R., & Kelzarkar, P. (1990). Reduction in pneumonia mortality and total childhood mortality by means of community-based intervention trial in Gadchiroli, India. *Lancet, 336*(8709), 201-206.

Chakravarty, A. (Ed.). (1961). *A Tagore reader.* Boston: Beacon.

Chou, C. P., Montgomery, S., Pentz, M. A., Rohrbach, L. A., Johnson, C. A., Flay, B. R., & MacKinnon, D. P. (1998). Effects of a community-based prevention program on decreasing drug use in high-risk adolescents. *American Journal of Public Health, 88*(6), 944-948.

Davis, F. (1991). *Moving the mountain: The women's movement in America since 1960.* New York: Simon & Schuster.

Ennett, S. T., Tobler N. S., Ringwalt, C. L., & Flewelling R. L. (1994). How effective is drug abuse resistance education? A meta-analysis of project DARE outcome evaluations. *American Journal of Public Health, 84,*(9), 1394-1401.

Farquhar, J. W., Maccoby, N., Wood, P. D., Alexander, J. K., Breitrose, H., Brown, B. W., Jr., Haskell, W. L., McAlister, A. L., Meyer, A. J., & others. (1994). Community education for cardiovascular health. In A. Steptoe & J. Wardle (Eds.), *Psychosocial processes and health: A reader* (pp. 316-324). Cambridge, UK: Cambridge University Press.

Flack, J. M., Amaro, H., Jenkins, W., Kunitz, S., Levy, J., Mixon, M., & Yu, E. (1995). Epidemiology of minority health. *Health Psychology, 14*(7), 592-600.

Freire, P. (1994). *Pedagogy of hope: Reliving pedagogy of the oppressed* (R. R. Barr, Trans.). New York: Continuum

Glazer, N. (1997). *We are all multiculturalists now.* Cambridge, MA: Harvard University Press.

Gotto, A. M., Jr. (1997). The Multiple Risk Factor Intervention Trial (MRFIT). A return to a landmark trial. *JAMA, 277*(7), 595-597.

Kar, S. (2000, April). *Women's health development: Imperatives for health and welfare systems.* Background paper and invited presentation for International Meeting on Women and Health, Sponsored by the World Health Organization, Kobe Center, Japan.

Kar, S., Jimenez, A., Campbell, K., Sze, F. (1998). Acculturation and quality of life: A comparative study of Japanese-Americans and Indo-Americans. *Amerasia Journal, 24*(1), 129-142.

Kar, S. B., & Alex, S. B. (1999). Public health approaches to substance abuse prevention: A multicultural perspective. In S. B. Kar (Ed.), *Substance abuse prevention in multicultural communities.* Amityville, NY: Baywood.

Kar, S. B., Pascual, C. A., & Chickering, K. L. (1999). Empowerment of women for health promotion: A meta-analysis. *Social Science & Medicine, 49,* 1431-1460.

Los Angeles County Department of Health Services. (1994). *LA County annual health risk assessment.* Information from data on CD-ROM. [Available from the LACDHS, 313 N. Figueroa St., Los Angeles, CA 90012]

Maccoby, N., & Altman, D. G. (1988). Disease prevention in communities: The Stanford Heart Disease Prevention Program. In R. H. Price, E. L. Cowen, R. Lorion, & J. Ramos-Mckay (Eds.). *Fourteen ounces of prevention: A casebook for practitioners* (pp. 165-174). Washington, DC: American Psychological Association.

Macera, L., & Oyola, T. (1997). *Empowering women: A critical analysis of community kitchens in Peru.* Unpublished term paper submitted to Professor Snehendu Kar for CHS 282: Communication in Health Promotion and Education, Winter 1997, UCLA/SPH.

National Center for Health Statistics. (1998, October 7). *AIDS falls from top ten causes of death; teen births, infant mortality, homicide all decline.* Press release, NCHS Public Affairs Office.

The Ottawa Charter for Health Promotion (17-21 November 1986). (1996). In *Health promotion anthology* (Scientific Publication No. 557). Washington, DC: World Health Organization, Pan American Health Organization.

Penn, N. E., Kar, S., Kramer, J., Skinner, J., & Zambrana, R. E. (1995). Ethnic minorities, health care systems, and behavior. *Health Psychology, 14*(7), 641-646.

Pentz, M. A. (1994). Directions for future research in drug abuse prevention. *Preventive Medicine, 23*(5), 646-652.

Piotrow, P. T., Kincaid, D. L., Rimon, J. G., & Rinehart, W. (1997). *Health communication: Lessons from family planning and reproductive health.* Westport, CT: Praeger.

Puska, P., Nissinen, A., Tuomilehto, J., Salonen, J. T., Koskela, K., McAlister, A., Kottke, T. E., Maccoby, N., & Farquhar, J. W. (1996). The community-based strategy to prevent coronary heart disease: Conclusions from the 10 years of the North Karelia Project. In *Health promotion: An anthology* (pp. 89-125). Washington, DC: Pan American Health Organization.

Rice, R. E., & Atkin, C. K. (Eds.). (1989). *Public communication campaigns* (2nd ed.). Newbury Park, CA: Sage.

Rogers E. M. (1973). *Communication strategies for family planning.* New York: Free Press.

Takeuchi, D. T., Sue, S., & Yeh, M. (1995). Return rates and outcomes from, ethnicity-specific mental health programs in Los Angeles. *American Journal of Public Health, 85*(5), 638-643.

Tew, S. (1998). *U.S. teenage pregnancy rate now lowest in two decades.* New York: Alan Guttmacher Institute.

Tocqueville, A. (1961). *Democracy in America.* New York: Schocken.

U.S. Bureau of the Census. (1990). *1990 census.* Retrieved from the U.S. Bureau of the Census Web site: http://www.census.gov

U.S. Bureau of the Census. (1993). *We the American . . . foreign born.* Washington, DC: Department of Commerce, Economics and Statistics Administration.

U.S. Bureau of the Census. (1996). *Estimate for 1996 US Population.* Retrieved from the U.S. Bureau of the Census Web site: http://www.census.gov

U.S. Bureau of the Census. (1998, April 9). *Foreign-born population reaches 25.8 million, according to Census Bureau.* Press release, Public Information Office.

U.S. Department of Health and Human Services. (1991). *Healthy people 2000: National Health promotion and disease prevention objectives* (DHHS Publication No. PHS 91-50212). Washington, DC: Government Printing Office.

World Health Organization/United Nations International Children's Emergency Fund. (1978). *ALMA-ATA 1978 primary health care: Report of the International Conference on Primary Health Care.* Geneva, Switzerland: Author.

Yunus, M. (1997, January). A bank for the poor: Bangladesh's Grameen Bank. *UNESCO Courier,* pp. 20-24.

Index

Acculturation:
    age and, 83
    biculturalism problems, 84
    culture and, 84
    defined, 82
    external factors in, 83
    findings analysis, 299
    health communication, 83
    index of acculturation measures, 298-
        299
    internal factors in, 83
    intervention impact, 299
    language preferences, 82-83
Adelaide Declaration, 8
Adolescent drug abuse prevention:
    abuse risk factors, 194-196
    Asian Indian Case Study, 197-207
    communication benefits, 194
    conclusions on, 207
    efficacy of, 194
    ethnic message differences, 196
    parent discussions on, 193-194
    problem importance, 193
Adolescent drug risk factors
    peer network correlation's, 195
    social interaction influences, 195-196
    socialization and, 195
    sources of, 195
Advocacy, health promotion and, 7-8

African Americans:
    child injury rates, 146-147
    death rates, 81
    death causes, 15, 149
    health information sources, 35, 341
    HIV knowledge, 241
    peer education programs, 344
    population composition, 11
    quality of life issues, 82
    South Carolina Study and, 153
    television viewing by, 36-37
Agenda-setting:
    hypothesis of, 128
    multicultural agendas, 128
    Aging populations, demographic
        changes, 11
AIDS:
    death rates, 341
    machismo culture and, 86
    new infection rates, 341-341
AIDS/HIV prevention, 317
Alan Guttmacher Institute, 342
Alcohol Addiction, 47
Alcohol, Tobacco, and Other Drugs
    Prevention Programs:
    California Model, 54
    goals of, 53
    other initiatives from, 54
    prevention elements of, 53-54

Alma Ata Declaration, 66
Alternative medicine, 32-34
    health care system and, 32-34
    JAMA articles, 33
    Landmark Healthcare Study, 32
    vs. traditional medicines, 32, 33
American Cancer Society, 123
Annenberg Foundation, 47
Arnold, Wendy, 222
Asian Americans:
characteristics of, 90
death causes for, 15, 149
death rates, 81
health care barriers, 90
health information sources, 35-36,
    341
"model minority" stereotype, 339
Mothers Clubs for, 346
paradoxes of, 17
population composition, 11
quality of life and, 82, 90-91
television viewing by, 36-38
See also Chinese Americans; Vietnam
    Americans
Asian cultural patterns:
    immigrant status, 88
    linguistic diversity, 88
    population growth, 88
    psychological distress sources, 88
    socioeconomic diversity, 88
    traditional value retaining, 88
Asian Indian Case Study:
    discussion on, 201-202
    drug use documentation, 198
    drug use periods, 198
    drug use prevalence, 199
    goals of, 197
    methods in, 197-198
    parent-child communications, 197
    policy implications, 202-207
    results of, 198-201
    sample criteria, 197
    sample description, 199
    semistructured survey questionnaire,
        198
    two-stage procedure, 197-198
Association of Schools of Public Health
    (ASPH), 57

BABES program, 54

Behavioral theories:
    group dynamic theories, 68
    health domains in, 68-69
    health field characteristics, 69
    See also Lewin, Kurt

California Department of Mental Health, 283
California parents study, 154-157
    Mexican parents' perceptions, 155
    white parents' perceptions, 155-157
California Smoking Control Programs for
    Targeted Populations, 129
California Wellness Foundation, 291-292
California *Wellness Guide* Distribution
    (WGD) Project, 282
Center for Health Policy Studies (CHPS), 167
Center for Media Education (CME), 38
Centers for Disease Control
    Health Promotion and Disease
        Prevention, 212
    proposed health outcomes, 312
Chi, 94
Child development:
    behavioral problems, 145-146
    males vs. females, 145
    preschoolers, 145
    school-aged children, 145
    task vs. ability, 145
    unintentional injuries, 145
Child injury cultural research:
    California parents study, 154-157
    child development, 150
    cultural attributes, 150-151
    "cultural scripts," 151-152
    culture recognition in, 150
    National SAFE KIDS Campaign, 153-
        155
    parental beliefs, 152
    parental safety barriers, 152
    South Carolina Study, 152-153
Childhood injuries:
    causes of, 142
    death rate from, 142
    fatal unintentional injuries, 143
    impacts from, 142
    injury rates, 142, 146-147
    risks for, 144-146
Childhood injury prevention:
    culturally informed prevention, 157-160
    culturally informed research, 152-157

culture and, 150-152
ethnic differences in, 146-149
injury problems in, 142-143
unintentional injuries, 141-142
Childhood physical environment, 144
Childhood social environment, 144-145
low-income families, 144
risk factors for, 144-145
Children:
global mortality rates, 5
health affordability gaps impacts, 31
"injury-prone," 145
television viewing risks, 38
"Children and People" program, 54
Chinese Americans:
etiology of, 94-95
growth of, 89
language barriers, 89
preferred treatment modalities, 95
women's health status, 89
Citizens Against a Radioactive Environment
(CARE), 347
Clinton administration, media violence and,
65
Collectivism, vs. U.S. culture, 91
Columbia University, 56
Commercial media:
children risk factors, 38
health promotion strategies, 40
health risk factors and, 38
media consolidations, 38-39
women's role in, 39-40
Communication, health issues using, 55
Communication effects:
ethnic differences, 296-298
hierarchy matrix domains, 316-317
Hispanic intervention impact, 298-299
individual level measurements, 315
multicultural communication factors,
315-316
See also Communication interventions
Communication evaluation:
information seeking, 294
self-efficacy, 295
self-reporting outcomes, 295
Communication interventions, 109-111, 242-
247, 295-296, 300-303
behavior changes, 300-301
conceptual considerations, 244-245
cultural competency, 246-247
health promotion findings, 302-303
implications of, 245

methodology considerations, 242-244
multiple channels use, 300
outcomes of, 301-302
peer health education, 247
positive impact reasons, 302
pretesting needs, 300
Project ABLE and, 242
vs. differential leaning rates, 303
Communication material development. *See*
Guía; Health Diary; Wellness Guide
Communication process, purpose of, 282-283
Communication research:
intervention concept, 229
policy implementations from, 228-229
theoretical underpinnings of, 228
Communication revolution:
characteristics of, 34
diversification of, 37-38
entertainment industry and, 34
health information sources, 35
health promotion campaigns, 34-35
health-related studies, 35-36
Internet as, 36
media expanding, 36-37
risk factors, 38-40
Communication studies, 46-47
Communication types:
approaches for, 99
cultural setting for, 98
message meanings, 98-99
personalismo in, 99
Community empowerment, health
promotion and, 7-8
See also Empowerment
Community Health Improvement Process
(CHIP) model:
communication intervention uses, 327
cycles in, 328
cycles interactions, 327-328
empowerment evaluation, 329
features of, 326
focus of, 327
health communication evaluations, 326-
329
participatory research importance, 327
Community involvement:
communication planners roles, 116
communication strategies from, 115
health issue analysis, 115
Community unification:
mobilization issues, 342
risks to children and, 342-343

saving children, 343
Community-based health promotion, 70-73.
    See also Health communication
    campaign design
Community-based organizations (CBOs), 96
Community-level theories:
    Diffusion of Innovations theory, 121
    social marketing model, 122-123
Condom use, 212-215, 244-245
    education approaches for, 214
    Project ABLE and, 244
    social influence modeling, 214-215
    STDs and, 212
    See also HIV risk reductions; Pregnancy
Cross-cultural frameworks, Healthy People
    2000 as, 340
Cultivation of Beliefs model, 125-126
Cultural acceptance:
    cultural competency and, 101
    importance of, 101
Cultural competency:
    barriers to, 98-100
    bilingual competency with, 100
    communication planning, 100
    defined, 100
    enhancing of, 345
    factors in, 345
    levels of, 101-104, 345
    Project ABLE and, 246-247
    models for, 102
    vs. language competency, 100-101, 345
Cultural etiology:
    Chinese culture and, 94
    concept of, 94
    difference areas in, 94-95
Cultural paradoxes, 81
    Asian paradoxes, 17
    French paradoxes, 17
    Latino paradoxes, 16-17
Cultural scripts:
    child injuries from, 151-152
    child-rearing rates, 151
Cultural understanding:
    cultural competency and, 101
    importance of, 101
Culturally informed prevention programs:
    criteria for, 160
    cultural differences, 157
    cultural issues studies, 157-159
    ethnic vs. cultural differences, 159-160
    injury prevention, 158
    injury risk unrecognized, 160

intervention success, 160
multicultural targeted research, 159
supervision vs. safety devices, 157-158
Culturally relevant communication:
    cultural competence recommendations,
        100
    "key information" use, 100
    qualitative methods for, 100
    relevant information for, 99-100
    semiology and, 100
    subjective culture analysis, 100
Culture:
    defined, 84, 100, 235
    personal health and, 81
    revealing of, 84

DARE Program, 334
    origin of, 53-54
De Madres a Madres, 346
Death rates:
    cardiovascular disease and, 27
    infectious disease contraction and, 26,
        28
    parasitic diseases, 26
    Demographic realities, 10-11
Department of Health and Human Services,
    origins of, 63
Diffusion of Innovation Theory:
    basis of, 121
    benefits of, 122
    components in, 121
    examples of, 121-122
    focus of, 121
Dual-epidemic period:
    cardiovascular diseases death rates, 27
    chronic disease problems, 25
    infectious diseases, 25-28
    mortality reduction goals, 25
    parasitic diseases death rates, 26

Ecological model of health, 112-113
    vs. individual behavior changes, 112
Ecological perspectives, 112-117
Empowerment:
    advocacy for, 130
    communication challenges, 111
    critical consciousness education, 131
    effects of, 348
    EMPOWER model, 132

evaluation of, 329
examples, 130-132
grassroots movement lessons, 130-131
health promotion as, 347-353
involvement as, 348
media synergy with, 353
resource mobilization, 131
social action model, 131
social capital mobilization, 131
Environment:
care health areas in, 68-69
health domains, 68
other issues as, 69
Ethnic group differences, 296-298
Ethnic injury rates:
allowances for, 147
deaths from falls, 149
epidemiological data, 146-147
ethnic differences, 148
Hispanic children, 148
motor vehicle injuries, 148-149
prevention research, 147
sports injuries, 149
swimming injuries, 149
unintentional injury categories, 148
Ethnic network microcommunicating, 341-
342
Ethnicity, defined, 236
Evaluation design:
experimental model for, 293
pre-and-posttest design, 293-294
questionnaire methods, 293
Evaluator:
purpose of, 322
qualifications for, 322
role of, 321

Fadiman, Anne, 128
Familísmo:
care of aging parents, 86
family vs. individual needs, 86
parenting roles, 86
Family planning:
communication reliance by, 55
contraception rate changes, 56
developing nation use, 55
success of, 55
Fatalism:
causes of, 92
ethnic groups with, 91

health promotion and, 91-92
Fatalismo:
defined, 91
health determent from, 92
Flavier, Juan, 315
Formative evaluations, health
communication and, 313
Framingham Heart Study:
chronic disease causes, 24
lifestyle analysis, 24
Freire's Method, uses of, 100
French paradoxes, wine drinking, 17

Gandhia movement, 130
Global village, defined, 36
Goldstick, Oliver, 237
Government, public health functions, 29-30
Government health institutions:
community-based campaigns, 70-71
development of, 64
funding of, 65-68
health promotion development, 68-70
importance of, 62-63
national agenda setting, 64-65
permanent health institutions, 63-64
Government role:
research investment, 65
tax subsidies, 65-66
Group attributes:
communication theories for, 113
disease etiology concepts of, 114
examples of, 113-114
health promotion, 113
message effectiveness, 115
target group communication needs, 115
target group cultural norms, 114
vs. target behaviors, 113
vs. translated materials, 115
Grumman Bank program, 346
Guía:
adaptations to, 290-291
development of, 288-290
examples of, 289-290
Guía distributions:
staff training for, 291-292
WIC clients and, 291

Halcolm's Evaluation Laws, 323
Harvard University, 56, 58

Health behavior reinforcements:
    examples of, 117
    importance of, 117
    vs. acculturation, 117
Health behaviors:
    cross-cultural framework, 93-94
    dimensions affecting, 92-93
    subgroup differences, 92
Health Belief Model, health promotion
    reasons, 50-51
Health care services:
    communicator cultural competency, 96
    competency basis, 97
    cross-cultural delivery models, 96-97
    cultural communication constructions,
        97-98
    ethnic minority barriers, 96
    lay health workers and, 97
    organizational domains, 68
    providers vs. advocates, 97
    public health paradigm and, 4
Health care system:
    affordability gaps, 31
    alternative medicine seeking, 32
    HMOs, 31
    managed care system, 30
    non-clinical prevention diseases, 31
    public health influences, 31
    vs. ethnic minority heath needs, 30-31
Health communication:
    academic degrees, 45
    government institutions strengthening,
        62-71
    health consciousness growth, 45
    HMO use, 49
    human relations research, 54-56
    implications of, 71-73
    importance of, 49
    interrelated development for, 45-46
    professional fields using, 49
    public health schools expansions, 56-62
    studies of, 46-47
    See also Health communication process
Health communication campaign design,
    283-292:
    effects of, 295-299
    evaluation, 293-295
    health intervention needs, 282
    intervention impact, 282
    intervention implications, 300-303
    minority inequalities, 281-282
    process of, 282-283

research strategy evaluation, 292
    theoretical framework, 292-293
Health communication campaigns:
    effectiveness elements, 336
    ethnic minorities focus, 335
Health communication evaluations:
    CHIP model, 326-329
    communication effects hierarchy, 315-
        317
    components of, 313
    dimensions in, 315
    evaluation model, 317-319
    failure of, 314-315
    improvement time period, 312
    indicator dimensions, 312-315
    indicator selection process, 312-313
    individual and community indicators,
        312
    methodology importance, 311
    outcome levels, 312-313
    physical health indicator ranking, 314
    purposes of, 313
    qualitative evaluations, 320-326
    quality of life indicators, 312
    socioeconomic factors, 312
    vs. cognitive changes, 312
Health communication process, 258-260,
    272-273
    culturally acceptable messages, 260
    "ethnic approval" as, 273
    feedback requirements, 272-273
    focus group use, 258, 258-259
    goals, 262
    marketing of, 258
    program design surveys, 261-262
    program implementation, 260
    program structure differences, 259
    survey feedback, 274
Health Communication Program:
    advisory council use, 256-257
    effects of, 262-272
    group outcomes, 257-258
    interventions for, 272-277
    lay community member input, 257-
        258
    problems with, 251-258
    process of, 258-262
    programs of, 256
    women-focused, 256
    See also Native American women;
        Samoan women
Health Diary, 166-186

benefits of, 185
clients' use of, 180
content, 166-167, 181-182, 187-188
distribution of, 176-177, 188
evaluation of, 167, 169-175, 177
fetal growth charts, 177
goals for, 166, 185
Healthy Start use of, 167-169
understandability of, 180-181, 185-186
prenatal assessments, 181
resources to supplement, 185
sample demographics, 175
sociodemographic characteristics, 178-179
summary of, 189-191
Health Diary data:
client impacts, 177
communication impact, 177-180
diary use, 180
health provider interactions, 181-182
health provider model, 184
helpfulness of, 181
lay staff model, 184
professional case manager's model, 184
provider diary usefulness, 186-185
staff changes, 186-188
staff training, 182-183
Health Diary sample, 173-174
factors in, 174
interview teams, 173-174
non-English clients, 173
size of, 173
staff interview process, 174-175
staff selection criteria, 175
Health and human services programs:
family planning, 55-56
health communication from, 55
international campaigns, 55
media techniques in, 54-55
problem with solution approaches, 55
Health maintenance organizations (HMOs):
cost effectiveness focus, 31
health communication use, 49
preventive care focus, 49
Health needs:
dual-epidemic period, 22, 25-29
infectious disease period, 22-24
lifestyle disease period, 24-25
public evolution, 21-22
Health objectives
communication on, 64
goals of, 64

national consensus for, 64
Health promotion:
community-based prevention, 66
concepts of, 67
education in, 67
expansion of, 66
intervention modality types, 66
key findings on, 353-355
medicine tasks and, 67
origin of, 66-67
Ottawa Charter, 7-8, 67-68
program evaluation, 355
See also Empowerment
Health promotion interventions:
communication analysis, 333-334
communication studies, 334-336
conclusions on, 355
effective implementations, 334
findings on, 353-355
health promotion empowerment, 346-353
multicultural health communication, 337-345
Health promotion messages:
multicultural population challenges, 110
structural constraints, 110
Health Resource and Services Administration (HRSA), 166
Health risks:
acculturation and, 82-84
"cultural paradoxes" in, 81
data reliability problems, 80-81
demographics changing in, 81-82
mortality rates, 81
quality of life issues, 82
structural determinates, 84-85
Healthy People 2000:
goals of, 340
national objectives, 340
targeted preventive efforts, 339
Healthy Start:
federal initiative for, 167
goals of, 167
Health Diary and, 168
populations in, 168-168
services within, 167-168
sites for, 168
Herbal remedies, sales of, 33
"Here's Looking at You" program, 54
Hispanic Americans:
child injury rates, 148

communication research, 228
cultural barriers to, 98
cultural communication for, 97
cultural competency and, 98
death causes, 15
death rates, 81
health information sources, 35, 340-341
HIV knowledge, 241
National KIDS SAFETY Campaign,
      153-155
peer education programs, 344
population composition, 11
quality of life issues, 82
television viewing by, 36-37
See also Latino paradoxes
Hispanic clients interventions:
   language variances, 298
   vs. acculturation, 298
Hispanic cultural patterns:
   core values of, 85-86
   familísmo, 86
   machismo, 86
   "outer directed" as, 87
   Spanish medial access, 87
   sympatía, 87
   women's health status, 87
Hispanic Health and Nutrition Examination
   Survey, women health status and, 87
Hispanic Smoking Cessation Project,
   Ecological Model and, 113
HIV/AIDS educational approaches
   celebrity participation, 54
   examples of, 214
   risk-taking behavior changes, 213-214
   theories for, 214
HIV/AIDS risk reduction:
   communication interventions, 242-247
   culture and, 235-236
   ethnicity, 236
   homeless youth and, 235-237
   peer education for, 236
   Project ABLE, 237-242
   STD risk shifting, 211
Homeless youth HIV risks
   estimates of, 236-237
   history of, 237
   women and, 237
Homicides, rates falling, 342
Human biology, health domains, 68
Human relations research:
   advertising messages tailoring, 48
   attitude changing, 48

communication importance, 48
group behavior impact, 47-48
health communication importance, 49
health determinants, 48
health psychology goals, 49
important studies in, 50-54
Human relations studies
   Alcohol, Tobacco, and Other Drugs
      Prevention Programs, 53-54
   HIV/AIDS Prevention, 54
   Minnesota Heart Heath Program, 52-53
   North Karelia Project, 52
   Pennsylvania County Health
      Improvement Program, 53
   Stanford Heart Disease Prevention
      Program, 51-52
   TB Screening Study, 50-51

Immigrants:
   health knowledge of, 338-339
   language barriers, 338
   sources of, 338
   stereotyping, 339
   vs. English care providers, 339
Individual-level theories:
   Planned Behavior Model, 120-121
   Social Learning Theory, 118-119
   Stages of Change Model, 119-120
Infant mortality:
   government reactions to, 166
   handbook development for, 166
   minority populations and, 165-166
   rates falling, 342
   rates of, 165
   See also Health Diary
Infectious disease period:
   large-scale epidemics battling, 22
   pathogen microbiology from, 22
   population changes from, 24
   sanitation work, 22
   smallpox vaccination campaign, 22
   typhoid fever and, 22-24
Institute of Medicine, 327
Internet:
   communication revolution, 36
   health promotion on, 36
   vs. television, 37
Intervention impacts
   additional information seeking, 296
   behavior changes from, 295-296

knowledge levels, 295
Project ABLE and, 245
IOX Assessment Associates, 292

Kaiser Family Foundation, 47
Kauffman Foundation, 47
Kellogg Foundation, proposed health
    outcomes, 312
Kelly, Marylea, 347
Kernell, Samuel, 48
King, Martin Luther, 130
Kitano, Harry, 323
KLAX, 127
Knowledge gaps
    examples of, 129
    widening of, 128-129
Knowledge seeking, hypothetical reactions,
    294
Knutson, Andie, 324
Koop, C. Everett, 64

Lalonde, Marc, 68
Landmark Healthcare Study, alternative
    medicine and, 32
Latino paradoxes:
    Latino characteristics, 16
    prenatal care, 16
    theories about, 16-17
    vs. African Americans, 16
Lay Health Start Staff Model:
    Health Diary integration, 184
    limitation of, 184
Lead poisoning, cultural scripts and, 151-152
Lewin, Kurt, 47, 54, 68
Life expectancy, 12
Lifestyle disease period:
    Framingham Heart Study, 24
    heart disease research, 24
    lifestyle changes, 24-25
Lifestyles, health domains, 68
Local health promoters (LHPs)
    at-risk gap bridging, 344
    health communications, 344-345
    minority health services, 96
    peer education, 344
Los Angeles County Department of Health
    Services, 340
Los Angeles Times, 33

Machismo:
    expectations of, 86
    sexual matters and, 86
    women's empowerment and, 350
MacLuhan, Marshall, 36
Madders de la Plaza Mayo, 346, 353
Mass communication theories:
    defined, 124
    health campaign issues, 124
    health promotion uses, 124
    media effects, 125-130
    multicultural populations and, 124
    technologies in, 124
Massachusetts Institute of Technology, 56, 58
Maternal and Child Health Bureau (MCHB),
    166
Mead, Margaret, 150
Media:
    communication objectives, 351-352
    communication role, 351
    empowerment benefits of, 352-353
    examples, 353
    grass-roots movement, 350
    health information dissemination, 340-
        341
    health promotion problems, 341
    Latino preferences, 340
    mainstream defined, 340
    methods for, 350-351
    minority groups effects from, 340
    public education, 352
    successful methods, 353
    synergy with, 353
    use objectives, 353
    See also Multilanguage media
Media advocacy
    defined, 123, 351
    goals of, 123
    types of, 352
Media dependencies:
    communication planners, 129-130
    focus of, 129
Media diversification
    ethnic viewing patterns, 37-38, 340
    fragmentation from, 37
Media effects:
    agenda setting, 128
    Cultivation of Beliefs Model, 125-126
    knowledge gaps, 128-129
    media dependencies, 129-130
    multilanguage media, 126-128

Media effects on dominant majority
    (MEDM):
    domain focus in, 334
    paradigm for, 336
    review categories, 334-335
    vs. ethnic group differences, 335
Media support:
    defined, 351
    types of, 351-352
Media violence, White House summit, 65
"Melting pot" theory, 338
Menchu, Rigoberta, 347
Messages about ethnic differences:
    family attitude perceptions, 196
    parents monitoring styles, 196
Methodological considerations
    causal validity threats, 242-243
    homoscedasticity lacking in, 243
    intervention vs. theoretical models,
        243
    sample size, 243
    sleeper effects testing, 243
    vs. cultural representatives, 244
Minnesota Heart Health Program:
    origin of, 52-53
    results in, 53
    techniques in, 53
Minorities:
    collectivism differences, 91
    fatalism and, 91-92
    fatalismo and, 91-92
    same group diversity, 91
Minority community partnerships:
    benefits from, 14
    community acceptance, 14-15
    strategy for, 14
Modality communication, language
    proficiency differences, 96
Model of Planned Behavior
    behavior defining, 120
    benefits of, 121
    focus of, 120
    self-efficacy in, 121
Mother's Against Drunk Driving, 346
Mother's Clubs, 346
Mother's prevention partnership:
    community participation, 343
    community priorities in, 343
    empowerment for, 343
    health professional challenges, 343
    mother's role in, 343-344
    parents roles in, 343-344

Multicultural group communication:
    community empowerment in, 337-338
    culturally conditioned risk behaviors,
        337
    findings on, 337
    foreign-born population increases, 337
Multicultural communicating:
    challenges in, 109-111
    community partnerships, 130-132
    conclusions on, 132
    ecological perspectives, 112-117
    mass communication theories, 124-130
    social behavior theories, 117-123
Multicultural communities
    determinate domains, 315
    factors affecting, 315-316
Multicultural demographic changes:
    Census data changes, 10
    communicating in, 13
    death causes, 15-14
    dual-epidemic period in, 13
    ethnic population composition, 11
    life expectancy, 12
    mainstream society perceptions, 10
    multicultural communities increasing,
        13
    partnership benefits with, 14
    public health implications, 10-13
    U. S. and, 9-10
Multicultural Evaluation Model:
    approaches to, 317
    "audience" empowerment, 318-319
    categories expanding, 319
    communicator cultural competency,
        319
    community-based campaigns, 317
    effective communication elements,
        319
    multicultural changes, 318
    program planning linking, 317
    public partnerships, 319
    success of, 317
Multicultural health communication:
    cultural competency, 345
    health behaviors and, 340
    local health promoters, 344-345
    mainstream media, 340-341
    microcommunications, 341-342
    mothers and, 343-344
    multiculturalism, 338-339
    threats to children, 342-343

Multicultural health paradigms, components of, 15-16
Multicultural research paucity:
  formative phase of, 322
  Halcolm's Evaluation Laws, 323
  knowledge lacking about, 322-323
  qualitative methods role, 322
Multicultural societies
  Asian cultural patterns, 88-91
  competency barriers, 98-100
  cultural diversity, 92-98
  ethnic mortality differences, 79-80
  health inequalities indicators, 80
  Hispanic cultural patterns, 85-88
  language and, 100-104
  minority variables, 91-92
  realities of, 79
  relative health risks in, 80-85
Multiculturalism:
  cultural diversity considerations, 339
  defined, 30
  health communication understanding, 30
  health promotion lacking, 339-340
  immigrants and, 338-339
  "melting pot" theory, 338
  minority population increasing, 338
  "rainbow" coalition, 338
  stereotyping, 339
Multilanguage media:
  English media, 127-128
  Hispanic media impact, 126
  Spanish language impact, 126
  Spanish radio, 127
Multiple Risk Factor Intervention Trial (MRFIT) project, 334

National Academy of Science, 327
National Agenda:
  health promotion and, 64
  president's influence, 64
National Cancer Institute, 47
National Center for Chronic Disease Prevention and Health Promotion
  health communication from, 64
  purpose of, 64
National Center for Health Statistics (NCHS), 341
National Commission to Prevent Infant Mortality, 166

National Fire Protection Association, 159
National Institute of Alcoholism, 47
National Institute of Drug Abuse, 47, 317
National Institutes of Health:
  origin of, 63
  research funding, 65
National SAFE KIDS Campaign:
  coalitions for, 159
  findings, 153-155
  focus of, 153
  parents telephone study, 153
  unintentional injury threats, 146
Native American women:
  baseline knowledge, 266
  chronic health developments, 252-253
  chronic risks types, 254-255
  cultural heritage maintaining, 255
  food adapting, 255
  general health attitudes, 269-270
  general health knowledge, 268-269
  general health practices, 271
  as lost group, 251-252
  migration history of, 252
  natural diet of, 255
  population status, 253-254
  prior research on, 254
  socioeconomic factors, 255
  stress linking, 255
  trends for, 271-272
  vs. Samoan women, 266
Native Americans:
  child injury rates, 146-14
  death causes, 15
  death from falls, 149
  death rates, 81
  fire arm deaths, 149
  house fire deaths, 149
  poisoning deaths, 149
  population composition, 11
New York Times, 83
Nielsen Media Research, 126
Nielsen's Hispanic Television Index, 126
North Karelia Project, 24, 333
  community-based approach, 52
  origin of, 52
  results of, 52

OMBUDSMAN program, 54
Ottawa Charter for Health Promotion, 343
  landmark document, 68

strategies of, 67
WHO principles, 67

Parent communication skills:
    importance of, 205-206
    message content, 205
    myths dispelling during, 205
    techniques for, 205
Parent management skills
    discipline consistency, 206
    drug abuse preventing, 206
    home nurturing, 206
Parent-child communication research:
    acculturation level differentials, 205
    acculturation process, 203
    conflict in views, 205
    ethnic group communication, 204
    family belief, 202-203
    family relationship findings, 203-204
    gender specific communicating, 204
    parent skills and, 204-206
    parents management skills enhancing,
        206
    risk factor understanding, 203
    societal consensus for, 204-205
Parenting practices:
    child safety understanding, 146
    risk factors in, 146
Parents and adolescent drug use:
    academic success importance, 202
    parent communication factors, 201
    parental concerns about, 200
    prevention communication
        components, 202
    users vs. nonusers, 199-200
Parks, Rosa, 346
Partnership for Drug Free America, 317
Peer Education Program of Los Angeles:
    demographic characteristics, 224
    educational approach effectiveness,
        222-223
    educator ratings, 227
    experimental design of, 223-224
    limitations of, 222
    presentation skills ratings, 225-226
    purpose of, 222
    results of, 223-225
    training and, 223, 226-227
Peer education programs:
    advantages, 217

benefits, 219
communication skills, 216
counseling approaches, 217
intervention success, 216
knowledge vs. behavior changes, 220
leadership training, 217
limitations of, 219, 219-220
peer credibility, 216
skill building in, 219
SNAPP, 218-219
STD/HIV prevention programs and,
    215-216
Teen Peer Outreach-Street Work
    Project, 218
vulnerable population reaching, 216
Peer education STD/HIV reductions
    benefit inconclusive, 227-228
    program effectiveness measures, 228
Peer educators:
    counselor training curriculum, 221-222
    interpersonal interaction skills, 221
    leadership training and, 217
    maintenance sessions for, 222
    selection criteria, 220-221
    site design, 221
    training criteria, 221
Peer health education, Project ABLE and,
    247
Pennsylvania County Health Improvement
    Program (CHIP)
    origin of, 53
    results of, 53
    techniques in, 53
Personal responsibility:
    cultures varying in, 95
    self-interest and, 95-96
Personalismo, media use of, 99
Pew Health Professions Commission, 102
Policy-level theories:
    examples of, 123
    medial advocacy, 123
    reframing benefits, 123
PRECEDE, defined, 238
Pregnancy:
    adolescent reduction risks, 213
    rates falling, 342
    STD infection and, 212-213
Prevention. See Culturally informed
    prevention programs
Professional Case Manager Model
    Health Diary integration, 184
    new doctor transitions, 184

Project ABLE:
    condom use, 241
    cultural competency, 246-247
    exposure impact of, 240-241
    hierarchical regressions, 241-242
    homeless evaluations, 239-240
    homeless youth play, 237
    impact of, 239
    males influences by, 241
    messages in, 238
    participant evaluations, 240
    peer actor perceptions, 239
    peer actor use, 238
    PRECEDE framework in, 238
    questionnaire results, 239
Project Adventure program, 54
Project CHARLIE, 54
Proposition 99 (California), 54
Public education:
    face-to-face programs, 352
    objective of, 352
Public health:
    communication implications, 40
    community partnerships with, 7
foundations, 58-62
    goal obtaining methods, 7
    strategic basis of, 7
Public health, global issues:
    aging populations, 6
    children mortality rates, 5
    communicable disease control, 6
    community-based prevention, 4
    "dual epidemic" era, 3-4
    health care costs, 4-6
    health promotion, 7-8
    industrial nations crisis, 4
    population control, 8
    public health from, 3-4
    public health legitimizing, 6
    quality of life and, 4-6
    training uniqueness for, 9
    United Nations efforts, 8
    vs. clinical medicine, 9
Public Health Model:
    communication implications, 40
    communication revolution, 34-40
    elements in, 29
    government functions, 29-30
    health care system and, 30-34
    health needs changing, 21-29
    mission of, 29-30

    multicultural health communication, 30
    preventive approach characteristics, 29
Public health needs:
    cultural paradoxes, 16-17
    global issues in, 3-9
    multicultural demographic imperatives, 9-15
    multicultural setting paradigms, 15-16
    summary of, 17-18
Public health schools
    accreditation core areas, 57
    communication importance to, 58-59
    disciplines within, 60
    emergence of, 57
    enrollment ethnicity projections, 62
    expansion of, 56-62
    graduate ethnicity, 60
    new enrollment ethnicity, 61
    origins of, 56-57, 58
    other disciplines from, 57
    purpose of, 57
    quantity of, 59
    student composition of, 59
    U. S. and, 57

Qualitative evaluations:
    defining of, 321
    design evaluation, 323
    evaluator role, 321-322
    measurement tools, 324-325
    research paucity, 322-323
    study populations access, 325-326
    vs. quantitative methods, 320-321
Quality of life:
    Asian Americans and, 90-91
    evaluation categories, 312
QUEST: Skills for Living, 54

Reciprocal relationships:
    cultural competency and, 101
    importance of, 101-102
Research design evaluation:
    elements in, 323
    examples of, 323
    problem matching, 323
Research measurement scales
    communication problem examples, 324

standardizing barriers, 324-325
standardizing scales, 324
Risk Watch, 159
Robert Wood Johnson Foundation, 47
Robinson, Jo Ann, 346
Rockefeller Foundation, 47
Rogers, Everett, 47

Sadik, Dr. Nafis, 8
Samoan women:
    advisory council for, 256
    baseline knowledge, 266
    chronic health developments, 252-253
    culture of, 254-255
    food adaptations, 255
    general health attitudes, 265-266, 269-
        270
    general health knowledge, 264-265, 268-
        269
    general health practices, 271
    lifecycles changes, 255
    as lost group, 251
    migration history of, 252
    natural diet of, 255
    population status, 253-254
    pre-and-posttesting attitudes, 264
    pre-and-posttesting knowledge, 262-264
    results of, 266
    risk factor types, 254
    stress linking to, 254
    trends for, 271-272
    vs. Asian Pacific Islanders, 253
    vs. Indian women priorities, 266
    Western socioeconomic factors, 255
Selection Model, cultural competency and,
    102
Self-efficacy:
    assistance-seeking, 295
    helplessness, 295
Semiology, use of, 100{
Sexually transmitted disease (STD)
    prevention:
    adolescent risk behavior, 211-212
    communication research, 228-229
    condom use, 212
    HIV risk shifting, 211
    Los Angeles Peer Education Program,
        222-227
    peer-based approaches, 215-217
    peer counselors, 222

peer education, 220-228
pregnancy rates, 212-213
sexual intercourse experiencing, 212
significance of, 212-213
social influences modeling, 214-215
strength and weakness of, 218-220
theoretical framework, 213-214
Sigerist, Henry, 66
Smoking:
    ethnic groups participating, 113-114
    Hispanic women and, 86
Smoking Cessation Project:
    community involvement in, 116
    Cultivation of Beliefs Model, 125-126
    cultural communication for, 97-98
Social behavior theories
    benefits from, 118
    change from, 118
    communication intervention goals, 117-
        118
    community-level theories, 121-123
    individual-level theories, 118-121
    media advocacy, 118
    policy-level theories, 123
    social marketing and, 118
Social influence modeling:
    behavior determinants from, 214-215
    denial and, 215
    mechanism for, 215
    peer influence, 214
    social norms influencing, 215
Social Learning Theory:
    audience targeting, 112
    benefits of, 118-119
    communication interventions, 119
    desired behavior skill leaning, 119
    entertainment format use, 119
    media intervention and, 119
    premise of, 119
Social Marketing Model
    characteristics of, 122-123
    defined, 122
    focus of, 122
    purpose of, 122
    stages in, 122
South Carolina Study:
    ethnic differences, 153
    findings of, 153
    focus of, 152
    risk perceptions vs. safety behaviors, 153
    safety behaviors in, 152-153

Southeast Asia American, cultural issues of, 90

Spanish International Communication Corporation, 126

Spanish International Network (SIN), 126

Spanish Katz Radio Group, 127

Spanish television
organizations in, 126
research from, 126-127

"Spiral of silence" effect, 128

Stages of Change Model
benefits of, 120
campaign focusing, 120
focus of, 119
stages in, 120

Stanford Heart Disease Prevention Program:
community vs. individual changes, 51
goal of, 52
origin of, 51
phases of, 51-52

Stanford project, 334

Structural determinants
access issues, 84-85
multicultural group impacts, 84
old vs. new country ways, 85

Study population access:
criteria for, 326
examples of, 325-326
structural problems with, 325
variables in, 325

Sudden infant death syndrome (SIDS), cultural scripts and, 151

Summative evaluation, health communication and, 313

Surgeon General's office
duties of, 63-64
healthy society strategy, 67
proactive role of, 64

Sympatía:
social interactions, 87
women's role, 87

TB screening study:
goal of, 50
health belief model, 50
health beliefs imparting, 51
media campaign, 50
target population, 50

Teen Peer Outreach-Street Work Project, 218

Skills and Knowledge for AIDS and Pregnancy Prevention (SNAPP), 218-219

Teleky, Ludwig, 6

Television
minority viewing habits, 36-37
popularity of, 36
vs. cable television, 36
vs. Internet, 37

Theoretical framework:
atheoretical evaluation, 292
information effectiveness, 293
knowledge gaps construct, 292-293

de Tocqueville, Alexis, 356

Training model, cultural competency and, 102

Treatment modality:
health communication programs, 95
traditional approaches, 95
Western system uses, 95

"Two-step" communication model, 47

2000 Program, 54

U. S. Public Health Service (USPHS):
creation of, 63
DHHS creating, 63-64
health communication, 64
health objective development, 64
health promotion and, 64-65
modern force developing, 63
national agenda of, 64
president's influence, 65
World War I role, 63

UNICEF, publications of, 7

University of California, 283, 347

University of Texas Health Science Center Campaign, 25

Univisión Group, 126

Vedic philosophy, 94

Vietnam Americans
characteristics of, 89
cultural aspects of, 89-90
cultural barriers to, 98
refugees as, 89
women's health status, 89

Vietnamese Americans, cultural competency and, 98

Wall Street Journal, 83
Weijts, Wies, 49
Wellness Guide:
    community-based approach, 283-287
    culture relevance of, 287
    development chronology, 284-286
    development process, 283-286
    expert-based model development, 283
    local focus group comments, 283
    purpose of, 287
Wellness Guide content
    checklist and, 288
    example of, 288
    layout standardization, 287
    life spans perspectives in, 287
    visual appearance, 288
    See also Guía
White, Ralph K., 68
Women:
    Chinese health status, 89
    community-based health promotion,
        347
    cultural competency and, 98
    cultural scripts for, 151
    empowerment, 343, 347-348
    empowerment model, 349
    Hispanic cultural and, 86-87
    immigrants health difficulties, 83
    media inequity, 39-40
    quality of life enhancing, 348
    Vietnam health status, 89
Woolworth, Dr. John, 63
World Health Organization (WHO)
    health promotion strategies, 67
    Ottawa Charter and, 67
    population aging trends, 6
    proposed health outcomes, 312
    publications of, 7

Yale University, 56
Youth Risk Behavior Surveillance System, 342

About the Contributors

Rina Alcalay, PhD, is Associate Professor of Communications and Rhetoric at the University of California at Davis and held a professorial position at the School of Public Health at UCLA for several years. She has had extensive experience in research, teaching, and consultations on issues of health communication with special reference to Hispanics and other underserved groups for over a decade. She is much sought after by national and international agencies for her established reputation as an expert in health communication in multicultural communities. She holds a doctorate degree in communication from Stanford University.

Shana Alex is Program Assistant at the UCLA Office of Public Health Practice. She is working on a master's degree in public policy at the University of California, Los Angeles, School of Public Policy and Social Research, focusing on health policy and the possibilities for reforming the health care system at the national level. Her other research interests include issues of multiculturalism and state and local regional issues facing California.

Robert A. Bell, PhD, is Professor of Communication at the University of California at Davis. He has expertise in communication theories and models for social and behavioral change. Among his recent projects are studies of social influence strategies for health promotion and investigations of the content and impact of direct-to-consumer drug advertising. He has worked with the Sacramento AIDS Foundation to develop strategies to overcome resistance to HIV testing among high-risk populations. He has been involved in evaluation research, including an evaluation of a social marketing intervention sponsored by The California Wellness Foundation and an evaluation of a physician-targeted medical education seminar on managed care. He is currently working in the role of co-principal investigator/analyst as part of an interdisciplinary team studying patients' requests, a project funded by the Robert Wood Johnson Foundation. His research has appeared in a variety of journals in public health, medicine, and communication. He earned his doctorate in communication from the University of Texas, Austin.

Gauri Bhattacharya, DSW, MSW, is a faculty member in the School of Social Work at the University of Illinois at Urbana-Champaign (UIUC). Her research interests and professional specialties include substance abuse prevention, the economics of substance abuse treatment, and access to health care services for HIV/AIDS. Current research projects focus on delineating the causal linkages of risk and protective factors to substance abuse (or no use) and examining the extent and the nature of the processes among adolescents in multicultural communities, and as the principal investigator on a number of projects funded by the National Institute on Drug Abuse (NIDA). She has developed community-based substance abuse prevention and intervention programs for adolescents. She has published on substance abuse prevention and health education on HIV prevention in peer-reviewed journals and authored several book chapters. She presents extensively at national scientific, public health, and medical meetings. She is a licensed and certified clinical social worker. Before joining in 1998, she was a principal investigator at the National Development and Research Institutes, New York. She received her DSW and MSW degrees from Adelphi University, Garden City, New York, and a master's degree in economics from Calcutta University, India.

Clifford Binder, MBA, coconducted the evaluation of the *Health Diary* for the Center for Health Policy Studies under contract with the Health Resources and Services Administration with James Wells. His research and evaluation activities include work for federal health care agencies, state health departments, and private health organizations. He is currently assessing Medicare contractor medical review activities and Medicaid network adequacy measures for the Health Care Financing Administration.

Linda Burhansstipanov, MSPH, DrPH, is Executive Director of Native American Cancer Initiatives, Inc., of Pine, Colorado. She is Western Cherokee (Tahlaquah, OK). She developed and implemented the Native American Cancer Research Program at the National Cancer Institute from 1989 to 1993. She was also the former director of the Native American Cancer Research Program of the AMC Cancer Research Center in Denver, Colorado. She was a full professor at California State University Long Beach and also taught part-time at UCLA. She has been the principal investigator of multiple Native American cancer research, service, and education grants.

Vicki J. Ebin, PhD, MSPH, is Assistant Professor at California State University, Northridge, in the Department of Health Sciences. Concurrently, she is the Project Director for the UCLA/CSULB Adolescent Tuberculosis Prevention Project. Her research interests include adolescent health, compliance issues, and community-campus partnerships. She received her degrees from the University of California, Los Angeles.

Deborah Glik, PhD, is Associate Professor at the UCLA School of Public Health and has also taught at the University of South Carolina. She is Co-Director of the UCLA Technical Assistance Group (TAG), which specializes in the assessment and evaluation of educational and community-based projects. Her expertise is in research on health behavior change, health communications, formative research, and program evaluation in community settings, having worked in both domestic and international settings. Substantive areas include evaluation and promotion of school and community immunization programs, infectious disease control, injury control, and evaluation of a broad range of programs and social interventions in schools and communities. She is currently conducting an evaluation of an immunization curriculum geared to sixth-grade students, a malaria curtains project in Malawi, and a child injury prevention project in South Central Los Angeles. Other recent evaluation projects include assessing the impact of Public Health Leadership training, WIC educational programs, and jobs training programs for inner-city and disadvantaged youth. Other current projects include development and evaluation of multimedia education in Latino communities, on topics such as immunizations, nutrition, and gestational diabetes, and research on the effectiveness of a teen theater program for U.S. adolescents sponsored by the Centers for Disease Control. She earned a doctorate in behavioral sciences and public health from Johns Hopkins University.

Fran Goldfarb, MA, CHES, is Director of Parent and Family Resources at the University of Southern California, Affiliated Program, Children's Hospital, Los Angeles. Her current research projects include Medical Home Project for Children with Special Needs and LA Connections: Improving Access to Primary and Preventive Care for Children With Special Needs. Previously, she was Director of the Community Action for Women's Health, Center for Healthy Aging (previously known as Senior Health and Peer Counseling). She did her graduate work in Family Life Education at Azusa Pacific College.

Snehendu B. Kar, MSc, DrPH, is Professor of Public Health at UCLA, where he's been since 1979. He is Director of the MPH Program for Health Professionals (MPHHP) in Health Promotion and Health Education and Codirector of Public Health Practice. His professional and research interests include acculturation and health, health communication in multicultural communities, empowerment and health education, and health promotion indicators. Previous positions include Associate Dean and Chair of the School and Department of Public Health (1984-1988), Head of the Behavioral Sciences and Health Education Division (1980-1984), and Chair of the Asian American Studies IDP (1980-1984) at UCLA; Associate Professor and Assistant Professor at the School of Public Health at the University of Michigan, Ann Arbor (1967-1978); and Deputy Assistant Director General (Research) at the Ministry of Health and Family Planning, Government of India, New Delhi. He received his MSc in psychology in 1958 from the University of Calcutta, India, and his master's and doctorate degrees in public health and behavioral sciences from the University of California at Berkeley.

Lené Levy-Storms, PhD, MPH, is Assistant Professor in the Department of Health Promotion and Gerontology and a Fellow of the Sealy Center on Aging at the University of Texas Medical Branch in Galveston, Texas. Her research interests include the social contexts of successful aging, long-term care use, and minority aging. Her current research focuses on how social networks influence self-care behaviors and the role of race, ethnic, and social factors on the use of formal care services among older adults. She holds a master's of public health in biostatistics and a doctorate in public health from the University of California, Los Angeles.

Angela Mickalide, PhD, CHES, is Program Director of the National SAFE KIDS Campaign, the only nationwide program for prevention of unintentional injuries among children ages 14 and under. She is an adjunct Associate Professor of

Prevention and Community Health at the George Washington University School of Public Health and Health Services and an Associate in the Department of Psychiatry and Behavioral Sciences at Johns Hopkins University School of Medicine. Prior to joining SAFE KIDS, she worked at the federal Office of Disease Prevention and Health Promotion, U.S. Public Health Service in Washington, D.C. Among her current public health leadership positions are as Governing Councilor for the American Public Health Association, Executive Board member of the International Society of Child and Adolescent Injury Prevention, and member of the Task Force on Injury Prevention for the American School Health Association. She earned a PhD degree in 1985 at Johns Hopkins University in Baltimore, Maryland, specializing in public health, psychology, and health education.

Donald E. Morisky, ScD, has worked at the UCLA School of Public Health since 1982, concurrently conducting research in Associate positions at the Johns Hopkins School of Hygiene and Public Health, the Charles R. Drew Post Graduate Medical School, and the UCLA Jonsson Comprehensive Cancer Center. From 1993-1994, he was chair of the Public Health Education Section of the American Public Health Association, and he has consulted extensively with the World Health Organization and other international health organizations. His current research focuses mainly on AIDS, particularly in the Filipina population. He received his doctorate degree from Johns Hopkins University in 1981 in behavioral sciences and health education.

Karen Thiel Raykovich, PhD, is a Senior Fellow in the Office of Planning, Evaluation and Legislation of the Health Resources and Services Administration where she directs the national evaluation of the Healthy Start Program. She has evaluated maternal, child, and adolescent health and social services programs at the federal, state, and local levels.

Lisa A. Russell, PhD, is Senior Research Associate with ETR Associates in Santa Cruz, California. Her research interests include health communication, health behavior, and mental health services. Specifically, she studies homelessness, child maltreatment, and mental health among youths and their families, and disaster communication, preparedness, and responses among adults. She received her PhD in public health from the University of California, Los Angeles.

Steven P. Wallace, PhD, is Associate Professor at the UCLA School of Public Health, Borun Scholar of the Anna and Harry Borun Center for Gerontological

Research at UCLA, and associate director for community programs of the UCLA Center for Health Policy Research. His research focuses on the impact of race and ethnicity on the use of long-term care and the consequences of public policies for the health and quality of life of racial and ethnic minority elderly. He has published widely on his research in journals such as *The Gerontologist, Journal of Gerontology: Social Sciences, American Journal of Public Health,* and *Journal of Aging Studies.* His current research includes projects on (a) determining the consequences of managed care on access to health care by racial/ethnic minority elderly; (b) better understanding how culture, economics, and racism shape the use of long-term care; and (c) evaluating the implementation of health and welfare policy in California. He received his PhD in sociology from the University of California, San Francisco.

James A. Wells, PhD, is a health services researcher and epidemiologist. He co-conducted the evaluation of the *Health Diary* for the Center for Health Policy Studies under contract with the Health Resources and Services Administration with Clifford Binder. In addition to maternal and child health, his experience includes work in HIV/AIDS, substance abuse treatment, managed care, bioethics, scientific productivity, and health education. He is currently a research consultant with the Gallup Organization, working in the Government and Education Research Division. He received his PhD in sociology from Duke University and completed a postdoctoral fellowship in epidemiology at the Yale University School of Medicine.

Trans Fats
Alternatives